D0317450

Other writings by Terry Lynch

Books:

Beyond Prozac: Healing Mental Distress, Ireland (2001 & 2005), Mercier Press.
UK (2004), PCCS Books.
Selfhood: A Key to the Recovery of Emotional Wellbeing, Mental Health and the Prevention of Mental Health Problems (2011), Mental Health Publishing.

Chapters in books:

"Understanding Psychiatry's Resistance to Change", in *Critical Psychiatry: The Limits of Madness,* Duncan Double (ed.), London & New York: Palgrave MacMillan, 2006, pps. 99-115.
"The Dominance of Drug-Based Mental Health Care in Ireland: A Personal Account of a General Practitioner Turned Psychotherapist", in *Power, Politics and Pharmaceuticals,* O'Donovan, O. & Glavanis-Grantham, K. (eds), Cork: Cork University Press, 2008, pps. 135-150.

Forewords:

Warning: Psychiatry can be Hazardous to your Mental Health, William Glasser MD, New York: HarperCollins, 2003.
Responding to a Serious Mental Health Problem: Person-Centred Dialogues, Richard Bryant-Jefferies, Oxon, UK: Radcliffe Publishing Ltd, 2005.
Soul Survivor: A Personal Encounter with Psychiatry, Mary & Jim Maddock, Stockport, UK: Asylum, 2006.

Terry's next book:

Depression: Its True Nature (working title), estimated publication date: mid-2016.

Sign up to Terry's newletter

Over the next decade, Terry Lynch intends to write 10-15 further books on important mental health topics including depression, anxiety, bipolar disorder, schizophrenia, OCD, eating disorders and suicide. To get news and updates, sign up for Terry's newsletter at www.doctorterrylynch.com.

"It is such an impressive book and it is so important to have this kind of very detailed setting out of the sheer scale of the deceit that is being practised on people, as well as, as you've also done, offering alternatives. It's an enormously useful resource both for people like me who are familiar with the arguments but don't have this level of detail easily available and also for 'ordinary' people to balance the weight of misinformation. There is a subtle and well orchestrated campaign here at the moment to re-establish the dominance of the medical model and it's good to be able to draw attention to books like yours as a counter to it–I shall recommend it wherever I can."

Mary Boyle, UK, clinical psychologist, Professor Emeritus at the University of East London, Fellow of the British Psychological Society and the Royal Society of Medicine, author of *Schizophrenia: A Scientific Delusion?*

"In challenging the very dangerous pseudo-scientific explanations of depression, Dr. Terry Lynch brings his medical background and his scientific integrity to bear on the issue. It was this powerful combination first seen in *Beyond Prozac* that attracted the interest and support of Dr. William Glasser, the creator of Reality Therapy and Choice Theory psychology, a long-time challenger of the chemical imbalance hypothesis. The *Depression Delusion* is essential reading for those who experience or deal with depression, one of the most painful of human conditions".

Brian Lennon, Ireland, psychologist, Founder of William Glasser International, guidance counsellor.

"In this book the courageous Irish physician Terry Lynch has taken on the fiction of 'chemical imbalances'. With no scientific evidence for this nonsense whatsoever, the psychiatric establishment, and the drug companies who own them, have been perpetrating an enormous fraud on the public. Doctor Lynch lays bare that this theory has no factual basis at all. I urge everyone concerned about the issue to read this important book."

Ted Chabasinski, USA, attorney, psychiatric survivor, anti-psychiatry activist.

"It was the delusion that a chemical brain imbalance could cause the problems I experienced for over two decades that actually caused me and my family severe distress. It was meeting and hearing Terry Lynch that helped me to find out the truth. It is the myth of the chemical brain imbalance theory that continues to give deceptive, coercive psychiatry the power to force psychotropic drugs and electroshock on vulnerable people. Terry Lynch's new book *Depression Delusion* will hopefully educate many, many others so that finally this myth will be exposed and eliminated. Everyone who wants to know the true facts will want to read this book."

Mary Maddock, Ireland, co-founder, MindFreedom Ireland, co-author of *Soul Survivor: A Personal Encounter with Psychiatry.*

"Dr. Terry Lynch in his book *Beyond Prozac* showed that he wasn't frightened to throw down the gauntlet and challenge the status quo within mainstream mental health care. In *Depression Delusion*, Dr. Lynch has surpassed this and thrown himself into the lion's den with gusto! Many mental health professionals, medical doctors, drug companies, members of the public and the mass media continue to propagate the 'chemical imbalance' theory of depression. Through extensive and valid research Terry takes the reader on an epic journey revealing why this myth needs to be eradicated. When this delusion is destroyed we will all need to decide how we view and deal with depression in the future. Terry continues to address these very important questions in detail. If you still hold to the belief that the world is flat, then *Depression Delusion* will rock your very foundations!"

Julie Leonovs, UK, MSc in Psychological Research Methods,
mental health activist, Gateshead, United Kingdom.

"I have never read a more accurate or frank account of the myths surrounding 'mental illness', or indeed the acknowledgement that these myths were (and are) pushed by psychiatry, the pharmaceutical industry and misinformed doctors. This fabulous book is a must for everyone who believes that they are suffering from a brain chemical imbalance. Terry's book is ground-breaking, brutally honest and totally unexpected – he pulls no punches. . . . Dr Terry Lynch takes one brave step for mankind – it remains to be seen whether this book will rock the very foundations of 'depression' and 'mental illness' as we know it, but I think that it just might.

Dr. Lynch is one very brave man to take on the so-called 'experts' in this forthright manner. It's a David and Goliath situation. Will the truth win out? Is this generation ready to see that the so-called 'experts' are in fact philistines? I sure hope so! Huge respect to Dr Terry Lynch for this much-needed exposé . . . *Depression Delusion Volume One: The Myth of the Brain Chemical Imbalance* is most definitely a keeper. . . . In my opinion it's just as brilliant as Robert Whitaker's *Anatomy of an Epidemic*, and the best thing to have come out of Ireland since *Pharmageddon*."

Leonie Fennell, Ireland, mental health activist.

"I am a big fan of Terry's first book *Beyond Prozac*, and *Depression Delusion* does not disappoint. A thorough, forensic examination of Western psychiatry's (mis)treatment of depression, and how doctors and mental health professionals are all too often misinformed about the facts concerning antidepressant treatment. When Terry describes his work with people suffering from depression, it is clear that what is required instead is compassion, empathy and gaining a real understanding about someone's story. Terry's insights into the reasons why we become depressed should form an integral part of all mental health training."

Nick Redman, UK, Survivor/Activist,
Member of Bristol Hearing Voices Network.

DEPRESSION DELUSION

VOLUME ONE

THE MYTH OF THE
BRAIN CHEMICAL IMBALANCE

DR. TERRY LYNCH

FOREWORD BY ROBERT WHITAKER

EDITED BY MARIANNE MURPHY

Mental Health Publishing

Published in 2015 by Mental Health Publishing.

Enquiries to:
Mental Health Publishing,
52 Wolfe Tone Street, Limerick, Ireland
Email: info@doctorterrylynch.com
Phone: +353.87.6592580.
www.doctorterrylynch.com

Printed by Lightning Source

ISBN 978-1-908561-01-5

Cover design by Thinkk Creative, 32 Cecil Street, Limerick, Ireland.

A CIP catalogue record for this book is available from the British Library.

ABOUT THE AUTHOR

Terry Lynch is a medical doctor, psychotherapist and author based in Limerick, Ireland. Terry qualified as a medical doctor in 1982 and worked as a general practitioner (GP) in Limerick, Ireland until 2000. He completed an MA in Humanistic and Integrative Psychotherapy at the University of Limerick in 2002.

Terry was appointed by the Irish Department of Health and Children to the Expert Group on Mental Health Policy (2003-6). This Expert Group's Report *A Vision for Change* (2006) forms the basis of mental health policy in Ireland. Terry was subsequently appointed by the Irish Department of Health and Children to the Independent Monitoring Group for *A Vision for Change* (2006-9). He was re-appointed by the Irish Department of Health and Children to the Second Monitoring Group for *A Vision for Change* (2009-12). Terry was also appointed by the Chief Executive Officer of the Irish Health Service Executive (HSE) to the HSE's Expert Advisory Group on Mental Health (2006-8).

Since 2002 Terry has provided a recovery-oriented mental health service in Limerick, Ireland. Since 2012 Terry has been joined in this practice by his wife, psychotherapist Marianne Murphy.

Terry's first book *Beyond Prozac* was published in Ireland in 2001. *Beyond Prozac* was published in Britain in 2004, and a second edition was published in Ireland in 2005. *Beyond Prozac* was short-listed for the UK Mind Book of the Year award in 2002, and reached number 3 in the Irish non-fiction best-sellers list in 2001. Terry's second book *Selfhood: A Key to the Recovery of Emotional Wellbeing, Mental Health and the Prevention of Mental Health Problems* was published in 2011.

ACKNOWLEDGEMENTS

To my wife Marianne, thank you for your unwavering support and enthusiasm for this project, and for your editing and your ideas. Thanks also to our children, Gary, David and Ciara, for your patience and encouragement.

To Robert Whitaker, thank you for your incisive and insightful foreword. My sincere thanks also to Peter Breggin, Joanna Moncrieff, Lucy Johnstone, Brent Slife, Kim Olver, Mary Boyle, Brian Lennon, Ted Chabasinski, Mary Maddock, Julie Leonovs, Leonie Fennell, Nick Redman, R. B. ("Truthman 30") and Ramo Kabbani for endorsing this book and for your enthusiasm for this project; to Patrice Campion and Patrick C. Coughlan for feedback on early drafts; to Sharon and Conleth for your ideas regarding the title; and to Thinkk Creative for the cover.

Thank you also to the many people who have supported me over the past thirteen years since the publication of *Beyond Prozac*. I am grateful to the people who have attended me over the years, from whom I have learned so much, including those who gave permission for their stories to appear in this book.

I would also like to acknowledge the many hundreds of people worldwide who continue to call for change in how emotional and mental health is understood and responded to, a necessary process of change that needs to be infused by truth, integrity and courage.

AUTHOR'S NOTE

No book can act as a substitute for individualized medical or psychological care. As it can be dangerous to reduce or stop medication abruptly, this should only be done with appropriate guidance and supervision.

CONTENTS

About the author vii

Acknowledgements viii

Author's note viii

Foreword xiii

Introduction 1

 The depression delusion 1

 Why it matters 6

 This book is pro-truth 7

 Logical fallacies 8

 Seminal moments 10

 What is real and what is not 12

 Book contents 12

 Notes to the Introduction 13

1. Crises in the camp 15

 The psychiatrist's bible 15

 Drug companies abandon psychiatry 23

 Worrying drug cycles 25

 Notes to Chapter One 27

2. There are no known brain chemical abnormalities in depression 31

 Depression and the *Diagnostic and Statistical Manual of Mental Disorders* 33

 The absence of evidence 34

 Fifty-year-old hypotheses, no facts 46

 The biochemical hypothesis: no scientific foundation 47

 A hypothesis based solely on deduction 48

 Serotonin breakdown products and depression 50

 What the medical textbooks say 51

 Notes to Chapter Two 57

3. A hypothesis discredited a long time ago 63

 The extraordinary complexity of the brain 63

 Serotonin depletion does not cause depression 67

Selective serotonin reuptake inhibition discredited years before Prozac 69

The timing of drug effects 71

"An astonishing betrayal of trust" 72

Notes to Chapter Three 74

4. There is a better way 77

The depression delusion and the repackaging of emotional distress 77

The core components of depression are *not* biological 79

Nine cases of depression 80

Notes to Chapter Four 89

5. Doctors promoting depression as a brain chemical imbalance 91

Psychiatry 92

The British Medical Association endorses the depression delusion 109

Family physicians (GPs) 111

The depression delusion, as seen on British TV 111

Dr. Greg's neurotransmitter nonsense 119

Other GPs promote the brain chemical imbalance delusion 125

Other physicians and brain chemical imbalances 130

Notes to Chapter Five 134

6. Drug companies, drug regulatory authorities and pharmacists 141

Eli Lilly 141

Lundbeck 143

GlaxoSmithKline 145

Forest Pharmaceuticals 148

Pfizer 150

Wyeth 152

Drug regulatory authorities 152

Pharmacists 155

Notes to Chapter Six 156

7. Psychology, psychotherapy and brain chemical imbalances 159

Psychology 160

Hook, line and sinker 160

Psychotherapy and counselling 172

Notes to Chapter Seven 175

8. Mental health organizations, the media and the general public 179

Mental health organizations 179

The media and the general public 185

Notes to Chapter Eight 208

9. The nutrition industry 215

Notes to Chapter Nine 223

10. Depression is a disease just like diabetes, right? 225

Notes to Chapter Ten 232

11. The prolonged promotion of a long-discredited theory 235

A perfect storm: why this falsehood survived and prospered 235

Antidepressants work, therefore brain chemical imbalances must exist 243

A useful metaphor or just plain lying? 243

We do it for the patients' sake 249

The drug companies are to blame 251

Assuming that what the experts say is objective and trustworthy 253

Biology is king 254

Collegiality before truth 256

A flawed disease model 263

Confusion about cause and effect 264

Notes to Chapter Eleven 266

12. The medical profession and the brain 271

Who treats brain diseases and disorders? 271

What do psychiatrists do? Are they brain experts? 271

Between a rock and a hard place 275

Do GPs generally treat treatable brain diseases and disorders? 279

Red herrings and the brain 282

Notes to Chapter Twelve 285

13. The depression delusion: what is real and what is not real 287

The experiences and behaviours of depression are very real 287

Delusion defined 287

The depression delusion 289

Groupthink, mass delusion and depression 291

Notes to Chapter Thirteen 298

14. Questionable practices and standards in high places 301

Depression is a flaw in chemistry not character, right? 301

Flawed perception 301

Flawed science 302

Propaganda, hegemony and sophistry 305

A perverse implantation 311

Notes to Chapter Fourteen 312

15. Future delusions 315

The delusion is dying, long live the next delusions 316

The National Institute of Mental Health forges ahead 319

Notes to Chapter Fifteen 325

16. The consequences of the depression chemical imbalance delusion 327

Exaggerated hope 331

Who benefits and who loses 332

Misinformed and manufactured consent 334

Notes to Chapter Sixteen 337

Conclusion 339

An appalling vista 340

Notes to the Conclusion 343

Index 345

FOREWORD

The notion that antidepressants fix a known chemical imbalance in the brain, and thus are like "insulin for diabetes," has had profound implications for society as a whole. This is a claim that, if true, tells of scientists discovering the molecular basis for our moods, and thus presents us with a new understanding of how the human brain works.

Indeed, the chemical imbalance story encourages us to think of ourselves as *governed* by the chemicals in our brains, with this chemical control seemingly disconnected from the many life events, that, at least according to past understandings of human nature, could be understood to dramatically alter one's moods. We are mechanistic machines, and if our mood molecules are out of balance, with this imbalance presented to us as a "disease," then it makes perfect sense to think that a solution must lie in a pill that fixes that imbalance.

But is the claim true? Did scientific investigations find that this is indeed so? Every society would do itself a favor if it publicly sought to answer that question.

In this book, Terry Lynch has done just that. And in so doing, he has told, step by step, how psychiatry and the pharmaceutical industry constructed and sold a false story to the public. By the end of this book, readers will be asking a new question: How could this falsehood have endured for so long?

As Terry Lynch writes, there was never good scientific reason to believe that antidepressants fixed a chemical imbalance in the brain. The hypothesis that this might be so arose from an understanding of how an antidepressant acted on the brain. Once researchers discovered that an antidepressant increased the activity of serotonin in the brain, they hypothesized that perhaps people suffering from depression had too little serotonin. However, researchers then investigated whether this was so, and discovered that it was not. Even by the early 1980s, researchers were saying that it didn't appear that a deficit in serotonin activity was a cause of depression.

Yet, when Prozac came to market in 1988, a drug touted as a selective serotonergic reuptake inhibitor, the public began to regularly hear about how it balanced serotonin in the brain. But by that time, the low-serotonin story was better described as a marketing slogan than a scientific claim. Researchers did continue to investigate serotonin function in depressed patients, but they never found it to be abnormal. Even so, academic psychiatrists, together with pharmaceutical companies, said otherwise. The new SSRIs fixed a chemical imbalance in the brain, like insulin for diabetes.

Terry Lynch provides an exhaustive, and even encyclopedic, review of this story in *The Depression Delusion*. He has combed through textbooks, media reports, educational brochures, websites and so forth to document, in extraordinary detail, the telling of this false story, with those making the claim often seen, by the public, as leading "experts" in this field. At the same time, he provides a thorough record of how a number of scientists, for the past 30 years, have been telling us that the story is false and that the science doesn't add up.

Yet, and this is the amazing thing, it is the false story that took hold in the public mind, rather than the scientific one that told of a hypothesis that doesn't pan out.

In this book, Terry Lynch also details what has been lost by societal adoption of this falsehood. That loss starts with societies not investing in non-drug therapies that might provide much more effective help for those struggling with depression. In this way, he makes a clear case for why society needs to put aside its delusion about chemical imbalances and seek to rethink what we do or don't know about depression and how to best treat people so diagnosed.

By the end, it is impossible to imagine anyone reading this book could believe in the chemical imbalance story. Terry Lynch, in this book, has given it a thorough burial.

Robert Whitaker, August 2014.

Robert Whitaker is an American journalist and author of the 2010 book *Anatomy of an Epidemic: Magic Bullets, Psychiatric Drugs and the Astonishing Rise of Mental Illness in America*, winner of the Investigative Reporters and Editors (IRE) best investigative journalism book of 2010. He is also the author of the 2001 book *Mad in America*. A 1998 Boston Globe article series he co-wrote on psychiatric research was a finalist for the 1999 Pulitzer Prize for Public Service. Articles co-written by Robert Whitaker won the 1998 George Polk Award for Medical Writing and the 1998 National Association of Science Writers' Science in Society Journalism Award for best magazine article.

INTRODUCTION

The world is engulfed in a mass delusion regarding depression. The widespread belief that brain chemical imbalances are present in depression has no scientific basis. In fact, this is a fixed belief that meets all the criteria of a mass delusion. If you are one of the millions of people who believe that biochemical brain imbalances are known to occur in depression, then you too have become seriously misinformed.

It may appear absurd to declare that the common understanding of depression as a brain chemical imbalance is misinformation, a delusion. You are probably familiar with the perception of depression as a chemical imbalance that is frequently referred to by doctors. You may accept this interpretation as truth, seeing no reason to question it. Doctors are viewed as honourable and knowledgeable experts. You may assume that their words are always accurate and trustworthy. These doctors are society's appointed experts after all. You may understandably have concluded that the interests of their patients is always their first priority.

I used to think that too. In my early years as a doctor, I fully believed in the medical approach to everything. That was before I expanded my horizons beyond the narrow confines of the medical understanding of depression I received from my medical training. Through my deliberations, work and research I have come to realize that important aspects of the medical approach to depression are indeed delusional. I have also come to realize that at times there is a greater priority for some doctors than the welfare of their patients; the protection and growth of their own ideologies and modus operandi.

The extent of the depression brain chemical imbalance delusion was accurately described in a March 2014 *Scientific American* article:

> Much of the public seems to have accepted the chemical imbalance hypothesis uncritically. For example, in a 2007 survey of 262 undergraduates, psychologist Christopher M. France of Cleveland State University and his colleagues found that 84.7 percent of participants found it "likely" that chemical imbalances cause depression. [1]

These results are similar to those of other surveys I mention in this book. Such results illustrate the extent to which the public have been misled by misinformation into believing that brain chemical imbalances are synonymous with depression.

I use the term "depression delusion" to describe a set of beliefs and heavily promoted ideas that have little or no grounding in science or logic, yet have become widely accepted as fact. The depression delusion applies across virtually every aspect of depression including its cause, nature, diagnosis, treatment and research. This delusion might be summed up as follows:

Depression is scientifically and reliably proven to be a medical illness; a disease like any other, characterized by known and measurable brain abnormalities; a brain disease caused by chemical abnormalities within the brain; a genetically inherited illness; antidepressants work by correcting chemical imbalances in the brain, especially imbalances in serotonin levels; antidepressants are highly effective and definitely not addictive; depression is the best way to interpret these people's experiences; doctors' understanding of and expertise in depression exceeds that of any other group.

The language of the medical profession can at times create an air of authority that in the case of mental health is not justified by the evidence. In this book I attempt to describe medical thinking in plain English.

The depression delusion has become accepted as truth in the eyes of those who believe in it. This delusion is regularly reinforced from many quarters. Aspects of the delusion regularly come up in everyday conversations and in the media. In this book I address the best known aspect of the delusion in detail; that depression is characterized and/or caused by brain chemical imbalances. The brain chemicals generally cited as the problem in depression are serotonin, noradrenaline and dopamine, serotonin being the most cited culprit. In some parts of the world including America, noradrenaline is referred to as norepinephrine. I address the other aspects of the depression delusion in future books.

The prevailing view for over half a century is that depression is caused primarily by biological brain abnormalities. For the past five decades and particularly since the arrival of the Prozac-type generation of drugs in 1988, people have been consistently fed the message that depression is caused by a brain chemical abnormality. Few people have not heard that a brain chemical imbalance is a known or believed characteristic of depression. The sources of this misinformation include trusted doctors; drug companies; television and radio programmes and in some countries, advertisements; websites; mental health organizations and books. Millions of people worldwide have been misinformed in doctors' offices that their depression is caused by a brain chemical abnormality. Medical doctors and drug companies have talked up chemical imbalances as a known characteristic of depression to their patients, colleagues and in the media for over half a century, putting the idea into people's heads and reinforcing it through repetition. Consequently most people are familiar with the notion that low serotonin causes depression and erroneously accept this as an established fact. It is hardly surprising that the prevailing medical view of depression has been accepted as truth by the general public.

But there is a problem, a major and inconvenient problem; *none of this is scientifically established to be true.* For more than fifty years the medical profession and the pharmaceutical industry have promoted the notion that biochemical brain abnormalities are at the heart of depression. This hypothesis remains unconfirmed despite many thousands of research projects undertaken to establish its veracity. This notion was actually discredited several years before Prozac was launched in 1988. Psychiatry has based much of its research upon the presumption that the assumed biological basis of depression is a foregone conclusion, aided and abetted by the pharmaceutical industry which has financed much of this research. Psychiatry does not seriously question—and does not welcome questioning of—the assumptions upon which their beliefs, practices and research are based; in particular, their unproven yet stubbornly-held conviction that there is a fundamental biological basis for depression.

The dominance of the flawed medical understanding of emotional and mental health including depression is one of the greatest crises of our time. The medical profession has become seduced into beliefs about depression that go well beyond and sometimes contradict scientific evidence, the depression brain chemical imbalance delusion being a major example. The vast majority of doctors who regularly diagnose depression and prescribe antidepressants are well-intentioned but they are seriously misguided. As a consequence, generations of people on medication have not been afforded sufficient opportunity to look at the emotional and psychological aspects of their distress, thereby reducing the potential for growth and recovery.

I am not suggesting that all of the promoters of the depression delusion debacle wilfully set out to deceive. Some have, but the majority are sincere people who mean well and are earnest in their efforts to ease the burdens of others. The desire to help can become intense and zealous, distorting objectivity and judgement. Hungarian mental health campaigner Gabor Gombos reminds us that good intentions do not always result in clear thinking or best outcomes:

> I remind myself that many of the mistakes in mental health care come from a helping attitude. But they want to help you without asking you, without understanding you, without involving you. [2]

A sizeable minority of people have seen through the depression delusion and have publicly express their concerns. Many are highly qualified scientists, doctors, psychologists, allied mental health professionals, journalists and users of the mental health system. They have become alarmed at the extent and the effects of the gross misinformation that pertains regarding depression and other psychiatric diagnoses. I include the words of some of these people in this book. I do so to illustrate the widespread nature of the depression delusion and to demonstrate that those who question the establishment are not a tiny bunch of disgruntled cranks who should be summarily dismissed. I include many references to demonstrate the considerable body of scientific knowledge that contradicts the depression brain chemical imbalance notion, demonstrating the woeful lack of scientific evidence for this widely believed delusion.

The comments of integrative medicine practitioner Chris Kresser accurately reflect the venerable status given to brain chemical abnormalities in depression:

> The idea that depression and other mental health conditions are caused by an imbalance of chemicals in the brain is so deeply ingrained in our psyche that it almost seems sacrilegious to question it. [3]

But if truth and real progress in mental health truly are our main priorities, then question it we must. The collapse of an idea that has formed an important part of the fabric of our way of understanding things can make us feel quite uncomfortable. We may be tempted to resist seeing the collapse of an idea we had assumed to be an important truth. The greater the part an idea plays in our life, the greater the temptation to resist seeing the truth, even if the collapse of the idea is right and necessary in the public interest.

Questioning the medical approach to depression is not merely a theoretical battle between opposing camps. This is not a debate between two equally legitimate positions. My position regarding the depression delusion is based on facts. There is no reliable scientific evidence behind assertions that brain chemical imbalances are known to be a feature of depression. The assumption that brain chemical imbalances occur or are likely to occur in depression is therefore not a legitimate position upon which to base the understanding of and responses to depression. As medicinal chemist Derek Lowe—who worked in drug development for a pharmaceutical company—wrote in his *In the Pipeline* blog:

> I worked on central nervous system drugs for eight years, and I can confidently state that we know slightly more than jack about how antidepressants work. [4]

American psychiatrist Daniel Carlat acknowledged this fact in his 2010 book *Unhinged: The Trouble with Psychiatry—A Doctor's Revelations About a Profession in Crisis*:

> The shocking truth is that psychiatry has yet to develop a convincing explanation for the pathophysiology of any illness at all. [5]

Pathophysiology is the study of functional changes in the body that occur in a disease.

Dr. Carlat is acknowledging an inconvenient and shocking truth. Psychiatry has yet to identify scientifically convincing evidence of abnormal structural or functional changes in the body for any psychiatric diagnosis treated primarily by psychiatry, depression included. Remarkably, despite this reality, the depression brain chemical imbalance delusion is firmly embedded within society. The medical approach to depression prescribes one way of explaining human pain and suffering as *the* right way to interpret human behaviour, experience and distress. Each of our lives is visited by struggle, loss, hurt, trauma, change and disappointment, to varying degrees. Experiencing distress is an unavoidable part of the human condition. Psychiatry is at the top of the mental health pyramid, entrusted with the authority to decide how our distress is to be interpreted. As physiology professor and lecturer Dr. Donald Gould, once editor of *World Medicine* and *New Scientist*, wrote in his 1985 book *The Black and White Medicine Show: How Doctors Serve and Fail their Customers*, what goes on in psychiatry impacts on us all in one way or another:

> It would therefore behove us well—public and politicians alike—to take an active interest in the welfare of our mentally disturbed compatriots, and not to leave their fate to the sole discretion of the experts. They are very far from being expert. And

the figures tell us there's a more than sporting chance that it will be you, or I, or our mother or brother or our daughter or our spouse who becomes a victim of their ignorance before too long. Medical paternalism can go too far, and we should beware of giving the medical establishment too much legal power. [6]

Dismantling this delusion will be no easy task, but it is essential if we are to create societies where people's emotional and psychological realities are properly understood and engaged with effectively. It is for this reason that I present many examples of the depression brain chemical imbalance delusion in this book in detail. Many health professionals refer to scientific evidence and evidence-based medicine as the backbone of their beliefs and practices regarding depression. How ironic that there is no evidence base whatsoever for the widely promoted notion that brain chemical imbalances are a characteristic feature of depression. Since this supposed "evidence" forms a core part of the depression delusion, I devote considerable space in this book to deconstructing fallacious claims made by those who have promoted the prevailing understanding of depression.

Sometimes the most important questions to ask are the ones that people assume have already been answered. In his 2013 book *The Book of Woe: The DSM and the Unmaking of Psychiatry*, American psychotherapist and author Gary Greenberg posed one such question:

> How much of our suffering should we turn over to doctors—especially our psychiatrists? . . . The inescapable a priori principle of psychiatry . . . is that our psychological suffering is *medical* . . . which . . . means located in body processes gone awry. [7]

Head of Mad Pride Ireland, John MacCarthy died in 2012. John had many years of contact with mental health services during his lifetime and considered himself a survivor of psychiatry. In his determined search for truth and justice for people experiencing emotional and mental distress, John asked many important questions about psychiatry and its practices. In his 2011 book *The Human Condition*, John asked:

> Is it time to decriminalize human emotions? Is it time to deconstruct the medical model of modern psychiatry that at its centre of complex language has nothing to substantiate its right to diagnose? Is it time to question every pill being dispensed as to the cause and effect behind that pill? Is it time to break down the barrier of fear that says it is dangerous to question your doctor? Is it time to demand time from your psychiatrist? Is it time that psychiatric nurses step forward and look to respecting their place on the pecking order, and to stop walking two paces behind their master? Is it time for other disciplines to get their house in order like social work, psychology, occupational therapy and finally take true leadership roles in multidisciplinary teams? Is it time to put the prescription pad into second place and to get back to holding and caring of people? Is it time for old fashioned love to be the first word to be written on a prescription pad? [8]

By deconstructing a key aspect of the depression delusion—that brain chemical imbalances are an established feature of depression—it is my hope that this book will contribute to the necessary changes articulated so well by this great campaigner.

At first glance, the depression brain chemical imbalance delusion sounds reasonable and familiar. As a book reviewer on amazon.co.uk wrote in 2013:

> If depression is not caused by a chemical balance, why after taking antidepressants do I feel so much better? [9]

People have been told for many years by their doctors that antidepressants work by correcting a brain chemical imbalance and this reviewer's comments reflect this. On reflection, it is clear that substances do not have to be correcting an imbalance to make people feel "so much better". After major bowel surgery in 2011, I was on a morphine drip for several days for pain relief. Not only did the drug relieve my pain; it made me feel so much better, almost euphoric. I wasn't suffering from a morphine deficiency at the time. A person may feel "so much better" when their splitting headache is relieved by paracetamol or their social anxiety is temporarily eliminated by a vodka or two. Few people in such circumstances would claim that these substances alleviated their situation because their chosen solutions corrected a pre-existing brain deficiency of paracetamol or alcohol respectively.

WHY IT MATTERS

In the minds of the vast majority of doctors and the public, brain chemical imbalances have become synonymous with depression. This is how depression has been framed for fifty years now, as a brain chemical imbalance for which chemicals that correct this imbalance are the most logical and appropriate treatment. This collective misrepresentation and misunderstanding of depression has diverted the search for greater understanding of depression way off course. As a consequence, the emotional and psychological aspects—which are the key aspects of depression—and detailed sustained research into these have been largely sidelined for half a century.

The consequences of this grossly distorted understanding and approach to depression have been catastrophic. The development of a comprehensive holistic understanding of depression has been thwarted by a virtually global error with equally global consequences. Perhaps more than any other phenomenon, the near-universal belief that brain chemical imbalances are a key characteristic of depression has greatly hampered developments that could have immense benefits for millions of people worldwide. I discuss the consequences of the dominance of the brain chemical imbalance delusion in chapter sixteen.

Public opinion has long been a powerful driver of change. Since the majority of the public believe that chemical imbalances occur in and probably cause depression, the natural public desire for answers regarding how and why people become depressed has for years been satisfied by the chemical imbalance falsehood. By becoming aware of the truth—that there is not and there never was any solid scientific basis to claims of brain chemical imbalances in depression—perhaps the sleeping giant that is public opinion will again awaken and demand more truthful answers.

A key objective of this book is to bring to public attention the complete lack of any direct evidence of brain chemical imbalances in depression. Antidepressants have been found to interfere with the reuptake of neurotransmitters in the nerve synapses, the spaces between brain cells. According to the fifty-year-old chemical abnormality theory of depression, because substances that increase neurotransmitter levels in brain synapses by interfering with neurotransmitter reuptake appear to help some people feel better, a deficiency of neurotransmitters is the likely cause of depression. That's it in a nutshell, the flimsy premise upon which the medical and pharmaceutical approach to depression has been based for more than fifty years.

Physician and pathologist Dr. Marcia Angell is a former editor-in-chief of the *New England Journal of Medicine* and Senior Lecturer in the Department of Global Health and Social Medicine at Harvard Medical School. In a 2011 *New York Review of Books* article Angell wrote the following about the depression brain chemical imbalance notion:

> The main problem with the theory is that after decades of trying to prove the chemical imbalance theory, scientists have come up empty-handed . . . Because certain antidepressants increase levels of the neurotransmitter serotonin in the brain, it was postulated that depression is caused by too little serotonin. Thus, instead of developing a drug to treat an abnormality, an abnormality was postulated to fit a drug. That was a great leap of logic. [10]

On 13 May 2013 in an unprecedented development, the British Psychological Society Division of Clinical Psychology issued a Position Statement in response to the publication of the latest edition of the *Diagnostic and Statistical Manual of Mental Disorders (DSM-5)* in which they called for a major review of mental health:

> It is timely and appropriate to affirm publicly that the current classification system as outlined in the *Diagnostic and Statistical Manual (DSM)* and the *International Classification of Diseases (ICD)* in respect of the functional psychiatric diagnoses, has significant conceptual and empirical limitations. Consequently, there is a need for a paradigm shift in relation to the experiences that these diagnoses refer to, towards a conceptual system not based on a disease model. The British Psychological Society calls for an approach that fully acknowledges the growing amount of evidence for psychosocial causal factors, but which does not assign an unevidenced role for biology as the primary cause, and that is transparent about the very limited support for the "disease" model in such situations. [11]

I fully support the position of the British Psychological Society Division of Clinical Psychology. Their claim of "an unevidenced role of biology as the primary cause" is accurate. There is no reliable corroborative evidence to support claims that depression is characterized by brain chemical abnormalities. I believe that exposing and deconstructing the depression delusion is an important step toward creating a new paradigm of understanding in emotional and mental health.

Many people report that they have been helped by medication. Medication has a place in the field of emotional and mental health. I prescribe medication, though less so than the majority of my colleagues. I and many others believe that medication is over-used. The widespread belief in the depression brain chemical imbalance delusion has contributed greatly to the over-reliance on medication in mental health.

LOGICAL FALLACIES

The study of correct and incorrect reasoning has a proud tradition, dating back to Aristotle and his teacher, Plato. Logical fallacies are long-established errors of logic and reasoning. Errors of both fact and logic are commonplace within the prevailing approach to depression. I include many references to logical fallacies in this book to demonstrate the degree to which psychiatric thinking and practice repeatedly contravenes basic principles of logic and reasoning. Flawed logic is a common characteristic of delusions, and the depression brain chemical imbalance delusion is no exception.

A logical fallacy is an invalid form of argument, an instance of incorrect reasoning. The *Oxford Dictionary* defines a fallacy as "a mistaken belief, especially one based on unsound arguments" and a logical fallacy as "a failure in reasoning that renders an argument invalid". [12] According to the Logicalfallacies website:

> Fallacious reasoning keeps us from knowing the truth, and the inability to think critically makes us vulnerable to manipulation by those skilled in the art of rhetoric". [13]

One would not expect to find logical fallacies within a discipline that publicly claims adherence to sound logical reasoning and scientific thinking. Such fundamental errors should have no place in any system that presents itself as fundamentally scientific. On the contrary, as you will see in this book, logical fallacies are a regular feature of the prevailing medical understanding of depression.

Two logical fallacies are worthy of mention at the outset. One of the themes of this book is to uncover the many fallacies that lie within the prevailing understanding of depression as an illness caused by brain chemical abnormalities. In doing so, I am mindful of the Fallacist's Fallacy. [14] This fallacy applies when a proposition is dismissed as false simply because some arguments in its favour are fallacious. In this book I describe the fallacies of the prevailing view of depression as a brain chemical imbalance. I do not dismiss the possibility that biological factors might be involved in depression. We cannot know the future, therefore it would be inappropriate for me to conclude that biological factors in depression will never be identified. Since the future is not ours to see, I confine myself in this book to the information we can usefully work with now, what is known and not known now.

As I discuss in chapter three, research is only beginning to discover the unfathomable complexity of the human brain. Scientists have increasingly realized that understanding the human brain is a far more challenging task than previously assumed. Rather than increase the likelihood of biological breakthroughs in the understanding of depression, the stark realization of the extraordinary complexity of the brain has if anything diminished the likelihood of identifying clear-cut biological abnormalities in depression. As I discuss in chapter one, the recent withdrawal and scaling down of psychiatric research by several pharmaceutical companies—previously psychiatry's greatest research allies—is evidence of the increasing realization that, in the opinion of many drug companies and many researchers, biological and chemical solutions are a great deal less likely than they seemed fifty years ago. At that time, drug companies were greatly increasing their investment in psychiatric research and drugs. They did so because they saw vast opportunities for growth and profits opening up for them. The wheel is turning full circle now.

In the event that biological abnormalities in depression are found at some point in the future, it would be a mistake to assume that any such abnormalities cause depression. As several people I refer to in this book have stated, any such abnormalities are at least as likely to be the result of the person's emotional and psychological state. Mainstream psychiatry has long had a blind spot in this regard, assuming that biology is generally *the* most important and influential aspect of the situation, even though biological abnormalities are never identified to exist in the patients with depression that they treat. Since the current situation is that no brain chemical abnormalities have been identified in depression, questioning whether brain chemical abnormalities are the cause or the consequence of depression is an entirely hypothetical discussion. In his 2000 book *Prozac Backlash: Overcoming the Dangers of Prozac, Zoloft, Paxil, and Other Antidepressants with Safe, Effective Treatments*, psychiatrist Joseph Glenmullen concluded:

> Eventually, scientists may discover real proof that a small percentage of patients have genetically determined, biological symptoms. But we are a long way from any such knowledge. When patients are told otherwise, they are being seriously misled. [15]

I also want to mention the Subjectivist Fallacy at the outset of this book. A subjectivist fallacy occurs when someone resists the conclusion of an argument by treating the conclusion as subjective when it is in fact objective. [16] This is typically done by labelling the arguer's conclusion as merely an opinion or perspective. Subjectivist fallacies feature regularly in the dismissal of those who disagree with the prevailing medical views on mental health. As I mentioned earlier in this chapter, the information I present in this book is not an *opinion* or *perspective*. It is based on *facts* and *truth*, and reflects the true state of scientific knowledge regarding brain chemical imbalances and depression.

Explanations for the other logical fallacies I refer to in this book are provided in the notes at the end of each chapter.

SEMINAL MOMENTS

As I reflect upon my journey from enthusiastic supporter of the medical approach to mental health to having little faith in it, many moments stand out. These include being repeatedly shocked upon reading psychiatrist Peter Breggin's *Toxic Psychiatry* [17] and many other books and articles expressing similar concerns; listening to many harrowing accounts of people attending GPs and psychiatrists whose stories, issues and needs regularly went unheard, unseen and unmet; and witnessing some people who attended me with major psychiatric diagnoses such as severe depression, bipolar disorder and schizophrenia make excellent recoveries—and reading many similar stories of recovery—that contradicted psychiatry's claim that these situations are chronic illnesses like diabetes from which recovery is not possible. Being contacted by American psychiatrist William Glasser, founder of Choice Theory and Reality Therapy, and being requested to write the foreword to his book *Warning: Psychiatry Can Be Hazardous To Your Mental Health* because he loved my book *Beyond Prozac* was another milestone for me. Meeting journalist Robert Whitaker, Pulitzer Prize finalist, author of *Mad in America* and *Anatomy of an Epidemic*—and now author of the foreword to this book—and speaking at a 28 February 2011 Mindfreedom Ireland conference in Cork, Ireland at which Robert was the keynote speaker, was another seminal moment for me.

Another milestone occurred in 1997. It involved an exchange in the Letters section of *Medicine Weekly* with psychiatrist Patricia Casey, professor of psychiatry at University College, Dublin, one of Ireland's most influential psychiatrists of the past forty years. By that time I had already developed many concerns about the principles and practices of psychiatry, concerns that were not alleviated by this exchange.

In 1997 Professor Casey wrote an article in *Medicine Weekly* titled "Prozac is now the scapegoat of the ignorant and the cruel". Something about this title unsettled me. I had many concerns about Prozac and its use, but I did not think that I was either ignorant or cruel. I do not think that many people who have attended me would have considered me to be ignorant or cruel either. By then I had read many books and articles that questioned the widespread enthusiasm for antidepressants. Rather than being ignorant and cruel, the vast majority of these authors appeared quite the opposite—well informed, caring and concerned for the welfare of people in distress. I wondered about the choice of words in the title of this article. At the time I was still working as a general practitioner.

In this article, Professor Casey asserted that depression was a "debilitative biological disorder", that "depressive illness is organic in nature". She referred to depression as "biological depression". [18] I felt from this article that Patricia Casey seemed convinced that depression was an organic, biological illness. To the best of my knowledge at the time—and I had researched the issue considerably by 1997—I was not aware of any definite scientific evidence that verified such assertions.

I wrote to Professor Casey through the Letters page of *Medicine Weekly*. I felt it reasonable and important that Patricia Casey provide valid reliable evidence to verify her claims. My request was straightforward and unambiguous:

On three occasions in this article, Professor Casey refers to the view that depression is biological in nature. I would be very grateful if, through the pages of your journal, Prof. Casey would outline the research (with references) which proves conclusively that the cause of depression is biological or biochemical. [19]

Published in the Letters page of *Medicine Weekly* on 14 January 1998, Professor Casey's reply was brief:

In his letter, Dr. Terry Lynch requests that I provide references to substantiate my statements relating to the biological nature of depressive illness. I suggest that he purchase any of the postgraduate textbooks on psychiatry, where he will find a myriad of references to same. [20]

I felt that she did not answer my question directly at all. Far from satisfied by this short reply, I wrote the following letter in response:

Dear Editor,
I refer to Prof. Patricia Casey's reply to my letter of 14th January in which I asked Prof. Casey to outline, with references, what conclusive evidence there is (if any exists) that the cause of depression is biological. Rather than tell me to go off and buy some psychiatry books, I had hoped that Prof. Casey would answer my question.
I am well aware that there are many references in psychiatry books to the view that depression is biological in origin. However, I have not come across any article in any journal which constitutes conclusive proof that depression is biological.
Many articles and much research has linked depression with biochemical changes in the brain. But these are not in themselves proof of a biochemical or biological cause for depression. While these biological changes could point towards a biochemical cause for depression, they could equally be the effect of the depressive state.
What is the current position? Do we have conclusive proof that the cause of depression is biological? If so, then I would love to hear precisely what that proof is. If we do not at this time have conclusive proof that the cause of depression is biological, then our belief in the biological causation of depression is not a proven fact; rather, it is a working hypothesis. The thing about a hypothesis is that while it may well be right, it may also be wrong. Which is it? Proven fact, or working hypothesis? [21]

At that time, *Medicine Weekly* was circulated weekly to around 6,500 doctors in Ireland. Neither Patricia Casey nor any other doctor replied to this letter.

I have learned much since I wrote those letters in the late 1990s. In my second letter, I mentioned that biochemical changes may just as likely be a consequence as a cause in depression, a point made by several people I refer to in this book. I now know that no biochemical abnormalities have been reliably scientifically identified in depression at all. Debate about whether biochemical changes are the cause or consequence of depression is therefore both a Begging the Question logical fallacy [22] and a Red Herring logical fallacy [23], but I did not realize that at the time.

In a sense, in this book I have done what Professor Casey recommended to me over sixteen years ago. As part of my research for this current book, I have researched many psychiatric books. I also researched many medical textbooks in other related medical disciplines. Far from providing conclusive proof that depression is a known biological disorder, there is a dearth of any such evidence in medical textbooks. As described in this book, many medical textbooks actually contradict the presumed chemical view of depression, particularly those with no affiliation to psychiatry.

WHAT IS REAL AND WHAT IS NOT

Not for one second does my questioning of the medical interpretation of depression mean that I do not appreciate the degree of heartbreak and unhappiness that people experience. On the contrary, I have been so acutely aware of the immense distress that many people experience that I gave up my thriving medical practice in 1999 to devote myself to becoming more effective at working in mental health. My medical training was woefully inadequate in this regard.

The experiences and behaviours that become labeled as depression are very real. Claims that these experiences and behaviours are characterized or caused by brain chemical imbalances are not based on fact or evidence. They are subjective interpretations, for which no verifying scientific evidence exists. I discuss what is real and what is not in detail in chapter thirteen.

BOOK CONTENTS

In chapter one I consider two current major crises facing psychiatry that are directly related to the depression brain chemical imbalance delusion—the validity of the *Diagnostic and Statistical Manual of Mental Disorders-5 (DSM-5)*, often referred to as the psychiatrist's bible, and the fact that in recent years many drug companies have withdrawn from psychiatric research. I also look at a recurring cyclical pattern that has occurred at an alarming rate regarding many psychiatric drugs to this day. I discuss the reality that there are no known brain biochemical abnormalities in chapter two. In chapter three I explore the fact that the hypotheses upon which the depression brain chemical imbalance delusion are grounded have been discredited for several decades. I discuss a better way of understanding and dealing with depression in chapter four. Also in chapter four, I summarise the stories of nine people who attended me with severe depression. In chapter five I examine the common practice of misrepresenting the brain chemical imbalance delusion as an established fact, as many psychiatrists and GPs have done for fifty years. In chapter six I describe the role of the manufacturers of antidepressants in promoting the depression brain chemical imbalance delusion, the failure of regulatory bodies to protect the public from false information from drug companies and the role of some members of the pharmacy profession. I explore how the brain chemical imbalance delusion has been incorrectly presented as a known fact by some psychologists and psychotherapists in chapter seven.

In chapter eight I discuss the depression brain chemical imbalance misinformation that regularly emanates from mental health organizations, the media and the general public. In chapter nine I look at misinformation regarding brain chemicals and depression that has on occasion emerged from the world of nutrition. I examine the appropriateness of comparisons between depression and diabetes in chapter ten. Chapter eleven involves a discussion on how a hypothesis that was suspect and discredited several decades ago has continued to be promoted as a fact to this day. In chapter twelve I examine the relationship between the medical profession and the brain. I consider which medical specialties actually have expertise in the brain and regularly examine this organ. In chapter thirteen I discuss the characteristics of a delusion. I examine whether the depression brain chemical imbalance notion meets psychiatry's own criteria for a delusion. Chapter fourteen contains a review of questionable practices and low standards that exist within psychiatry in relation to the brain chemical imbalance delusion. In chapter fifteen I consider recent ideas being promoted within psychiatry that will likely replace the brain biochemical imbalance depression delusion. I look at the key role of the U.S. National Institute of Mental Health in the process of replacing current delusions with new ones. I discuss the major consequences of the widespread belief in brain chemical imbalances in depression in chapter sixteen. Notes are included at the end of each chapter. The book contains an extensive index.

This is the first of three books I am writing about depression. The purpose of this series is to contribute as much as I can to the urgent need for a paradigm shift regarding how depression is understood and responded to. My next book will address two further aspects of the depression delusion—whether or not depression is a biological disease like any other, and the often-claimed genetic nature of depression. That book will be published approximately twelve months after the publication of this book. I will then publish a book that sets out what in my experience are the core aspects of what is commonly known as depression. I refer to these briefly in chapter four of this book. Unlike supposed chemical brain abnormalities, for which no hard evidence of their existence has been identified despite over fifty years of intensive research, these features are right there in the story, experiences and behaviour of people who become diagnosed with depression, if one has the ability and the willingness to see them. I intend to approach bipolar disorder, schizophrenia, obsessive compulsive disorder, eating disorders, anxiety and suicide in similar fashion in future books.

NOTES TO THE INTRODUCTION

1. Hal Arkowitz & Scott O. Lilienfeld, "Is Depression Just Bad Chemistry?" *Scientific American*, 01 March 2014, http://www.scientificamerican.com/article/is-depression-just-bad-chemistry/, accessed 15 September 2014.
2. Gabor Gombos, Hungarian mental health rights activist, *Mental Illness: The Neglected Quarter*. Summary Report, Amnesty International, 2002.
3. Chris Kresser, "The 'chemical imbalance' myth", http://chriskresser.com/the-chemical-imbalance-myth, accessed 24 February 2014.

4. Derek Lowe, quoted in Begley, Sharon, in "Some Drugs Work to Treat Depression, But It Isn't Clear How", 18 November 2005, *Wall Street Journal*, http://online.wsj.com/news/articles /SB11 3226807554400588, accessed 07 May 2014.
5. Daniel Carlat, Unhinged: The Trouble with Psychiatry—a Doctor's Revelations about a Profession in Crisis, London: Free Press, 2010, p. 9.
6. Donald Gould, *The Black and White Medicine Show: How Doctors Serve and Fail their Customers,* Trafalgar Square Publishing, 1985.
7. Gary Greenberg, *The Book of Woe: The DSM and the Unmaking of Psychiatry,* London: Scribe Publications, 2013, pps. 21, 126.
8. John MacCarthy, *The Human Condition,* Elizabeth Press, 2011, p. 134.
9. A member of the public—using the name "Neagley"—in a 2013 review on amazon.co.uk of Dorothy Rowe's book *Depression: The Way out of Your Prison.* http://www.amazon.co.uk/ product-reviews/158391286X/ref=cm_cr_pr_btm_link_next_5?ie=UTF8&pageNumber =5&showView points=0&sortBy=byRankDescending, accessed 08 August 2014.
10. Marcia Angell, "The Epidemic of Mental Illness: Why?", *The New York Review of Books*, 23 June 2011, http://www.nybooks.com/articles/archives/2011/jun/23/epidemic-mental-illness-why/ ?pagination=false, accessed 15 February 2014.
11. British Psychological Society, http://dxrevisionwatch.files.wordpress.com/2013/05/position-statement-on-diagnosis-master-doc.pd, accessed 16 April 2014.
12. http://www.oxforddictionaries.com/definition/english/fallacy, accessed 13 November 2013.
13. http://www.logicalfallacies.info/, accessed 10 November 2013.
14. http://www.fallacyfiles.org/fallfall.html, accessed 02 January 2014.
15. Joseph Glenmullen, Prozac Backlash: Overcoming the Dangers of Prozac, Zoloft, Paxil and Other Antidepressants with Safe, Effective Alternatives, New York: Simon & Shuster, 2001, p. 203.
16. http://www.logicalfallacies.info/presumption/subjectivist/, accessed 02 January 2014.
17. Peter Breggin, *Toxic Psychiatry,* London: HarperCollins, 1993.
18. Psychiatry professor Patricia Casey, "Prozac is now the scapegoat of the ignorant and the cruel", *Medicine Weekly,* 17 December 1997.
19. Terry Lynch, letter, *Medicine Weekly,* 04 February 1998.
20. Patricia Casey, psychiatry professor, letter, in *Medicine Weekly,* 14 January 1998.
21. Terry Lynch, letter, *Medicine Weekly,* 04 February 1998.
22. The Begging the Question logical fallacy is an argument or other statement that merely assumes or re-states its own position as truth rather than provide relevant supportive evidence and logical arguments. An argument begs the question when it assumes as a fact any questionable point not conceded by the other side. A premise is presented as though it were a fact, in order to support one's position. If the premise is questionable, the argument is not solid. Presenting the premise as though it were a fact gives the false impression that the argument is based on solid ground.
    http://www.kspope.com/fallacies/fallacies.php, accessed 02 January 2014.
    http://www.fallacyfiles.org/begquest.html, accessed 02 January 2014.
    http://grammarist.com/rhetoric/begging-the-question-fallacy/, accessed 02 January 2014.
23. A Red Herring logical fallacy occurs when issues are raised that mislead or distract from the real issue. Red Herring logical fallacies involve an attempt to divert attention and to redirect the argument to another issue to which the person doing the redirecting can better respond. In this case, the focus is on whether brain biochemical abnormalities cause or are caused by depression. This is a red herring, taking the focus away from the inconvenient truth that no biochemical abnormalities have been identified in depression.
    http://www.redherringexamples.com/#sthash.WQJ55K7N.dpuf, accessed 12 May 2014.
    http://www.logicallyfallacious.com/index.php/logical-fallacies/151-red-herring, accessed 12 May 2014.

1. CRISES IN THE CAMP

Mainstream psychiatry presents a largely united front regarding its core beliefs. Regarding their understanding of and approach to depression and other mental health issues, psychiatrists and general practitioners regularly present their thinking and practices in a fashion that is favourable to their own position. This generally means presenting psychiatry as a medical specialty like any other, solidly grounded in a trustworthy bed of science. Beneath the surface a different story rumbles, one in which real scientific evidence plays little part. This reality applies to the notion of the depression brain chemical imbalance, and to two related topics that I discuss in this chapter; the *Diagnostic and Statistical Manual of Mental Disorders*, and the exodus by many drug companies from research into depression and other mental health problems. Both are directly linked to the absence of evidence of identified brain chemical abnormalities.

THE PSYCHIATRIST'S BIBLE

The creation of the American Psychiatric Association and often referred to as the psychiatrist's bible, the *Diagnostic and Statistical Manual of Mental Disorders (DSM)* is the flagship of psychiatry, the main psychiatric diagnostic reference along with the *International Classification of Diseases (ICD)*. The following comments made in books published in 2012—the first by a psychologist, the second by the authors of a psychiatry textbook—illustrate the efforts made within psychiatry to minimise the differences between the *DSM* and the *ICD*:

> Both diagnostic manuals are revised to keep up with research and treatment advances in mental illness, and are designed to work in concert with each other. [1]

According to the authors of the 2012 psychiatry textbook *The Shorter Oxford Textbook of Psychiatry*, the most recent editions of the *DSM (DSM-5)* and *ICD (ICD-10)* have been:

> Developed in parallel, and to avoid unnecessary differences there was close consultation between the working parties preparing the two documents. [2]

The *DSM* has become widely accepted within society as a trustworthy scientific manual, regularly used not only by psychiatrists and the rest of the medical profession, but also by insurance companies, hospitals, courts, prisons, schools, researchers and government agencies. Known as the *DSM-5*, the fifth edition was published in May 2013.

Over recent decades, an aura of scientific authority has developed around the *Diagnostic and Statistical Manual of Mental Disorders*. According to the American Psychiatric Association, the creators of the *DSM*:

The *Diagnostic and Statistical Manual of Mental Disorders (DSM)* is the handbook used by health care professionals in the United States and much of the world as the authoritative guide to the diagnosis of mental disorders. *DSM* contains descriptions, symptoms, and other criteria for diagnosing mental disorders. [3]

The following quote from the Allaboutdepression website illustrates the deference in which the *DSM* is generally held:

> The clinical usefulness of the *DSM* is much more than a tool for making diagnoses. It is used by mental health professionals and physicians as a guide for communicating about mental health conditions. When two clinicians discuss a diagnosis such as "major depressive disorder, single episode, severe with psychotic features", they both have the same conceptualization of the condition. The *DSM* also allows mental health professionals to reach consensus on which symptoms or groups of symptoms should define which disorders. Such decisions are based on empirical evidence—research results—usually by a multidisciplinary staff of professionals. Further, the *DSM* is used as an educational tool and a reference for conducting all types of research, e.g., clinical trials, prevalence studies, outcome research. [4]

Beneath this veneer of supposed science and authority, major points of concern arise in regard to the *Diagnostic and Statistical Manual of Mental Disorders*. The *DSM* is created by a group of American psychiatrists who spend years debating and arguing about which aspects of human experience and behaviour they consider to be "abnormal" and therefore authoritatively declared as illnesses to be diagnosed by doctors. The first *DSM* was published in 1952 and alluded to one hundred and six disorders. Each of the subsequent revisions included a significant increase in the number of disorders. Published just over forty years later in 1994, the *DSM-4* referred to 365 disorders, a 350% increase compared to the first *DSM*. The latest edition of the *Diagnostic and Statistical Manual of Mental Disorders—DSM-5*—was published in 2013. This edition contained 15 new mental disorders and many other changes to existing diagnoses including the elimination of some.

Mental disorders are deemed to exist by consensus agreement in the absence of any objective scientific verification. In no other medical specialty does anything like this occur. No other medical specialty meets intermittently to manufacture consensus on what are deemed to be illnesses. The entire psychiatric process depends on doctors' interpretations of people's experiences and behaviours. Without any confirmatory physical signs or investigations, the diagnostic process is fundamentally subjective, lacking scientific consistency and reliability.

The absence of supporting evidence of illness can lead to dubious practices. Diagnoses are added, removed or changed at a rate unparalleled in any other medical specialty. Two of the more dubious at various points in history have been the labelling of homosexuality and masturbation as mental illnesses. Homosexuality was included in the *Diagnostic and Statistical Manual of Mental Disorders* as a mental disorder until the early 1970s. Protests and lobbying by gay rights activists and evidence from Alfred Kinsey led to the removal of homosexuality from the *DSM-4* in 1974. Alfred Kinsey was the co-author of the Kinsey Reports that helped to transform the understanding of human sexuality. Prior to the abolition of homosexuality as a mental illness, many people were subjected to various forms of aversion therapy such as electric shocks and nausea-inducing drugs in an attempt to "cure" their "mental illness". Among the changes made in the 2013 *DSM-5* was the reduction of grief as a valid entity from two months to just two weeks, after which grief and bereavement can now be considered to be depression and treated as such.

The *DSM*-creating process consists primarily of debate among mainly American psychiatrists. Eventually they come to some sort of consensus, which then forms the basis of the manual. This caucus-like approach to establishing psychiatric diagnostic categories is unparalleled in medicine. In every other medical specialty, there is little need for debate or consensus regarding what constitutes illness. Psychiatry is the only medical specialty in which testing for biological abnormalities that are known to occur in specific illnesses—known as biological markers—plays virtually no part in diagnosis and management.

While an air of controversy has surrounded the *DSM* for decades, this has risen to unprecedented levels following the publication of the *DSM-5* in 2013. Several heavy hitters within mainstream psychiatry have expressed grave concern about the manual and the manner in which it was constructed. Four of the most influential psychiatrists of the past twenty years have been highly critical of the *DSM*; the current director of perhaps the world's most powerful mental health organization—the National Institute of Mental Health (NIMH)—and his predecessor, and the lead psychiatrists for the two previous *Diagnostic and Statistical Manual of Mental Disorders, DSM-3* and *DSM-4*.

In an unprecedented development that illustrates a growing crisis within psychiatry, in April 2013 the National Institute of Mental Health—a United States federal agency—moved to distance itself from the then soon-to-be-published *DSM 5*. According to a statement issued by Thomas Insel, director of this institute on 29 April 2013:

> At best, the *DSM* is a dictionary, creating a set of labels and defining them. The weakness is its lack of validity . . . Unlike our definitions of ischaemic heart disease, lymphoma or AIDS, the *DSM* diagnoses are based on consensus about clusters of clinical symptoms, not any objective laboratory measures. In the rest of medicine, this would be equivalent to creating diagnostic symptoms based on the nature of chest pain or the quality of fever. Indeed, symptom-based diagnosis, once common in other areas of medicine, has been largely replaced in the past half-century as we have understood that symptoms alone rarely indicate the best choice of treatment. Patients with mental disorders deserve better. [5]

In a May 2013 *New York Times* article Thomas Insel stated:

> As long as the research community takes the *DSM* to be a bible, we'll never make progress . . . People think that everything has to match *DSM* criteria, but you know what? Biology never read that book. [6]

My understanding of Insel's cryptic final sentence above is that it is a reference to the fact that the *DSM-5* was created largely with few references to biology or biological abnormalities. This is not surprising, since there are no identified biological abnormalities in psychiatric disorders, with the exception of known organic conditions such as dementia. Organic disorders are not generally considered to be psychiatric conditions. Dementia is fundamentally a neurological disorder characterised by known characteristic degenerative changes in the brain. More on this in chapter twelve and in my next book.

Also during the weeks before the publication of the *DSM-5*, in April 2013 psychiatrist Steven Hyman, Insel's predecessor as Director of the National Institute of Mental Health, expressed major reservations regarding the current state of psychiatry, the *DSM* in particular. In a May 2013 *New York Times* article titled "Psychiatry's Guide is Out of Touch with Science, Experts Say", Dr. Hyman said that the model chosen by the creators of the *DSM:*

> Is totally wrong . . . In fact, what they have produced is an absolute scientific nightmare. [7]

Further concerns regarding the *DSM-5* have been expressed in 2013 by leading American psychiatrist Allen Frances who chaired the process involved in the formation of the *DSM-4,* the predecessor of the *DSM-5,* which was published in 1994. In an article in *Psychology Today* titled "Price gouging", Frances described the price of 199 dollars for a hardback copy of the *DSM-5* and 149 dollars for a paperback copy as "incredible", "ridiculously expensive", involving the "rigging of prices". [8] He stated that the *DSM-5* cost 25 million dollars to create, whereas its predecessor *DSM-4* published less than twenty years previously cost just five million to produce. Regarding this 25 million dollars, Frances wrote, "God only knows where the money went". He referred to the fact that the American Psychiatric Association is "in deficit and rapidly losing membership dues and drug company funding" and "desperately needs all the publishing profits it can pull from *DSM-5* to bridge its budgetary gap".

Dr. Allen Frances expressed other concerns regarding the *DSM-5.* He wrote that the process involved in creating the *DSM-5* was "flawed". He described the *DSM-5* itself as "reckless". He wrote that "*DSM-5* boycotts are sprouting up all over the place" and that even before it is published, the *DSM-5* "has been discredited as unsafe and scientifically unsound". He referred to the "gross incompetence of *DSM-5*". I mentioned earlier that psychiatry was alone in medicine in that the foundation of its diagnostic process was flimsily based on consensus rather than on any verified scientific evidence. According to Dr. Frances, even the consensus approach to psychiatric diagnosis is in the process of collapsing. He lamented that psychiatrists "will no longer have a consensus method of making psychiatric diagnoses". In the 26 June 2009 issue of *Psychiatric Times* Frances wrote that the emerging *DSM-5* would be:

> A bonanza for the pharmaceutical industry but at huge cost to the new false positive patients caught up in the excessively wide *DSM-5* net. [9]

One might understandably assume that the definition of mental disorder is well established and reliable, particularly since the term actually features in the title of the *Diagnostic and Statistical Manual of Mental Disorders*, the manual which the American Psychiatric Association described as the "authoritative guide to the diagnosis of mental disorders". [10] In fact, major reservations about the term "mental disorder" have been expressed by high-level mainstream psychiatrists including the aforementioned head of the *DSM-4* Allen Frances and by Darrel A. Regier, vice-chair of the *DSM-5*. In an interview with British psychologist James Davies, Allen Frances acknowledged that the mental disorders listed in the 1980 *DSM-3* in which he was also involved were created arbitrarily, without solid supporting scientific evidence. [11] In a 2010 interview, psychotherapist and author Gary Greenberg asked Frances if a good definition of mental disorder would clarify those who were ill from those who were not. [12] Frances replied:

> There is no definition of a mental disorder. Its bullshit. I mean, you can't define it ... these concepts are virtually impossible to define precisely. [13]

Psychiatrist Darrel A. Regier was vice-chair of the *DSM-5*, published in 2013. In a 2012 publication, Regier admitted that the broad definitions of "mental disorder" were "almost impossible to test". [14] Given this lack of clarity regarding what the term actually means, it seems remarkable that the expression "mental disorder" nevertheless remains both in the title of this highly influential manual and as a largely unquestioned system of labelling millions of people worldwide.

James Davies also interviewed Robert Spitzer, the lead psychiatrist behind the creation of the *DSM-3*—the predecessor of the *DSM-4*—published in 1980. This psychiatrist was frank in his recollections. According to Davies, Spitzer told him that the *DSM-3* was the product of consensus; that there were no biological markers available for any of the mental disorders they listed in the *DSM-3*. Spitzer added:

> It is certainly true that the amount of research validating data on most psychiatric disorders is very limited indeed. There are very few disorders whose definition is the result of specific research data. Rarely could you say that there was research literature supporting the definition's validity. [15]

James Davies' research led him to conclude (italics his):

> The *DSM* committee did not *discover* mental disorders ... they *contrived* them. [16]

Regarding the secretive approach and potential conflicts of interest involved in the creation of the *DSM-5*, lead *DSM-3* psychiatrist Robert Spitzer severely criticised the methods adopted by the creators of the *DSM-5* in a 2008 *New York Times* article:

> When I first heard about this agreement, I just went bonkers. Transparency is necessary if the document is to have credibility, and, in time, you're going to have

people complaining all over the place that they didn't have the opportunity to challenge anything. [17]

Members of the professions of psychology and psychotherapy have expressed major concerns about the validity of the *Diagnostic and Statistical Manual of Mental Disorders* and the assumed biological nature of depression, including the brain chemical imbalance notion. In the introduction I mentioned the 2013 British Psychological Society Division of Clinical Psychology Position Statement in regard to the newly-published *Diagnostic and Statistical Manual of Mental Disorders*. [18] In 2011 Don W. Locke—then president of the American Counseling Association—wrote to the president of the American Psychiatric Association on behalf of his association's 120,000 members. Don Locke expressed many concerns regarding the process of creating the *DSM*, including the lack of empirical evidence. Locke wrote:

> The current evidence does not fully support a biological connection for all mental disorders. We therefore request that the definition of mental disorder be amended to indicate that mental disorders may not have a biological component. [19]

Don Locke requested that the American Psychiatric Association include four recommendations, reflecting the American Counseling Association's concerns about the quality and validity of the *DSM*. These recommendations included:

> Make public all empirical evidence submitted to the *DSM-5* Scientific Review Work Group, as well as the Group's evaluations and recommendations . . . Submit all evidence and data (from work groups and field trials) for review by an external, independent group of experts in evidence-based decision-making and make the results of this review public. [20]

Mentioning the fact that half a million non-psychiatric professionals in the United States alone refer to the *DSM* in their work, Locke concluded:

> To produce a credible diagnostic manual, it is essential that the *DSM-5* be based on research that involves rigorous, systematic, and objective procedures; an open process; and independent, objective scientific review. [21]

That the president of the American Counseling Association felt the need to express such concerns—on behalf of the association's 120,000 members, many of whom had voiced similar concerns—is itself alarming. Given the repeated claims by psychiatrists that psychiatry is a solidly evidence-based discipline, it is noteworthy that the American Counseling Association had grave doubts about the scientific validity of the emerging *DSM-5*. In his reply, president of the American Psychiatric Association John Oldham declined to agree to any of the recommendations of the American Counseling Association. [22]

Dr. Paula Caplan Ph. D. is an American clinical and research psychologist and social justice and human rights activist. She was previously professor of psychology, assistant professor of psychiatry and head of the Center for Women's Studies at the University of Toronto. Caplan has received much recognition for her work including an Eminent Woman Psychologist award in 1996 from the American Psychological Association, a 1995-96 Presidential Citation for Contributions as Chair of Sexism in Diagnosis Task Force, and a Distinguished Career Award in 2008 from the Association for Women in Psychology. Paula Caplan was a consultant to two committees appointed by the *DSM-4* Task Force's lead psychiatrist Allen Frances to adjudicate on what should be included in the *DSM-4* which was published in 1994. Caplan was shocked by what she witnessed during the process involved in contriving this manual:

> I resigned from these committees after two years because I was appalled by the way I saw that good scientific research was often being ignored, distorted, or lied about and the way that junk science was being used as though it were of high quality . . . if that suited the aims of those in charge. [23]

In the preface to her 1995 book *They Say You're Crazy: How the World's Most Powerful Psychiatrists Decide Who's Normal*, Caplan wrote:

> I have written this book with a very limited purpose in mind: to help people see how decisions are made about who is normal . . . As a former consultant to those who construct the world's most influential manual of alleged mental illness, the American Psychiatric Association's *Diagnostic and Statistical Manual of Mental Disorders (DSM)*, I have had an insider's look at the process by which decisions about abnormality are made. As a longtime specialist in teaching and writing about research methods, I have been able to assess and monitor the truly astonishing extent to which scientific methods and evidence are disregarded as the handbook is being developed and revised . . . Although my focus is on the *DSM*, I could not attempt in a single book to address the vast array of its biases, examples of sloppiness and illogical thinking, and just plain silliness [24] . . . Mental disorders are established without scientific basis or procedure. The low level of intellectual effort was shocking. Diagnoses were developed on the majority vote on the level we would use to choose a restaurant. Then it's typed into the computer. It may reflect on our naiveté, but it was our belief that there would be an attempt to look at things scientifically. [25]

Caplan described the experience of fellow psychologist Lynn Rosewater, who attended a meeting during the process of the creation of the *DSM-3*. This meeting was chaired by the lead psychiatrist for the *DSM-3*, Robert Spitzer:

> They were having a discussion for a criterion about Masochistic Personality Disorder and Bob Spitzer's wife says "I do that sometimes", and he says, "Okay, we'll take it out". [26]

Psychologist and author Dorothy Rowe wrote about the *Diagnostic and Statistical Manual of Mental Disorders* in her 2010 book *Why We Lie:*

Apart from where it deals with demonstrable brain injury, the *DSM* is not a valid document. None of the mental disorders included in the *DSM* have been shown to have a demonstrable physical cause. Psychiatrists might talk about "chemical imbalance in the brain" and genes that cause depression or schizophrenia, but there is no scientific evidence to support these ideas. The *DSM* is a collection of opinions. When the committee of psychiatrists change their opinions, a mental disorder might be removed from the *DSM* and some new one included. [27]

It is perhaps no coincidence that the *Diagnostic and Statistical Manual of Mental Disorders* is frequently referred to as the psychiatrist's bible, since it is largely a faith-based rather than an evidence-based manual. As Dorothy Rowe wrote in 2010:

Believing in the *DSM* is much the same as believing in, say, the doctrines of the Presbyterian Church . . . neither can point to evidence that supports the doctrine that lies outside the doctrine itself . . . When our ideas are supported by evidence, we can regard them as truths. Ideas unsupported by evidence are fantasies. [28]

Physician and pathologist Dr. Marcia Angell, a former editor-in-chief of the *New England Journal of Medicine* and Senior Lecturer in the Department of Global Health and Social Medicine at Harvard Medical School, had some important things to say about the *Diagnostic and Statistical Manual of Mental Disorders* and the process of psychiatric diagnosis in a 2009 *New York Review of Books* article:

Diagnostic criteria are pretty much the exclusive province of the current edition of the *Diagnostic and Statistical Manual of Mental Disorders*, which is the product of a panel of psychiatrists, most of whom had financial ties to the pharmaceutical industry. Given its importance, you might think that the *DSM* represents the authoritative distillation of a large body of scientific evidence . . . it is instead the product of a complex of academic politics, personal ambition, ideology and, perhaps most important, the influence of the pharmaceutical industry. What the *DSM* lacks is evidence. [29]

In a 2011 *New York Review of Books* article, Dr. Angell expressed further concerns about the *DSM*:

The problem with the *DSM* is that in all of its editions, it has simply reflected the opinions of its writers. Not only did the *DSM* become the bible of psychiatry, but like the real Bible, it depended a lot on something akin to revelation. There are no citations of scientific studies to support its decisions. That is an astonishing omission, because in all medical publications, whether journal articles or books, statements of facts are supposed to be supported by citations of scientific studies. [30]

In this article, Angell explained that books referred to within the *DSM* as "sourcebooks" that are occasionally referred to as providing the rationale for decisions, but these sourcebooks do not match the standard required of scientific publications; specific references to published scientific studies. Psychiatrist Daniel Carlat described an important consequence of the widespread practice of labeling within the *Diagnostic and Statistical Manual of Mental Disorders* and within psychiatry:

> It has de-emphasised psychological-mindedness, and replaced it with the illusion that we understand our patients when all we are doing is assigning them labels. [31]

Since a deficiency in brain serotonin levels has never been identified, it is not surprising that the *DSM* does not list serotonin depletion, or an imbalance of any other brain chemical, as the cause of depression or any other psychiatric disorder.

DRUG COMPANIES ABANDON PSYCHIATRY

The pharmaceutical industry has been at the forefront of the movement to persuade the public that depression is caused by brain chemical imbalances. As you will read later in this book, drug companies have placed a great deal of misinformation into the public arena about depression and brain chemicals. Some continue to do so to this day. In recent years, many drug companies have been quietly distancing themselves from research into mental health. In a 2013 article titled "Psychiatric Drug Development: Diagnosing a Crisis", psychiatrist and former director of the National Institute of Mental Health Steven Hyman wrote:

> During the past three years the global pharmaceutical industry has significantly decreased its investment in new treatments for depression, bipolar disorder, schizophrenia and other psychiatric disorders. Some large companies, such as GlaxoSmithKline, have closed their psychiatric laboratories entirely. Others, such as Pfizer, have markedly decreased the size of their research programs. Yet others, such as Astra-Zeneca, have brought their internal research to a close and are experimenting with external collaborations on a smaller scale. [32]

Steven Hyman outlined an apparent paradox in this development:

> This retreat has happened despite the fact that different classes of psychiatric drugs have been among the industry's most profitable products during the past several decades—and despite the fact that . . . one in five American adults now takes at least one psychiatric drug. [33]

Hyman provided the following explanation for this major development:

> As the expiration of patents on blockbuster drugs squeeze budgets, companies perceive their withdrawal from psychiatry as an unfortunate but rational reallocation of research resources. This withdrawal reflects a widely shared view

that the underlying science remains immature and that therapeutic development in psychiatry is simply too difficult and too risky. [34]

Hyman added that the absence of evidence of brain chemical abnormalities has contributed significantly to the pharmaceutical company exodus from psychiatric research:

> The molecular and cellular underpinnings of psychiatric disorders remains unknown; there is broad disillusionment with the animal models used for decades to predict therapeutic efficacy; psychiatric diagnoses seem arbitrary and lack objective tests; and there are no validated biomarkers with which to judge the success of clinical trials. As a result, pharmaceutical companies do not see a feasible path to the discovery and development of novel and effective treatments. [35]

Dr. Hyman's comments are correct, with one exception. He referred to "molecular underpinnings" of psychiatric disorders as if such underpinnings were a certainty, a given to be assumed despite the absence of any verifying scientific evidence for this major assumption. He neglected to even consider that the underpinnings of mental health problems might be emotional or psychological in origin. In so doing, Steven Hyman inadvertently committed a Begging the Question logical fallacy. [36] This assumption is common within psychiatry, a reflection of the gross underestimation and lack of awareness within psychiatry of the emotional and psychological aspects of the human being, and of psychiatry's major need to see all mental health problems as fundamentally biological.

The decline in drug company involvement in psychiatry and psychiatric research has been commented upon by other prominent psychiatrists. In the aforementioned 2013 article published in *Psychology Today* titled "Price Gouging: Why Will *DSM-5* Cost $199 a Copy?", lead *DSM-4* psychiatrist Allen Frances referred to the reduced pharmaceutical funding of psychiatry:

> The American Psychiatric Association is in deficit and rapidly losing membership dues and drug company funding. [37]

In a 2013 interview Richard Friedman, professor of clinical psychiatry at Weill Cornell Medical College in New York stated:

> The companies seem to have concluded that developing new psychiatric drugs is too risky and too expensive . . . There is very little in the pipeline. [38]

In the same article psychiatrist Steven Paul, professor of psychiatry at Weill Cornell Medical College, also expressed concern at this development. Steven Paul described the drop in research and development as "very significant":

> It has to be at least half of what has been invested 10 to 15 years ago. [39]

In a 2012 *Spectator* interview, journalist and author Robert Whitaker, author of several books on mental health including the 2010 *Anatomy of an Epidemic: Magic Bullets, Psychiatric Drugs and the Astonishing Rise of Mental Illness in America* also referred to this recent major development:

> A number of pharmaceutical companies have shut down their research into psychiatric drugs and they are doing so because, as they note, there is a lack of science providing good molecular targets for drug development. Even the drug companies are moving away from the chemical-imbalance theory, and thus, what we are seeing now is the public collapse of a fabrication, which can no longer be maintained, putting the blame instead on the drug companies. [40]

How ironic that after decades of seeking to persuade the general public that brain chemical imbalances are as much a characteristic of depression as raised blood sugar in diabetes, drug companies are pulling out of psychiatric drug research because of the lack of any such evidence or the prospect of it in the foreseeable future. Medical enthusiasts for a fundamentally biological understanding of depression confidently claim that brain research has greatly progressed the understanding of depression and will continue to do so. This optimism is clearly no longer shared by a significant section of the pharmaceutical industry. Many authors acknowledge that brain research has demonstrated how extraordinarily complex this organ is. While this research has provided no reliable answers regarding brain abnormalities in depression, it has raised a myriad of questions and mysteries. It appears that several drug companies, whose first duty is generally to their shareholders, have decided that further investment in psychiatric research is unlikely to be fruitful.

WORRYING DRUG CYCLES

A cyclical pattern has been a characteristic of many psychiatric drugs over the past one hundred years or so. Typically the cycle lasts in the region of thirty years, give or take a few. In his 2001 book *Prozac Backlash: Overcoming the Dangers of Prozac, Zoloft, Paxil and Other Antidepressants with Safe, Effective Alternatives*, American psychiatrist Joseph Glenmullen referred to this cycle as the "10-20-30 Year Pattern". [41] The drugs rise on an upward curve during the first ten years, aggressively marketed as "revolutionary breakthroughs, remarkable scientific advances over their predecessors". [42] This tends to plateau at a high pitch after about ten years. Then, between ten and twenty years:

> Signs of problems appear . . . Pharmaceutical companies and drug proponents deny the problems, adopting the strategy of defending the medication to the last . . . it is typically only after the twenty-year mark that enough data has accrued for the problems to be undeniable and for a significant number of physicians to begin sounding the alarm. Still another ten years or more elapse before professional organizations and regulatory agencies actively take steps to curtail prescribing. Thus, the cycle from miracle to disaster typically takes thirty years or more. [43]

This has been the pattern with benzodiazepine tranquillizers, barbiturates, meprobamate, the bromides, amphetamine, the opiates and cocaine. In his 1992 book *Power and Dependence: Social Audit on the Safety of Medicines*, Charles Medawar of Social Audit UK described the inglorious history of these and other substances initially hailed as wonder drugs for emotional and mental distress, only to be belatedly found out to cause major problems, often including addiction. [44] Medawar wrote that it took the medical profession nearly fifty years to fully acknowledge the addictive nature of barbiturates. [45] Millions of drug addicts to prescribed medication were thus created.

Benzodiazepines are a recent example of this cycle. The limited effectiveness and the major addiction problems associated with these drugs are now well known. Benzodiazepine withdrawal clinics are now a reality in many cities. Yet for years the medical profession and the manufacturers of these substances were very reluctant to see and to acknowledge these problems. For example, at a roundtable discussion on Valium sponsored by Roche who manufactured this drug, held sixteen years *after* these substances became available, acknowledged expert on and enthusiast for benzodiazepines Dr. David Greenblatt stated that dependence on these substances was:

> An astonishingly unusual event . . . unusual enough to be a medical curiosity worthy of a medical case report or of being picked up by the press . . . I have never seen a case of benzodiazepine dependence. [46]

Charles Medawar concluded:

> The evidence suggests that the providers of medicine keep making the same mistakes, mainly because they have been allowed to deny how badly things have gone wrong. Virtually every anti-anxiety drug and sleeping pill ever prescribed has proved to be a drug of dependence—yet each one has been prescribed, often for many years, as if the risk did not exist. This pattern of error has been established over the past 100 years or more, and continues to this day. [47]

When the truth about benzodiazepines was finally accepted within the medical profession, treating anxiety with these substances for longer than a month became frowned upon within the profession. Conveniently at this time, a new group of drugs were emerging—the selective serotonin reuptake inhibitors, the SSRIs. Perhaps relieved at having a brand new group of drugs and a new focus—depression rather than anxiety—doctors quickly endorsed and increasingly prescribed the SSRIs. These quickly became promoted as the "good drugs", allowing doctors to refer to benzodiazepines as "bad drugs" in an effort to move on from the benzodiazepine debacle as quickly as possible.

However, the story of the SSRI antidepressants has closely followed this cycle also. Prozac and the SSRIs are approaching the end of their cycle. This reality makes the need for a new seductive idea to replace the fading brain biological brain imbalance notion all the more urgent for those with vested interests. Given the dramatic withdrawal of many drug companies from psychiatric research, doctors may struggle to come up with a credible bright new alternative this time around.

Unfortunately, thirty years is also long enough for us to forget past disasters, thus increasing the possibility that we may allow the same mistakes to occur all over again.

NOTES TO CHAPTER ONE

1. Deborah Serani, Living with Depression: Why Biology and Biography Matter Along the Path to Hope and Healing, Lanham, Maryland: Rowman & Littlefield, 2012, p. 22.
2. Philip Cowen, Paul Harrison and Tom Burns, *The Shorter Oxford Textbook of Psychiatry*, Oxford: Oxford University Press, 2012, p. 32.
3. American Psychiatric Association website, "*DSM-5* Frequently Asked Questions", http://www-.dsm5.org/about/pages/faq.aspx, accessed 12 July 2014.
4. http://www.allaboutdepression.com/dia_01.html, accessed 03 December 2013.
5. Thomas Insel, "Director's Blog: Transforming Diagnosis", National Institute of Mental Health, 29 April 2013, http://www.nimh.nih.gov/about/director/2013/transforming-diagnosis.shtml, accessed 10 July, 2014.
6. Pam Bullock and Benedict Carey, "Psychiatry's Guide is Out of Touch with Science, Experts Say", *New York Times*, 06 May 2013, http://www.nytimes.com/2013/05/07/health/psychiatrys-new-guide-falls-short-experts-say.html? pagewanted=all, accessed 12 July 2014.
7. Pam Bullock and Benedict Carey, "Psychiatry's Guide is Out of Touch with Science, Experts Say", *New York Times*, 06 May 2013, http://www.nytimes.com/2013/05/07/health/psychiatrys-new-guide-falls-short-experts-say.html?pagewanted=all, accessed 12 June 2014.
8. Allen Frances, "Price Gouging: Why Will DSM-5 Cost $199 a Copy?", *Psychology Today*, 23 January 2013, http://www.psychologytoday.com/blog/dsm5-in-distress/201301/price-gouging-why-will-dsm-5-cost-199-copy, accessed 26 November 2014.
9. Allen Frances, "A Warning Sign on the Road to DSM-V: Beware of its Unintended Consequences", *Psychiatric Times*, 26 June 2009, http://www.psychiatrictimes.com/articles/warning-sign-road-dsm-v-beware-its-unintended-consequences, accessed 10 July 2014.
10. American Psychiatric Association website, "*DSM-5* Frequently Asked Questions", http://www.-dsm5.org/about/pages/faq.aspx, accessed 12 July 2014.
11. James Davies, *Cracked: Why Psychiatry is Doing more Harm than Good*, London: Icon Books Ltd, 2013, pps.45-51.
12. Gary Greenberg, *The Book of Woe: The DSM and the Unmaking of Psychiatry*, London: Scribe Publications, 2013, p. 23.
13. Gary Greenberg, "Inside the Battle to Define Mental Illness", *Wired* Magazine, January 2011, http:-//www.wired.com/magazine/2010/12/ff_dsmv/, accessed 22 March 2014.
14. Darrel A. Regier, "Diagnostic Threshold Considerations for DSM-5". In *Philosophical Issues in Psychiatry II: Nosology*, eds. Kenneth S. Kendler and Josef Parnas, pps. 285-97. New York: Oxford University Press, 2012, pps. 285-97.
15. James Davies, Cracked: Why Psychiatry is Doing more Harm than Good, London:Icon Books Ltd. 2013.
16. James Davies, *Cracked: Why Psychiatry is Doing more Harm than Good*, London: Icon Books Ltd., 2013, p. 36.
17. Benedict Carey, "Psychiatrists Revise the Book of Human Troubles", *New York Times*, 17 December 2008.
18. British Psychological Society, http://dxrevisionwatch.files.wordpress.com/2013/05/position-statement-on-diagnosis-master-doc.pd, accessed 16 April 2014.
19. Don W. Locke, president of the American Counseling Association, in a letter dated 08 November 2011 to John Oldham, president of the American Psychiatric Association, http://www.counseling.org/resources/pdfs/aca_dsm-5_letter_11-11.pdf, accessed 01 August 2014.

20. Don W. Locke, president of the American Counseling Association, in a letter dated 08 November 2011 to John Oldham, president of the American Psychiatric Association, http://www. counseling.org/resources/pdfs/aca_dsm-5_letter_11-11.pdf, accessed 01 August 2014.
21. Don W. Locke, president of the American Counseling Association, in a letter dated 08 November 2011 to John Oldham, president of the American Psychiatric Association, http://www. counseling.org/resources/pdfs/aca_dsm-5_letter_11-11.pdf, accessed 01 August 2014.
22. John Oldham, 21 November 2011, "DSM-5: APA Responds to American Counseling Association Concerns", http://www.psychiatrictimes.com/dsm-5-0/dsm-5-apa-responds-american-counseling-association-concerns#sthash.3IkH4IxX.dpuf, accessed 02 August 2014.
23. Paula Caplan, "The Great 'Crazy' Cover-up: Harm Results from Rewriting History", 17 February 2014, http://www.madinamerica.com/2014/02/great-crazy-cover-harm-results-rewriting-history-dsm/, accessed 12 July 2014.
24. Paula J. Caplan, *They Say You're Crazy: How the World's Most Powerful Psychiatrists Decide Who's Normal,* New York: Addison-Wellesley Publishing Company, 1995, preface.
25. Paula J. Caplan, *They Say You're Crazy: How the World's Most Powerful Psychiatrists Decide Who's Normal,* New York: Addison-Wellesley Publishing Company, 1995, p. 90.
26. Paula J. Caplan, *They Say You're Crazy: How the World's Most Powerful Psychiatrists Decide Who's Normal,* New York: Addison-Wellesley Publishing Company, 1995, p. 91.
27. Dorothy Rowe, *Why We Lie,* London: Fourth Estate, 2010, p. 130.
28. Dorothy Rowe, *Why We Lie,* London: Fourth Estate, 2010, pps. 131, 296.
29. Marcia Angell, "Drug Companies and Doctors: A Story of Corruption", *New York Review of Books,* 15 January 2009, accessed 19 December 2013.
30. Marcia Angell, "The Illusions of Psychiatry", *New York Review of Books,* 14th July 2011, accessed 20 December 2013.
31. Daniel Carlat, *Unhinged: The Trouble with Psychiatry—a Doctor's Revelations about a Profession in Crisis,* 2010, London: Free Press, p. 60.
32. Steven Hyman, "Psychiatric Drug Development: Diagnosing a Crisis", 02 April 2013, The DANA Foundation Website http://www.dana.org/cerebrum/2013/psychiatric_drug_development__diagnosing_a_crisis/, accessed 14 July 2014.
33. Steven Hyman, "Psychiatric Drug Development: Diagnosing a Crisis", 02 April 2013, The DANA Foundation Website, http://www.dana.org/cerebrum/2013/psychiatric_drug_development__diagnosing_a_crisis/, accessed 14 July 2014.
34. Steven Hyman, "Psychiatric Drug Development: Diagnosing a Crisis", 02 April 2013, The DANA Foundation Website, http://www.dana.org/cerebrum/2013/psychiatric_drug_development__diagnosing_a_crisis/, accessed 14 July 2014.
35. Steven Hyman, "Psychiatric Drug Development: Diagnosing a Crisis", 02 April 2013, The DANA Foundation Website, http://www.dana.org/cerebrum/2013/psychiatric_drug_development__diagnosing_a_crisis/, accessed 14 July 2014.
36. The Begging the Question logical fallacy is an argument or other statement that simply assumes or re-states its own position as truth rather than provide relevant supportive evidence and logical arguments. An argument begs the question when it assumes as a fact any questionable point not conceded by the other side. A premise is presented as though it were a fact, in order to support one's position. If the premise is questionable, the argument is not solid. Presenting the premise as though it were a fact gives the false impression that the argument is based on solid ground. http://www.kspope.com/fallacies/fallacies.php, accessed 02 January 2014. http://www.fallacyfiles.org/begquest.html, accessed 02 January 2014. http://grammarist.com/rhetoric/begging-the-question-fallacy/, accessed 02 January 2014.
37. Allen Frances, "Price Gouging: Why Will DSM-5 Cost $199 a Copy?", *Psychology Today,* 23 January 2013, http://www.psychologytoday.com/blog/dsm5-in-distress/201301/price-gouging-why-will-dsm-5-cost-199-copy, accessed 26 November 2014.
38. "Big pharmaceutical cuts investment in depression meds", 27 November 2013, news.com.au, http://www.news.com.au/lifestyle/health/big-pharmaceutical-cuts-investment-in-depression-meds/story-fneuzlbd-1226769133716, accessed 14 July 2014.
39. "Big pharmaceutical cuts investment in depression meds", 27 November 2013, news.com.au http://www.news.com.au/lifestyle/health/big-pharmaceutical-cuts-investment-in-depression-meds/story-fneuzlbd-1226769133716, accessed 14 July 2014.

40. Bruce Levine, "Psychiatry Now Admits It's Been Wrong in Big Ways—But Can It Change?", *Truthout*, 05 March 2014, http://truth-out.org/news/item/22266-psychiatry-now-admits-its-been-wrong-in-big-ways-but-can-it-change-a-conversation-with-investigative-reporter-robert-whitaker, accessed 12 March 2014.

41. Joseph Glenmullen, *Prozac Backlash: Overcoming the Dangers of Prozac, Zoloft, Paxil and Other Antidepressants with Safe, Effective Alternatives*, Simon & Shuster, 2001, p. 12.

42. Joseph Glenmullen, *Prozac Backlash: Overcoming the Dangers of Prozac, Zoloft, Paxil and Other Antidepressants with Safe, Effective Alternatives*, Simon & Shuster, 2001, p. 12.

43. Joseph Glenmullen, *Prozac Backlash: Overcoming the Dangers of Prozac, Zoloft, Paxil and Other Antidepressants with Safe, Effective Alternatives*, Simon & Shuster, 2001, p. 12.

44. Charles Medawar, *Power and Dependence: Social Audit on the Safety of Medicines*, London: Social Audit Ltd, 1992.

45. Charles Medawar, *Power and Dependence: Social Audit on the Safety of Medicines*, London: Social Audit Ltd, 1992, p. 62.

46. K. Fruensgaard, "Withdrawal Psychosis: a Study of 30 Consecutive Cases", *Acta Psychiat Scand*, 1976, 53, 105-118.

47. Charles Medawar, *Power and Dependence: Social Audit on the Safety of Medicines*, London: Social Audit Ltd, 1992, p. 5.

2. THERE ARE NO KNOWN BRAIN CHEMICAL ABNORMALITIES IN DEPRESSION

Despite what you may have heard, no chemical imbalances have been found in the brains of people diagnosed with depression. Fifty years of intensive research designed to detect brain chemical imbalances has not yielded any reliable scientific proof of chemical abnormalities in depression. The widespread belief that brain chemical abnormalities cause depression is based not on any solid direct evidence but on fifty-year-old discredited hypotheses that have erroneously become widely accepted as facts. As psychologist and author Gary Greenberg wrote in his 2010 book *Manufacturing Depression: The Secret History of a Modern Disease:*

> It would be nice to hear psychiatrists acknowledge in public that even though they've been telling the public for two decades that they know what the underlying pathology of depression is, they really don't. [1]

Brain serotonin levels cannot be measured. Blood levels of serotonin can be taken but they never are measured by doctors in the context of depression, because they add nothing to our understanding of brain serotonin. Ninety-five per cent of serotonin in the body is in the gastrointestinal tract and other tissues apart from the brain. *Blood* serotonin levels provide no insight into *brain* levels of serotonin.

Many commentaries from mental health experts confirm the fact that there never have been any known brain chemical abnormalities in depression. Many of these statements were made up to twenty-five years ago and more, yet the depression brain chemical imbalance delusion remains alive and well to this day, still being touted in many quarters as a scientifically established fact. I now present some of these commentaries in chronological order. I include further examples in "The absence of evidence" section later in this chapter.

In 1989 psychiatrist Z. J. Lipowski acknowledged in the *Canadian Journal of Psychiatry* that telling people they had biochemical imbalances was about as helpful and as profound:

> As if you said to the patient, "you're alive", since as long as we are alive, our bodies are in a constant state of flux, reaction and change. [2]

Psychiatrist David Kaiser of Northwestern University Hospital, Chicago wrote in a 1996 *Psychiatric Times* article:

> Modern psychiatry has yet to convincingly prove the genetic/biologic cause of any single mental illness. Patients have been diagnosed with "chemical imbalances" despite the fact that no test exists to support such a claim, and there is no real conception of what a correct chemical balance would look like ... Yet conclusions such as "depression is a biochemical imbalance" are created out of nothing more

than semantics and the wishful thinking of scientists/psychiatrists and a public that will believe anything now that has the stamp of approval of medical science.[3]

Professor Emeritus of Neuroscience Elliot Valenstein wrote in his 1998 book *Blaming the Brain: The Truth About Drugs and Mental Health:*

> Although it is often stated with great confidence that depressed people have a serotonin or norepinephrine deficiency, the evidence actually contradicts these claims. [4]

Just a reminder; norepinephrine is the name given in some parts of the world to the chemical that is referred to elsewhere as noradrenaline. Experienced science writer John Horgan wrote in his 2000 book *The Undiscovered Mind: How the Brain Defies Replication, Medication and Explanation:*

> Given the ubiquity of a neurotransmitter such as serotonin and the multiplicity of its functions, it is almost as meaningless to implicate it in depression as it is to implicate blood. [5]

Psychiatrist Edward Drummond M.D., Associate Medical Director at Seacoast Mental Health Center in Portsmouth, New Hampshire stated in 2000 (brackets mine):

> First, no biological etiology (cause) has been proven for any psychiatric disorder in spite of decades of research. So don't accept the myth that we can make "an accurate diagnosis". Neither should you believe that your problems are due solely to a "chemical imbalance". [6]

Psychologist and author Bruce Levine Ph.D. wrote in his 2003 book *Commonsense Rebellion: Taking Back your Life from Drugs, Shrinks, Corporations, and a World Gone Crazy:*

> Remember that no biological marker has been found for depression. [7]

Stanford psychiatrist and professor of psychiatry David Burns, the 1975 winner of the A.E. Bennett Award given by the Society of Biological Psychiatry for his research on serotonin metabolism, wrote in his 2006 book *When Panic Attacks:*

> Many neuroscientists no longer consider a chemical imbalance theory of depression valid . . . We still don't know the relationship between biology and the mental disorders. [8]

Psychiatrist and author Professor Thomas Szasz wrote:

> The more progress scientific medicine actually makes, the more undeniable it becomes that "chemical imbalances" and "hard wiring" are fashionable clichés, not evidence that problems in living are medical diseases. [9] Nobody has yet

measured, demonstrated or created a test to show that somebody has a chemical imbalance in their brain. Period! [10]

According to psychiatrist Daniel Carlat in his 2010 book *Unhinged: The Trouble with Psychiatry—a Doctor's Revelations about a Profession in Crisis*, the chemical imbalance idea is a "myth". [11] In answer to his own question posed in his 1995 book *Beyond Prozac: Brain Toxic Lifestyles, Natural Antidotes and New Generation Antidepressants*, "How long should you take Prozac?" American psychiatrist Michael Norden's answer is, "It depends". [12] Not for a genuine chemical imbalance it doesn't; you take treatment for a chemical imbalance for as long as the imbalance is demonstrated by investigations to be there, generally for life.

DEPRESSION AND THE *DIAGNOSTIC AND STATISTICAL MANUAL OF MENTAL DISORDERS*

For about ten years after I qualified as a medical doctor, I accepted the medical approach to depression without question. The more contact I had with real people in my work as a general practitioner and listened to their stories, the more I came to question the validity of the medical approach to depression. By 2001, when my book *Beyond Prozac: Healing Mental Distress* was first published, I had developed serious misgivings about the prevailing understanding of and approach to depression. I set out these concerns in *Beyond Prozac*. The method by which doctors arrive at a diagnosis of depression was one of the issues I discussed in that book, issues that if anything are more worrying now than when I wrote that book.

Science plays no part in the diagnosis of depression. The *Diagnostic and Statistical Manual of Mental Disorders (DSM)* lists nine criteria which psychiatrists have decided provide evidence of depression. Neither laboratory investigations nor physical findings specific to depression receive a mention in any of these nine criteria:

Criterion 1 describes the mood in a major Depressive Episode as "depressed, sad, hopeless, discouraged", or "down in the dumps", feeling "blah", having no feelings or feeling anxious, irritability, and bodily experiences such as aches and pains.
Criterion 2 refers to loss of interest or pleasure, including a loss of interest in hobbies.
Criterion 3 describes changes in eating habits, either an increase or a decrease in appetite or weight.
Criterion 4 refers to sleep disturbance such as insomnia or oversleeping.
Criterion 5 describes bodily expressions of distress including "agitation, e.g. the inability to sit still . . . or retardation e.g. slowed speech, thinking or bodily movements".
Criterion 6 refers to decreased energy, tiredness and fatigue.
Criterion 7 includes a "sense of worthlessness or guilt, unrealistic negative evaluations of one's worth", and "guilty preoccupations or ruminations" about the past.

Criterion 8 describes people's reported "inability to think, concentrate or make decisions", appearing "easily distracted", or "memory difficulties".
Criterion 9 speaks of "thoughts of death, suicide ideation, or suicide attempts".

The *Diagnostic and Statistical Manual of Mental Disorders* asserts that a diagnosis of a Major Depressive Episode can be made when the severity and duration of a person's mood meets *Criterion 1* and the person is experiencing four of the remaining eight criteria. In *Beyond Prozac: Healing Mental Distress*, I questioned many aspects of the diagnostic approach to depression, including the following:

Why did the American Psychiatric Association select five criteria as the magic figure? What is the difference between a person who meets six criteria—and is therefore diagnosed as having a Major Depressive Episode and needing antidepressant treatment—and one who meets four criteria, and therefore receives no psychiatric diagnosis or treatment? Why five criteria? Why not three? Or seven? How valid are these criteria? [13]

In his 2010 book *Unhinged: The Trouble with Psychiatry—A Doctor's Revelations about a Profession in Crisis*, psychiatrist Daniel Carlat asked similar questions. Carlat interviewed Robert Spitzer, lead psychiatrist of the *DSM-3*, the edition of the *DSM* in which this approach to depression was first set out as *the* way to diagnose depression. Here is an extract from that interview: [14]

Carlat: How did you decide on five criteria as being your minimum threshold for depression?
Spitzer: It was just consensus. We would ask clinicians and researchers, "How many symptoms do you think patients ought to have before you would give them a diagnosis of depression?" And we came up with the arbitrary number of five.
Carlat: But why did you choose five and not four? Or why didn't you choose six?
Spitzer: Because four just seemed like not enough. And six seemed like too much.

Carlat commented that "Spitzer smiles mischievously" as he uttered the last sentence above. This is the quality of the "science" upon which the diagnosis of depression is based.

THE ABSENCE OF EVIDENCE

One of the great ironies of psychiatry is that while psychiatrists and GPs regularly claim to practice evidence-based medicine, there is no evidence base whatsoever for a cornerstone upon which the psychiatric understanding of depression has been built; the notion that biochemical imbalances occur in depression. Despite decades of talking up a role for neurotransmitter abnormalities in depression, a phenomenon referred to in 2013 by psychiatrist and historian of psychiatry Edward Shorter as "neurotransmitter chatter", [15] no reliable evidence of neurotransmitter abnormalities has been uncovered.

In a 2003 article psychiatrist Joanna Moncrieff wrote:

> Psychiatry as an institution has long been obsessed with identifying biological causes of mental disorders and with the narrow technical solutions that flow from such a paradigm. The pharmaceutical industry has helped to reinforce this approach by the promotion of drug treatments, funding biological research and by promoting claims that psychiatric disorders are caused by simplistic biological notions such as "chemical imbalances". [16]

Seeking to identify that depression might be characterized by brain chemical abnormalities—as blood glucose abnormalities are a core feature of diabetes—has been a major driving force behind depression research for over fifty years. It is not difficult to see why. Reliably identifying chemical abnormalities in depression would reap enormous rewards for the two most powerful and invested groups involved in depression research—psychiatry and the pharmaceutical industry. Psychiatrists would be immediately vindicated as real doctors treating real diseases, a status sought desperately by psychiatry for over a century. Any such identified abnormalities would legitimize depression as a medical illness like any other. Such discoveries would contribute greatly to legitimizing psychiatry as a medical specialty treating real physical diseases with a level of scientific validation equal to other medical specialties. The position of drug companies would similarly be validated as the producers of treatments for these diseases.

As I outline in chapter twelve under the heading "Between a rock and a hard place", there is another twist to this. If brain abnormalities were ever found in depression, the medical status of depression would change to a known neurological disorder. Care of patients would shift from psychiatry to neurology, a scenario not likely to be welcomed with open arms by psychiatrists. In chapter twelve I describe how the current situation—where abnormalities are widely believed to be there but have not been established to exist—is actually ideal for psychiatry.

In spite of this massive effort to identify biochemical brain abnormalities as known features of depression, not a single item of reliable scientific evidence confirming any such findings exists. It was obvious at an early stage to some realistic psychiatrists and scientists that the chemical imbalance theory of depression was highly suspect.

Low levels of neurotransmitters such as serotonin, noradrenaline and dopamine have never been identified in depression. It is not even possible to measure these chemicals in the brains of living people. Brain chemical abnormalities are regularly assumed and claimed to be present in depression, but their existence is never confirmed. The fact that clinical tests for chemical imbalances, neurobiological problems and brain disorders including brain-imaging scans play no part in the assessment, diagnosis and ongoing management of depression, other than to rule out known organic brain diseases, speaks volumes.

I now present commentaries by experienced mental health professionals that confirm the absence of scientific evidence of brain chemical abnormalities in depression. To illustrate that these commentaries originate from a wide range of mental health professionals over a prolonged period of time, I present these in chronological order. Bear in mind that Prozac, the first of the new generation of antidepressants, was launched in 1988. As long ago as 1978, psychiatrist L. Ratna wrote (brackets mine):

> Although it is stated by practically all the (psychiatric) textbooks that the aged are more prone to depression of an endogenous nature (that is, arising from within the person rather than in response to external triggers, generally assumed to be biologically caused) . . . we believe that the unhappiness which is misdiagnosed and treated as an endogenous illness is a legitimate response to the plight that many of the aged find themselves in . . . The so-called depression therefore, is not primarily due to a biochemical upset but an understandable reaction to the alienation, rejection, isolation and social stress that the aged are subject to. [17]

According to a 1990 textbook described in the *New England Journal of Medicine* as "a 'bible' . . . a most valued volume" [18] published two years after the launch of Prozac, the data for the neurotransmitter hypothesis of mood disorders such as depression:

> Are inconclusive and have not been consistently useful either diagnostically or therapeutically. [19]

Governments, health authorities, the medical profession and the drug industry knew or should have known for decades that there was no identified correlation between brain chemical deficiency and depression. The U.S. Congress Office of Technology assembled a panel of experts in the field in the early 1990s. In 1992 these experts reported to the Congress Office of Technology that:

> Prominent hypotheses concerning depression have focused on altered function of the group of neurotransmitters called monoamines, particularly norepinephrine and serotonin . . . studies . . . have found no specific evidence of an abnormality to date. Currently, no clear evidence links abnormal serotonin receptor activity in the brain to depression . . . the data currently available do not provide consistent evidence either for altered neurotransmitter levels or for disruption of normal receptor activity. [20]

In his 1993 book *Toxic Psychiatry* American psychiatrist Peter Breggin wrote:

> Scientific reviews of the biochemistry of depression have failed to identify a consistent biochemical basis. The most recent psychiatric textbooks review the biochemistry of depression, sometimes in detail, as if a great deal must be known about the subject; but they end up admitting that the theories are conflicting and remain speculative. [21]

Colin Ross M.D., Associate Professor of Psychiatry at Southwest Medical Center, Dallas, wrote in his 1995 book *Pseudoscience in Biological Psychiatry:*

There is no scientific evidence whatsoever that clinical depression is due to any kind of biological deficit state. [22]

At a 1997 Harvard Medical School conference, Harvard professor and director of the depression research programme at the Massachusetts General Hospital Dr. Andrew Nierenberg discussed the disease model of depression. He then said:

> The dark side of all this is that we have many elegant models but the real fact is that when it comes to the exact mechanisms by which these things work, we don't have a clue. [23]

Professor Emeritus of Psychology and Neuroscience at the University of Michigan Elliot Valenstein wrote in his 1998 book *Blaming the Brain:*

> It may surprise you to learn that there is no convincing evidence that most mental patients have any chemical imbalance. Yet many physicians tell their patients they are suffering from a chemical imbalance despite the reality that there are no tests available for assessing the chemical status of a living person's brain . . . The truth is that we still do not know what causes any mental disorder or how drugs sometimes help patients get better. Yet, despite this, the theory that mental disorders arise from biochemical imbalance is widely accepted. [24]

Valenstein added that such ideas "are simply an unproven hypothesis", yet they have "enormous implications". He wrote that claims that psychiatric drugs such as antidepressants "correct a chemical imbalance also rests on a shaky scientific foundation". [25]

Thomas J. Moore, Senior Fellow in Health Policy at George Washington University Medical Centre, wrote in 1998:

> The chemical imbalance theory has not been established by scientific evidence.[26]

Ross Baldessarini, a senior research psychiatrist at the McLean Hospital said in 1998:

> We have pursued fads in much of biological psychiatry, including grossly over-valuing our partial understanding of the pharmacodynamics of some drugs as a putative route to clarifying the pathophysiology of psychiatric illnesses. [27]

Pharmacodynamics is the effect of drugs on the body, and pathophysiology is the study of functional changes in the body that occur in response to disease or injury. Baldessarini spoke of:

> The largely fruitless efforts to support a dopamine hypothesis of schizophrenia or mania, a norepinephrine or serotonin deficiency in major depression, a serotonin deficiency hypothesis in obsessive-compulsive disorder, and so on. [28]

Then Clinical Associate Director of Psychiatry and Behavioural Sciences at the Stanford University Hospital of Medicine, psychiatrist David Burns wrote in his 1999 book *The Feeling Good Handbook:*

> Some psychiatrists appear to confuse theory with fact. They tell depressed patients that they have chemical depressions that must be treated with antidepressants. I would prefer that psychiatrists not do this, because it creates an impression of certainty in the patient's mind that is not justified by current scientific evidence. [29]

In a 2000 textbook used to teach medical students about psychiatric medications, psychiatrist Professor Stephen M. Stahl wrote:

> So far, there is no clear and convincing evidence that monoamine deficiency accounts for depression; that is, there is no "real" monoamine deficit. [30]

Monoamines are the chemical group to which serotonin and other brain chemicals claimed to be imbalanced belong. Psychiatrist Professor Steven Hyman, then Director of the U.S. National Institute of Mental Health, wrote about the chemical imbalance notion in a 2000 World Health Organization bulletin:

> Too simple was the concept . . . that abnormal levels of one or more neurotransmitters would satisfactorily explain the pathogenesis of depression or schizophrenia. [31]

American psychiatrist Joseph Glenmullen, Clinical Instructor of Psychiatry at Harvard Medical School, wrote in his 2001 book *Prozac Backlash: Overcoming the Dangers of Prozac, Zoloft, Paxil and Other Antidepressants with Safe, Effective Alternatives:*

> A serotonin deficiency for depression has not been found . . . there has been no shortage of alleged biochemical explanations for psychiatric conditions . . . not one has been proven. Quite the contrary. In every instance where such an imbalance was thought to have been found, it was later proven false . . . Still, patients are often given the impression that a definitive serotonin deficiency in depression is firmly established. [32]

In his 2001 book *The Rape of the Soul: How the Chemical Imbalance Model of Psychiatry has Failed its Patients,* clinical psychologist and author Ty C. Colbert Ph.D. wrote:

> Biopsychiatrists have created the myth that psychiatric "wonder" drugs correct chemical imbalances. Yet there is no basis for this model because no chemical imbalance has even been proven to be the basis of a mental illness. [33]

In his foreword to the 2001 edition of my book *Beyond Prozac,* Irish psychologist and author Dr. Tony Humphreys wrote:

In spite of 200 years research, no enduring evidence has emerged to substantiate the medical model of psycho-social distress. Indeed, there is no evidence that conditions such as bipolar depression, schizophrenia, personality disorder, obsessive-compulsive disorder and endogenous depression have any genetic, biochemical, biological or hereditary basis. [34]

Dr. Thomas Szasz, then Professor Emeritus of Psychiatry at the New York University Medical School, Syracuse, wrote in 2002:

There is no blood or other biological test to ascertain the presence or absence of mental illness, as there is for most bodily diseases. If such a test were developed . . . then the condition would cease to be a mental illness and would be classified, instead, as a symptom of bodily disease. [35]

In 2003 Ireland's drug regulatory body the Irish Medicines Board banned drug company GlaxoSmithKline from stating on its patient information leaflet that Seroxat "works by bringing serotonin levels back to normal". Irish Medicines Board officials concluded:

There is no scientific investigation to measure what are normal serotonin levels in the human brain receptors. As such, claiming that a particular medicinal product works by bringing serotonin levels back to normal is not accurate. [36]

As I was involved in this situation, more about this later. Psychologist and author Bruce Levine, Ph.D. wrote in his 2003 book *Commonsense Rebellion: Taking Back your Life from Drugs, Shrinks, Corporations, and a World Gone Crazy*:

No biochemical, neurological, or genetic markers have been found for Attention Deficit Disorder, Oppositional Defiant Disorder, Depression, Schizophrenia, Anxiety, compulsive alcohol and drug abuse, overeating, gambling or any other so-called mental illness, disease, or disorder. [37]

Stanford psychiatrist David Burns again, in 2003:

I spent the first several years of my career doing full-time brain research on brain serotonin metabolism, but I never saw any convincing evidence that any psychiatric disorder, including depression, results from a deficiency of brain serotonin. In fact, we cannot measure brain serotonin levels in living human beings so there is no way to test this theory. Some neuroscientists would question whether this theory is even viable, since the brain does not function in this way, as a hydraulic system. [38]

In a 2004 article, neuroanatomy professor Jonathan Leo wrote:

Never has a theory with so little scientific evidence been so well accepted by the American public. [39]

Leo made the following suggestion to people told by doctors that they had a chemical imbalance:

If a psychiatrist says you have a shortage of a chemical, ask for a blood test and watch the psychiatrist's reaction. The number of people who believe that scientists have proven that depressed people have a low serotonin is a glorious testament to the power of marketing. [40]

New York psychiatrist Ron Leifer suggested a similar approach:

There's no biological imbalance. When people come to me and they say, "I have a chemical imbalance", I say "Show me your lab tests". There are no lab tests. So what's the chemical imbalance? There is no such thing as a chemical imbalance, and any psychiatrist that you talk to, if you ask them that question, they'll all admit it in private but they won't admit it in public. It's a scandal. [41]

Dr. Darshak Sanghavi, clinical fellow at Harvard Medical School said in 2004:

Despite pseudoscientific terms like "chemical imbalance", nobody really knows what causes mental illness. There's no blood test or brain scan for major depression. [42]

Psychiatrist Kenneth Kendler, then co-editor-in-chief of *Psychological Medicine*, wrote in a review article in 2005:

We have hunted for big simple neurochemical explanations for psychiatric disorders and have not found them. [43]

Psychiatrist Joanna Moncrieff, senior lecturer in psychiatry at University College London, said in a 2005 interview that:

The pharmaceutical industry has managed to convey a misleading picture. I speak to quite a few journalists, and they are quite shocked to hear that the link between serotonin and depression is very tenuous and the research conflicting and not convincing. The psychiatric profession and academic researchers are probably also partly to blame for glossing over the weakness of the research. [44]

Gordon McCarter PhD is assistant professor of biological sciences at the College of Pharmacy at Tuoro University in Vallejo, California. In a 2005 interview, McCarter acknowledged that the evidence for an imbalance of neurotransmitters in depression was:

Circumstantial . . . more and more tenuous. Stating that depression is caused by a chemical imbalance is extremely simplistic. [45]

In a 2005 article, professor of neuroanatomy Jonathan Leo and social work professor Jeffrey Lacasse wrote:

> During the past fifty years, a steady stream of researchers have attempted to identify direct evidence for the monoamine theory of depression, of which the serotonin hypothesis is one aspect . . . They have consistently failed to do so. Indeed, as many scientific researchers have demonstrated, most of the evidence they found either directly contradicted or did not support this theory . . . Contemporary neuroscience research has failed to confirm any serotonergic lesion in any mental disorder, and has in fact provided significant counterevidence to the explanation of a simple neurotransmitter deficiency. Modern neuroscience has instead shown that the brain is vastly complex and poorly understood. While neuroscience is a rapidly advancing field, to propose that researchers can objectively identify a "chemical imbalance" at the molecular level is not compatible with the extant science. In fact, there is no scientifically established ideal "chemical balance" of serotonin, let alone an identifiable pathological imbalance. To equate the impressive achievements of neuroscience with support for the serotonin hypothesis is a mistake. [46]

Following the publication of this Leo and Lacasse 2005 article and a 2005 *Wall Street Journal* article by Sharon Begley, [47] an article by the Alliance for Human Research Protection illustrated the degree to which the chemical abnormality notion had become synonymous with depression:

> One after another of psychiatry's theoretical constructs and therapeutic armamentarium have been knocked down and relegated to the dust-heap of pseudoscientific history. None of psychiatry's claims have withstood the test of scientific scrutiny. The very core upon which psychiatry's practice guidelines— using drugs to restore a "chemical imbalance" in the brain—has been shown to be nothing but unsubstantiated speculation. [48]

Psychiatrist and psychopharmacologist Professor David Healy of the University of Wales is former secretary of the British Association for Psychopharmacology and a historian on the SSRI antidepressants. In his 2006 book *Let Them Eat Prozac: The Unhealthy Relationship between the Pharmaceutical Industry and Depression*, Healy wrote:

> It is now widely assumed that our serotonin levels fall when we feel low . . . but there is no evidence for any of this, nor has there ever been . . . No abnormality of serotonin in depression has ever been demonstrated. [49]

Psychiatrist David Burns again, in his 2006 book *When Panic Attacks: The New Drug-Free Anxiety Therapy that can Change your Life*:

In the 1970s my colleagues and I did a variety of experiments to test the theory that depression results from a deficiency of serotonin in the brain. Our results were simply not consistent with this theory. I also reviewed the scientific literature on brain serotonin but couldn't find one shred of compelling evidence that a deficiency of serotonin, or any other chemical imbalance in the brain, causes depression, anxiety or any other psychiatric disorder. To this day, I am not aware of any studies that have validated the chemical imbalance theory. If I tell you that your depression or your panic attacks result from a chemical imbalance in the brain, then I'm telling you something that cannot be proven, because there is no test for a chemical imbalance in the human brain. [50]

Also in 2006 psychiatrist Joanna Moncrieff and Professor of Social Work David Cohen wrote:

Antidepressants are believed to exert their therapeutic effects by acting on brain monoamines, which are believed to be important determinants of mood. However, in a circular chain of logic, the monoamine theory of depression was itself formulated primarily in response to observations that early antidepressants increased monoamine levels. Independent evidence has not confirmed that there is a monoamine abnormality in depression. For example, the findings of brain imaging studies of serotonin abnormality are contradictory. [51]

In a 2007 *Newsweek* article psychiatrist Thomas Insel, head of the U.S. National Institute of Mental Health was quoted as saying:

A depressed brain is not necessarily underproducing something. [52]

American psychiatrist Peter Breggin again, in 2007:

Despite more than two hundred years of intensive research, no commonly diagnosed psychiatric disorders have been proven to be either genetic or biological in origin, including . . . major depression. At present there are no known biochemical imbalances in the brain of typical psychiatric patients. [53]

In a 2007 article, Australian British-based psychologist and author Dorothy Rowe wrote:

There never has been any evidence that any brain chemical was depleted when a person was depressed. However, psychiatrists kept hoping that one day their hypothesis that depression was caused by a chemical imbalance would be proved to be right. Now, thirty years after the hypothesis was first introduced, the Royal College of Psychiatrists and the Institute of Psychiatry have accepted that depression isn't caused by a chemical imbalance. But you will find this out only if you visit their websites. They haven't issued a press release saying "We were wrong". On the Institute of Psychiatry's website there is a lengthy notice about an important conference on depression to be held in April 2007. The preamble to this notice reads, "Depression cannot be described any longer as a simple disorder of the brain". The website of the Royal College of Psychiatrists has dropped all references to chemical imbalance causing depression. [54]

Commenting on experiences of his patients that clearly did not fit into the narrow medical model, Irish psychiatrist Professor Ivor Browne wrote in his 2008 book *Music and Madness:*

It was experiences like this which taught me how bogus is the concept of "clinical depression". The idea that there is a chemically mediated form of depression which is an "illness", quite separate from the sadness and depression which are part of the slings and arrows of ordinary life, is manifest nonsense. [55]

In his 2009 book The *Emperor's New Drugs: Exploding the Antidepressant Myth,* psychologist, researcher and author Professor Irving Kirsch wrote:

During the last 50 years researchers have tried to find more direct evidence for the monoamine theory of depression, but by and large they have failed. Instead of finding confirmation, much of the evidence they have found is contradictory or runs counter to the theory . . . The evidence did not really fit the story, but few doctors had the time to carefully sift through the data . . . There is no simple direct correlation of serotonin or norepinephrine levels in the brain and mood. [56]

British psychiatrist Joanna Moncrieff wrote in her 2009 book *The Myth of the Chemical Cure: A Critique of Psychiatric Drug Treatment:*

Summarizing the evidence reviewed so far reveals that there are no grounds for considering antidepressants to be a disease-centred treatment. Evidence about serotonin and noradrenaline levels in people with depression is inconsistent and confusing. Overall, there is little evidence that there is a characteristic in either of these systems that is associated with depression. [57]

In a 2009 *New York Review of Books* article Dr. Marcia Angell wrote that some of the biggest blockbuster drugs of all time have been psychoactive drugs such as SSRI antidepressants:

The theory that psychiatric conditions stem from a biochemical imbalance is used as justification for their widespread use, even though the theory has yet to be proved. [58]

In a 2009 letter to the *Irish Times,* Irish psychiatrist Michael Corry referred to the delusional nature of the brain chemical imbalance notion and summarized a far more accurate understanding of depression than that presented by the majority of psychiatrists and GPs:

Psychological distress is a valid human experience and no one is immune. It has a context, a time-line, and represents a legitimate response to life's difficulties. Depression is an emotion not a disease. It is a reflection of loss, grief, broken hearts, chronic anxiety, panic attacks, sexual abuse, bullying, difficult relationships, financial problems, overwhelm, and the impact of having life fired at you point blank. To regard depression as a chemical imbalance, something pathological, is in my view deluded. It has, in reality, no basis in science; it takes away the need for understanding, compassion, healing psychotherapy, prevention, and in particular educational modules in schools based on wellness and human sustainability. [59]

In his 2010 book *Unhinged: The Trouble With Psychiatry—a Doctor's Revelations about a Profession in Crisis*, psychiatrist Daniel Carlat comes clean about not coming clean with his patients. Regarding having just informed a patient that the antidepressant Lexapro worked by increasing serotonin levels in the brain, he admitted:

I didn't tell her that, despite my training at Harvard's Massachusetts General Hospital, I have no idea how Lexapro works to relieve depression, nor does any psychiatrist. There is no direct evidence of a disorder of reduced serotonin. [60]

Psychologist Jonathan Rottenberg Ph.D., Associate Professor of Psychology at the University of South Florida, wrote in a 2010 *Psychology Today* article that:

As a scientific venture, the theory that low serotonin causes depression appears to be on the verge of collapse. [61]

Australian psychiatrist and author Niall McLaren stated in a 2010 recording:

People are being told, "you have a chemical imbalance in the brain which is genetically determined, and you've got it for life. And there's nothing you can do about it". [62]

McLaren described this as part of the psychiatric "catastrophe that needs to be exposed". [63] Professor of Social work and psychiatry at New York University Jerome Wakefield stated in 2012:

We've thrown tens of billions of dollars into trying to identify biomarkers and biological substrates for mental disorders . . . The fact is we've gotten very little out of all that. [64]

Psychiatrist Vivek Datta studied medicine and psychology at the University of London. He was a Research Fellow in Psychological Medicine at the Institute of Psychiatry at the Maudsley in London. He obtained a Masters in Public Health from Harvard University. In an article titled "Chemical Imbalances and Other Black Unicorns" published on the Mad in America website on 25 June 2012, Datta wrote:

The notion that mental illnesses are caused by chemical imbalances is neither true, nor helpful. Worse still, the idea of mental illnesses as chemical imbalances is making us ill . . . It provides a simple explanation during a time when individuals crave certainty, and is packaged in the respectable veneer of pseudo-medical jargon . . . It was supposed to be a beautiful narrative. A previously well person becomes depressed, feels too listless and tired to live. A chemical imbalance is identified as the perpetrator. The "chemical imbalance" is corrected with an antidepressant, and the patient is restored to her previous self. It is a story of restitution. It is a story where medicine is the hero and bad biochemistry the villain. It is a story with no basis in reality. Instead, we have convinced individuals that they are in some way defective and in need of lifelong treatment. [65]

Dr. Steven Reidbord is a board-certified psychiatrist with a full-time office practice in San Francisco. His internet blog is titled "Reidbord's Reflections". On 29 April 2012 he published an article on his blog titled "Chemical imbalance—Sloppy thinking in psychiatry 1". Dr. Reidbord wrote:

There's a lot of sloppy thinking in my field. This troubles me . . . "Chemical imbalance" is a phrase used by psychiatrists and laypeople alike. When a mental problem seems to arise from within instead of without, it is said to be due to a chemical imbalance. In truth, however, no chemical imbalance, nor any structural abnormality in the brain, has ever been found to account for anything we currently consider a psychiatric disorder. [66]

According to a 2012 research article, brain serotonin deficiency (brackets mine):

Has been theorized to be a core pathogenic factor in depression for half a century . . . However, whether such (antidepressant) drugs indeed correct a primary deficit remains unresolved. [67]

In his 2013 book *How Everyone Became Depressed*, Canadian psychiatrist and historian of psychiatry Edward Shorter wrote:

There is no biological marker for depression, major or not . . . Nor has any psychiatric illness been convincingly attributed to a shortage of any particular transmitter. [68]

A biological marker is an identifiable biological abnormality that consistently and reliably demonstrates the presence of a particular disease.

Irishwoman Mary Maddock has been a leading figure in the Irish and international movement for mental health change. Along with her husband Jim, Mary is co-founder of Mindfreedom Ireland. She is on the board of directors of Mindfreedom International, an international mental health support group. Mary has had considerable personal experience of psychiatry and considers herself a survivor of psychiatry. The author of *Soul Survivor*, for which I was honoured to write the foreword, Mary's experience of psychiatry was profoundly traumatic. After many years of being diagnosed with bipolar disorder, Mary has been very well and off all medication for over ten years. In a 2014 YouTube video about Mindfreedom Ireland, Mary Maddock correctly stated:

> Psychiatry is the only form of medicine that diagnoses you without having any physical test . . . if there is something wrong with my brain, and I have a tumour or I have something else, you will be able to see that I have a tumour. You will be able to know there is something wrong with it . . . Their whole basis is that people who are in need of psychiatry have a chemical imbalance in their brain and they need drugs to fix it. Well there is no test, there is nothing to be able to say that you have a broken brain or that you have anything wrong with your brain. No doctor can say that one brain is supposed to be normal and another brain is supposed to be different when it comes to psychiatry. And yet they are going on that false premise all the time. [69]

FIFTY-YEAR-OLD HYPOTHESES, NO FACTS

The chemical imbalance notion has been floating around within psychiatry since the mid-1950s, gathering a head of steam in the early 1960s. In an attempt to understand depression, two related hypotheses emerged within psychiatry in the 1960s. In 1965 Joseph Schildkraut proposed that problems with the recently discovered neurotransmitter noradrenaline (known as norepinephrine in America) might cause depression. [70] This proposal became known as the catecholamine hypothesis. Schildkraut's article became one of the most cited in the history of psychiatry. Two years later, brain serotonin deficiency was proposed as a possible cause of depression. [71] These two propositions became the bedrock of the medical approach to depression. Since these two substances and other considered culprits such as dopamine are described chemically as monoamines, these hypotheses became known as the monoamine theory of depression.

Emeritus Professor of Psychiatry at Cambridge University, psychiatrist Eugene Paykel received the British Association for Psychopharmacology Lifetime Achievement Award in 2000 and the European College of Neuropsychopharmacology Award for Clinical Neuroscience in 2001. He was editor of *Psychological Medicine* until 2006. In 1985, three years *before* the first SSRI was launched upon the public, Paykel wrote:

> Is the amine hypothesis of depression dead? Diabetes comes down very clearly to a relative deficiency of insulin. Fifteen years ago depression was like that. We thought it was a clear-cut deficiency of noradrenaline or serotonin in a particular neurotransmitter system in the brain. But it is not as simple as that. [72]

Pakel, then professor of psychiatry at the University of London, was widely recognised at the time as one of the most distinguished leaders in the international field of psychiatry.

Despite over fifty years of intense research on the subject, these hypotheses remain as unproven now as they were when first proposed. Indeed they have been largely disproven. There is no direct evidence that a deficiency of any neurotransmitter is involved in depression or any other condition, despite thousands of studies that sought to identify such a deficiency. It is true that antidepressants interfere with levels of neurotransmitters in brain synapses, but there is no evidence to support the notion that neurotransmitter levels are deficient to begin with.

If a vulnerable and distressed person craving answers and hope is told by a doctor they trust that the doctor believes or thinks they have a chemical imbalance or that depression is caused by a chemical imbalance, this will usually be enough to convince the person that they do indeed have a brain chemical imbalance.

A sentence from a 2011 psychiatry textbook illustrates how consensus rather than science drives psychiatric thinking. Regarding the monoamine hypothesis of mood disorders, the authors wrote that this hypothesis "now emphasizes the role of serotonin, rather than just noradrenaline. [73] The authors provided no scientific evidence to support this position, no detail and no specific supportive information. Since no role for serotonin has been established scientifically, if accuracy was the authors' first priority, they would have replaced "the role of serotonin", which implies that serotonin is known to have a role, with "the postulated role of serotonin".

Psychologist John Grohol wrote the following in a 2014 article on the popular Psych Central website (brackets his):

> One of the leading myths that unfortunately still circulates about clinical depression is that it is caused by low serotonin levels in the brain (or a "chemical imbalance"). This is a myth because countless scientific studies have specifically examined this theory and have come back universally rejecting it. So let us put it to rest once and for all—low levels of serotonin in the brain don't cause depression. [74]

THE BIOCHEMICAL HYPOTHESIS: NO SCIENTIFIC FOUNDATION

The hypothesis that problems with brain serotonin levels cause depression is largely based upon the observation that SSRI antidepressants raise serotonin in brain tissue of rats. Not living rats with fully functioning brains at the time of testing; in killed rats, whose brains are removed, smashed to bits and blenderized; fragments of dead rats' brains, assessed in a test tube. The level of credibility of claims that conclusions can be drawn from such experimentation that reliably apply to the living human being is anyone's guess.

As two psychiatrists pointed out in 2000, assuming one form of abnormality without supporting evidence and basing the understanding and treatment of depression upon this assumption is a highly questionable practice:

> Some have argued that depression may be due to a deficiency of norepinephrine or serotonin because the enhancement of noradrenergic or serotonergic neurotransmission improves the symptoms of depression. However, this is akin

to saying that because a rash on one's arm improves with the use of a steroid cream, the rash must be due to steroid deficiency. [75]

In a letter to the *New York Times* in 2002, American psychiatrist and author of *Listening to Prozac* Peter Kramer wrote:

I argued that the theories of brain functioning that led to the development of Prozac must be wrong or incomplete. [76]

In his 2009 book *The Emperor's New Drugs: Exploding the Antidepressant Myth*, psychologist and researcher Irving Kirsch wrote:

Considering all of the data together, I have come to the conclusion that the chemical imbalance theory is completely implausible. It now seems beyond question that the traditional account of depression as a chemical imbalance in the brain is simply wrong. [77]

A HYPOTHESIS BASED SOLELY ON DEDUCTION

It is over fifty years since the chemical imbalance theory of depression was first promoted by psychiatry and the pharmaceutical industry. Given the absence of any scientific evidence of brain chemical abnormalities associated with depression, the entire hypothesis is based solely on deduction, as psychiatrist Daniel Carlat acknowledged in his 2010 book *Unhinged: The Trouble with Psychiatry—a Doctor's Revelations about a Profession in Crisis*:

The neurotransmitter deficiency notion derives from deduction, from reasoning backwards from the apparent action of antidepressants. [78]

Deducing that brain chemical deficiencies exist because substances that raise the levels of these chemicals seem to ease some of the features of depression is the extent of the "evidence" that brain chemical abnormalities are a known feature of depression. In a 2005 article, social work professor Jeffrey Lacasse and professor of neuroanatomy Jonathan Leo described the obvious shortcomings of such reasoning:

With direct proof of serotonin deficiency in any mental disorder lacking, the claimed efficacy of SSRIs is often cited as indirect support for the serotonin hypothesis. Yet, this ex juvantibus line of reasoning—i.e. reasoning "backwards" to make assumptions about disease causation based on the response of the disease to a treatment—is logically problematic. The fact that aspirin cures headaches does not prove that headaches are due to low levels of aspirin in the brain. [79]

The tenuous basis for the biochemical imbalance notion was outlined by New York psychiatrist James W. Hicks in his 2005 book *50 Signs of Mental Illness: A Guide to Understanding Mental Health* (italics mine):

> The medications that treat mental illness have complex effects on certain molecules in the brain, particularly those involved in the communication between brain cells. Scientists *speculate* that abnormal levels of these molecules may cause the underlying illness. That is why psychiatrists often talk about a chemical imbalance in the brain. [80]

Regrettably many psychiatrists and GPs do not make it clear that they are speculating when they refer to biochemical abnormalities in depression. Psychology professor and author Richard Bentall PhD wrote in his 2009 book *Doctoring the Mind: Why Psychiatric Treatments Fail:*

> Both the dopamine and serotonin theories are based on indirect evidence, often from animal experiments, mainly on the effects of drugs on the brains of animals that would be killed for the purposes of science. Researchers realized that direct observation of abnormal biochemistry in living patients would be necessary to firm up their theories . . . direct support for the serotonin hypothesis has remained elusive to this day. [81]

Psychiatrist Daniel Carlat explained the psychiatric rationale in his 2010 book *Unhinged: The Trouble with Psychiatry—a Doctor's Revelations about a Profession in Crisis:*

> The idea that depression is a "chemical imbalance" derives from how the drugs seem to work. We have come to the theory through a process of deduction, reasoning back from the effects antidepressants have on neurotransmitters. Antidepressants increase levels of neurotransmitters in the synapses, and they treat depression. Ergo, depression must be caused by a deficiency of such neurotransmitters . . . The theory makes intuitive sense, explaining its enduring popularity. But the problem is that there is no direct evidence that a serotonin or norepinephrine deficiency is involved, despite thousands of studies that have attempted to demonstrate such a deficiency . . . the problem is that getting precise measures of brain neurotransmitters has proven devilishly tricky. [82]

Carlat's last sentence becomes more accurate by replacing "has proven devilishly tricky" with "has not been achieved". Also in his book, this psychiatrist acknowledged the weakness in the medical position of assuming that because antidepressants ease symptoms in some people, a brain chemical deficiency must be the cause:

> By this same logic one could argue that the cause of all pain conditions is a deficiency of opiates, since narcotic pain medications activate opiate receptors in the brain. [83]

The weakness of this position is rendered even more fragile when the true effectiveness of antidepressants is taken into account. In his 2009 book The *Emperor's New Drugs: Exploding the Antidepressant Myth*, psychologist, researcher and author Professor Irving Kirsch wrote:

A half-century has passed since the chemical imbalance theory of depression was introduced, and the presumed effectiveness of antidepressants remains the primary evidence for its support. But as we have seen, [84] the therapeutic effects of antidepressants are largely due to the placebo effect, and this pretty much knocks the legs out from under the biochemical theory . . . During the last 50 years researchers have tried to find more direct evidence for the monoamine theory of depression, but by and large they have failed. Instead of finding confirmation, much of the evidence they have found is contradictory or runs counter to the theory . . . The evidence did not really fit the story. [85]

SEROTONIN BREAKDOWN PRODUCTS AND DEPRESSION

Since levels of brain neurotransmitters cannot be measured directly, researchers have looked elsewhere in their attempts to measure brain serotonin function. [86] Commenting on the results of this research, British psychiatrist Joanna Moncrieff wrote in 2009:

Research on noradrenaline is highly inconsistent, with studies showing increased, decreased and normal levels in depressed patients compared with controls. Research on serotonin is similarly confusing. [87]

Many supporters of the biological notion of depression have claimed that levels of breakdown products of neurotransmitters provide evidence of abnormal brain neurotransmitter levels. The truth is that this research has not borne any fruit, but it has served to further reinforce the depression delusion within the public mind. Many scientists and doctors have raised concerns regarding research into the breakdown products of serotonin. In 1998 neuroanatomy professor Elliot Valenstein wrote that attempts to find abnormal metabolite levels of serotonin and norepinephrine in people diagnosed to be depressed "have not been encouraging". [87] The metabolites Valenstein was referring to are the breakdown products of serotonin and norepinephrine in the cerebrospinal fluid—the fluid that surrounds and circulates within the brain and spinal cord—and the urine.

American psychiatrist Daniel Carlat wrote about this in his 2010 book *Unhinged: The Trouble With Psychiatry—a Doctor's Revelations about a Profession in Crisis*:

You can't just put a syringe into a living brain and draw out fluid without damaging brain tissue, and even if you could, levels of serotonin in a brain humming with neural activity are likely to ebb and flow unpredictably. Thus, scientists have had to settle for indirect measurements, such as the breakdown products in the blood, urine or cerebrospinal fluid. Another indirect, if more gruesome, method entails removing brains from bodies after death, grinding up the neurons, and measuring levels of neurotransmitters postmortem . . . all these studies thus far have been inconclusive. [88]

Award-winning journalist Robert Whitaker addressed the issue of breakdown products of serotonin in his 2010 book *Anatomy of an Epidemic*. Whitaker wrote (brackets mine):

In 1969, Malcolm Bowers of Yale University became the first to report on whether depressed patients had low levels of serotonin metabolites in their cerebrospinal fluid. In a study of eight depressed patients, all of whom had been previously exposed to antidepressants, he announced that their 5-HIAA levels (a chemical product of serotonin breakdown within the body) were lower than normal, but not "significantly" so. Two years later, investigators at McGill University said that they, too, had failed to find a "statistically significant" difference in the 5-HIAA levels of depressed patients and normal controls, and that they also had failed to find any correlation between 5-HIAA levels and severity of depression symptoms. In 1974, Bowers was back with a more finely tuned follow-up study: Depressed patients who had not been exposed to antidepressants had perfectly normal 5-HIAA levels. The serotonin theory of depression did not seem to be panning out. [89]

This conclusion was confirmed in research published in 2008 in a prestigious medical journal, a study referred to by psychiatrist Daniel Carlat as "the most recent definitive review of all basic antidepressant research", [90] in which the authors concluded:

Numerous studies of norepinephrine and serotonin metabolites in plasma, urine and cerebrospinal fluid, as well as post-mortem studies of the brains of patients with depression, have yet to identify the purported deficiency reliably. [91]

The Shorter Oxford Textbook of Psychiatry, a 2012 psychiatry textbook, confirmed the lack of reliable evidence regarding breakdown products of serotonin in depression and suicide. Regarding studies of cerebrospinal fluid, the authors wrote:

Overall the data do not suggest that drug-free patients with major depression have a consistent reduction of 5-HIAA, the main metabolite of serotonin formed in the brain . . . Overall, there is little consistent evidence that depressed patients dying from natural causes or suicide have lowered brain concentrations of serotonin or 5-HIAA". [92]

WHAT THE MEDICAL TEXTBOOKS SAY

What medical textbooks say—or don't say—about brain chemical imbalances in depression is revealing. I have found that the most objective medical textbooks in this regard are often those that deal with areas of medicine other than psychiatry.

With some exceptions—such as some medical textbooks that contain a chapter on psychiatry as part of a comprehensive overview of all branches of medicine—these branches of medicine generally have little or no vested interest in maintaining psychiatry's dominant position in mental health or in prioritizing allegiance to their psychiatrist colleagues above truth. Textbooks on the basic medical sciences such as biochemistry are particularly objective in this regard. The Merriam-Webster on-line dictionary defines biochemistry as:

> Chemistry that deals with the chemical compounds and processes occurring in living organisms; the chemical characteristics and reactions of a particular living system or biological substance. [93]

Substances such as serotonin and noradrenaline that are claimed to be out of balance in depression are biochemical substances. If scientifically identified abnormalities or imbalances of these chemicals were known to be associated with depression, they would be presented and discussed in detail in medical biochemistry books. With this in mind, in 2014 I checked the most up-to-date medical biochemistry textbooks in the University of Limerick library. This library contains a wide range of books for the use of the university's medical school.

The biochemical abnormality hypotheses upon which the medical approach to depression is based have been around since the mid-1960s. If there were any biological evidence for these notions, it would be clearly set out in recent biochemistry textbooks. I also compared and contrasted how depression is dealt with relative to diabetes, a known biochemical abnormality condition to which depression is frequently compared.

Lecture Notes on Clinical Chemistry was published in 1988, the year Prozac was launched amid widespread claims of serotonin deficiencies in depression that were corrected by Prozac. This book contains just one index entry for depression, a reference to "depressive illness or any cause of stress to the patient" as a potential cause of raised cortisol levels.[94] In contrast, there are 20 references to diabetes, 28 entries for glucose and 9 for insulin. There is no discussion of the chemistry of depression in this book. This book's only reference to serotonin is in relation to carcinoid syndrome, a very rare condition caused by a form of tumour arising mainly in the digestive system.[95]

Biochemistry: Molecules, Cells and the Body is a comprehensive medical textbook of 592 pages published in 1995, seven years after the launch of Prozac. This book contains no index entries for depression, which is not discussed in the book. There are no index entries for SSRIs or antidepressants. There is one index entry for serotonin, which amounts to four lines in the text. This brief passage contains no mention of depression, the brain, or brain serotonin balance or imbalance. However, three pages in this book are devoted to the biochemistry of diabetes. There are four index entries for diabetes, 19 for glucose and ten for insulin. [96]

Clinical Chemistry: Principles, Procedures and Correlations, 3rd edition is a substantial 773-page medical biochemistry textbook. [97] It was published in 1996, eight years after the launch of Prozac. By this time, the notion of brain chemical imbalances in depression had been widely promoted and accepted as an established fact. The chemistry of diabetes is discussed in detail in this book, evidenced by 27 index entries for glucose, 11 for diabetes and 14 for insulin, including two pages on laboratory tests for diabetes. The chemistry of depression is not discussed at all in this book. There is no entry for depression in the index. This book contains just one index entry for serotonin. In the corresponding section in this book, the biochemistry of serotonin is discussed without a single mention of depression or reference to serotonin and depression. [98]

Medical Biochemistry is a comprehensive 1,106-page medical textbook published in 2002, fourteen years after Prozac was launched. This book contains 36 index entries for diabetes, 32 for glucose and 36 for insulin. There is not a single index entry for depression. There are 7 index entries for serotonin, which is to be expected since serotonin is present across many areas of the body. In none of these references in the text does a discussion on the biochemistry of brain serotonin deficiency or brain chemical imbalances in depression occur. [99]

Medical Biochemistry is also the title of a 2005 medical textbook comprised of 693 pages. The index contains 73 entries for diabetes. There are seven index entries for depression, four of which are about possible links with vitamin deficiencies of thiamine, pyridoxine, biotin, and excess levels of selenium, none of which receive much attention in everyday medical practice. There is no reference to the biochemistry of depression in this book, whereas the biochemistry of diabetes is discussed in detail. [100]

Mark's Basic Medical Biochemistry: A Clinical Approach is an extensive 2005 medical biochemistry text of 977 pages. The index contains five entries for diabetes, nineteen for blood glucose and none for depression. Insulin—often quoted by doctors as the diabetes equivalent of neurotransmitters such as serotonin—has 42 index entries compared to just one index entry for serotonin. This one entry concerns the synthesis of serotonin in the body, which amounts to just two brief paragraphs. The book contains no reference to any neurotransmitter abnormalities or any illnesses that might be related to brain serotonin or other neurotransmitters. [101]

The *Textbook of Biochemistry with Clinical Correlations* is a comprehensive 2006 biochemistry textbook of 1208 pages. There are 29 index entries for diabetes and 64 for insulin. Depression does not appear in the book's index. In the section on serotonin, "some types of depression are associated with low brain levels of serotonin" is the only reference to depression. [102] One might reasonably expect a comprehensive biochemistry textbook to elaborate in detail upon such a statement and explain what "associated" means, if any such details were known. There is no elaboration, and serotonin is not discussed further anywhere in the book.

Lecture Notes: Clinical Biochemistry is a 2006 medical textbook of 21 chapters. This book contains a full chapter on diabetes. The index contains 19 entries for diabetes, 11 for glucose, 10 for insulin, but none for either depression, serotonin, SSRIs or antidepressants. [103]

In summary; a review of the most recent biochemistry books in the University of Limerick library, which serves the University of Limerick medical school, identifies plenty of evidence of the abnormal biochemistry of diabetes, but no evidence whatsoever of scientifically verified chemical abnormalities in depression.

The 2012 medical textbook *Histology and Cell Biology: An Introduction to Pathology* includes a detailed description of cell and tissue biology, physiology, biochemistry and cell signaling and associated pathways, as structure and function are inter-related. [104] This book contains a substantial 32-page chapter on nervous tissue in which a wide range of brain diseases are dealt with in detail including multiple sclerosis, Guillian Barre syndrome and many others. There is no reference to depression in this chapter. The book also contains a 22-page chapter on the neuroendocrine system, in which there is not a single reference to depression. There is no mention of depression in the book's index. In contrast, there are three references to diabetes and 12 references to insulin in the index. Serotonin gets one mention in the book as a neurotransmitter. There are no references to neurotransmitter imbalances or abnormalities in the book or to structural or functional changes relating to neurotransmitters.

Neuroscience is regularly referred to by doctors as an area that has provided and that will continue to provide evidence of biological abnormalities and markers for depression. *Neuroscience in Medicine* is a 2008 eBook that contains a full chapter on chemical messengers which includes considerable detail on neurotransmitters. A clinical correlation is presented after each chapter. There is no mention of serotonin in relation to depression in this book. [105]

The remarkable complexity of the brain and the implications of this fact are acknowledged in the 2004 neuroscience textbook *Functional Neuroanatomy: An Interactive Text and Manual.* This book contains no discussion of or index entries for depression. There is no reference to either depression or to brain serotonin deficiency in the three-page section on serotonin. Discussing drugs that act on serotonin within the body, the authors acknowledged:

> Understanding their complete mechanism of action is complicated by the overwhelming forest of receptor subtypes that they may affect in addition to their unique but overlapping anatomic distributions. [106]

The lack of evidence for the biochemical brain abnormality notion in depression surfaces in many other medical textbooks. *Principles of Anatomy and Physiology* is a comprehensive 2006 medical textbook of over 1,200 pages. The anatomy and physiology of diabetes are discussed in some detail in this book. The only reference to depression in the text is as "a downward movement of a part of the body". [107] This book contains just one index entry for serotonin. This entry refers to four lines in the "Neurotransmitters" section of the book, in which there is no mention of serotonin deficiency or abnormality, or depression. [108]

The 2007 medical textbook *Memorizing Medicine: A Revision Guide* is written by a neurologist. This book contains ten chapters, covering the range of medical specialties including cardiology, respiratory medicine, gastroenterology, infectious diseases, rheumatology, neurology, endocrinology, clinical chemistry, renal medicine and haematology. There is no chapter on psychiatry and no mention of psychiatry anywhere in the book. There is no mention of depression in any of the chapters including the neurology chapter, which is revealing since the author is a neurologist attached to the Imperial College in London and would have specialist knowledge in neurology and the brain. Depression, psychiatry, neurotransmitters and serotonin are not mentioned in the index. In the 26-page chapter on clinical chemistry there is no mention of brain chemical imbalances, serotonin or any other neurotransmitter. [109]

Medical Sciences is a detailed 2009 medical textbook comprised of 895 pages. The first-named editor is a Fellow of the Royal College of General Practitioners. The only reference to serotonin and depression in this biologically detailed book is one sentence, in which there is no reference to any scientifically established facts:

> This treatment (with SSRI antidepressants) is based on possible correlations between reductions in serotonergic transmission and clinical depression. [110]

Having considered all of the so-called evidence including neurotransmitters and all forms of scans, the authors of the 2009 *American Textbook of Psychiatry* concluded:

> The central question of what variables drive the pathophysiology of mood disorders remains unanswered. [111]

Pathophysiology is the study of changes in functioning within the body that occur in response to disease or injury.

Medical textbooks that have no allegiance to psychiatry sometimes inadvertently give the game away by articulating mainstream medical thought and principles rather than those of mainstream psychiatry. *Essentials of Preventive Medicine* is a 1984 medical textbook written by a community physician and a general practitioner/clinical reader attached to the University of Oxford. Depression is considered not under any section on prevention of brain diseases or biological disorders, but under the heading "Prevention of Emotional Disorders". The authors are correct in doing so, but one can see why psychiatrists much prefer the term "mood disorders" to "emotional disorders", the former having a far more impressive impact than the latter. Published just over three years before the Prozac bandwagon hit the headlines and almost 20 years after the monoamine hypothesis began to sweep through psychiatry as either a fact or so-close-to-a-fact-that-makes-no-difference, the authors stated:

> It is still thought that there is a type of depression caused by a chemical disorder. Research into the biochemical and neuropharmacological causes of depression continues but no cause has been found, so the main scope lies in the prevention of depression that is simply a more severe degree of the type of feeling we all experience. [112]

The last sentence could be a little clearer. Research into possible biological and neuropharmacological abnormalities and causes has continued, but neither biological abnormalities nor biological causes have been found. This primitive state of understanding is reflected in the author's comments regarding how little can be done to prevent depression by approaching depression through the lens of biology.

As I researched through many medical textbooks, I came across some books that had fallen victim of the brain chemical imbalance delusion. Given how pervasive this delusion has become within the medical profession and beyond, this is not surprising. *The Human Brain: An Introduction to its Functional Anatomy* is a one such book. This 720-page textbook was published in 2009. Conditions with known brain abnormalities such as multiple sclerosis are discussed in detail. There is no discussion in this book of depression as an illness or disease entity, yet the authors deemed it appropriate to include the following heading:

Neurochemical Imbalances are Involved in Certain Forms of Mental Illness. [113]

The following appears in the text beneath this headline:

Drugs commonly used as antidepressants enhance the effectiveness of transmission at norepinephrine and serotonin synapses. Observations like these, coupled with our current ability to map out the cells, axons and synaptic endings that use a neurotransmitter, have contributed to a better understanding of these disorders . . . Although there are few disorders in which malfunction of a single neurotransmitter system accounts for all findings, there is a growing number of examples in which one transmitter plays a major role. [114]

Many problems arise here. There is no scientific justification for the heading. Since brain neurochemical imbalances have never even been identified in any form of mental illness, unequivocal claims that neurochemical imbalances are involved in certain forms of mental illness are highly inappropriate. It has not been scientifically established that "antidepressants enhance the effectiveness of transmission" of neurotransmitters. This is misinformation, a Wishful Thinking logical fallacy. [115]

All that has been established with any degree of scientific reliability is that these substances interfere with neurotransmitter function. However, no reliable scientific evidence has demonstrated that neurotransmitter function is in need of such interference. The fact that science has made some progress in mapping out brain cells and neurotransmitters has not added to "better understanding of these disorders" at all. As I discuss in chapter twelve under the heading "red herrings and the brain", this is a red herring that is often trotted out to impress, without informing the reader that all of this is irrelevant since no brain chemical abnormality has been identified in depression. The final sentence of the above passage is very problematic. The authors either know or should know that no "malfunctions" of any neurotransmitter system have been identified. It is therefore wrong and misleading to claim that "a growing number of examples in which one transmitter plays a major role" when no role at all has been directly identified scientifically in the case of any neurotransmitter.

Laboratory Tests and Diagnostic Procedures, 6th edition, is a 2013 book devoted to the range of laboratory investigations available for medical diagnostic purposes. In the section titled "Laboratory Tests and Diagnostic Procedures", serotonin is listed as a blood test. Depression is the first-named condition in which this level is decreased. The authors also include a long list of other conditions in which they claim that serotonin is known to be decreased. Yet they state that a serotonin blood test is only used to test for one condition:

This test is used to confirm the diagnosis of carcinoid tumours . . . this test is used to screen for carcinoid tumours. [116]

The authors acknowledge that blood serotonin samples are "unstable". Having mentioned depression, they provide no further information regarding depression and serotonin. Nor do they clarify that, as I mentioned earlier, a serotonin blood test provides no insight regarding brain serotonin levels.

The Science of Laboratory Diagnosis is a comprehensive 2005 medical textbook that deals with all areas of laboratory diagnosis. Unlike the book just mentioned above, the content in relation to serotonin is all accurate. The only reference to serotonin and its measurement is in relation to carcinoid tumours. There is no mention of brain serotonin in relation to depression to be found anywhere in this textbook of laboratory diagnosis. [117]

MedlinePlus is the official U.S. National Institutes of Health website created as a trustworthy source of information for the general public. MedlinePlus contains a webpage titled "Serum serotonin level" in which it is also stated that carcinoid syndrome is the only condition for which blood serotonin levels have any clinical application:

> The serotonin level is a blood test to measure the amount of serotonin in your body . . . This test may be done to diagnose carcinoid syndrome. Many patients with carcinoid syndrome have high levels of serotonin in blood and urine . . . The normal range is 101-283 nanograms per milliliter (ng/mL) . . . A higher-than-normal level may indicate carcinoid syndrome. [118]

NOTES TO CHAPTER TWO

1. Gary Greenberg, *Manufacturing Depression: The Secret History of a Modern Disease*, London: Bloomsbury, 2010, p. 345.
2. Z. J. Lipowski, "Psychiatry: Mindless, Brainless, Both or Neither?", *Canadian Journal of Psychiatry* 34, 1989, pps. 249-54.
3. David Kaiser, "Commentary: Against Biologic Psychiatry", *Psychiatric Times*, 01 December 1996 Vol. XIII, Issue 12 mnhttp://psychiatry#sthash.buCwo5Qp.dpuf, accessed 28 February 2014.
4. Elliot S. Valenstein, *Blaming the Brain: The Truth About Drugs and Mental Health*, New York: The Free Press, 1998.
5. John Horgan, *The Undiscovered Mind: How the Brain Defies Replication, Medication and Explanation*, London: Weidenfeld, 2000, p. 37.
6. Edward Drummond, *The Complete Guide to Psychiatric Drugs*, New York: John Wiley & Sons, 2000.
7. Bruce Levine, *Commonsense Rebellion: Taking Back your Life from Drugs, Shrinks, Corporations, and a World Gone Crazy*, Bloomsbury Academic, 2003.
8. David Burns, *When Panic Attacks: The New Drug-Free Anxiety Therapy that can Change your Life*, Harmony, 2006.

9. Thomas Szasz, *Coercion as Cure: A Critical History of Psychiatry,* Transactions Publishers, 2007, http://www.bible.ca/psychiatry/psychiatry-mental-illness-myths-chemical-imbalances.htm, p. viii, accessed 27 February 2014.

10. Thomas Szasz, http://www.anxietycentre.com/downloads/Chemical-Imbalance-Theory-is-False.pdf, accessed 25 March 2014.

11. Daniel Carlat, *Unhinged: The Trouble with Psychiatry—a Doctor's Revelations about a Profession in Crisis,* London: Free Press, 2010.

12. Michael J. Norden, *Beyond Prozac: Brain Toxic Lifestyles, Natural Antidotes and New Generation Antidepressants,* New York: Regan Books, 1995, p. 155.

13. Terry Lynch, *Beyond Prozac: Healing Mental Distress,* Ross-on-Wye: PCCS Books, 2004, p. 103.

14. Daniel Carlat, *Unhinged: The Trouble with Psychiatry—A Doctor's Revelations about a Profession in Crisis,* London: Free Press, 2010, pps. 53-4.

15. Edward Shorter, *How Everyone Became Depressed,* Oxford: Oxford University Press, 2013, p. 152.

16. Joanna Moncrieff, "Is Psychiatry for sale?: An Examination of the Influence of the Pharmaceutical Industry on Academic and Practical Psychiatry", June 2003, http://www.critpsy-net.freeuk.com/pharmaceuticalindustry.htm, accessed 05 March 2014.

17. L. Ratna, 'Crisis intervention in Psychogeriatrics: A Two-Year Follow-up Study', in L. Ratna, L., (ed.), *The Practice of Psychiatric Crisis Intervention,* 1978, Hertfordshire: League of Friends, Napsbury Hospital.

18. Solomon H. Snyder "Book Review—*Goodman and Gilman's The Pharmacological Basis of Therapeutics*", *New England Journal of Medicine,* 28 February 1991; 324:636-637, http://www.nejm.org/doi/full/10.1056/NEJM199102283240919, accessed 18 May 2014.

19. A. Gilman, T. Rail, A. Nies, and P. Taylor, P (eds.), *Goodman and Gilman's The Pharmacological Basics of Therapeutics,* 8th edition, New York: Pergamon Press, 1990, p. 1811.

20. "The Biology of Mental Disorders", U.S. Government Printing Office, 1992.

21. Peter Breggin, *Toxic Psychiatry,* London: HarperCollins, 1993, pps. 173-5.

22. Colin Ross, *Pseudoscience in Biological Psychiatry,* New York: John Wiley & Sons, 1995, p. 111.

23. A. Nierenberg, "Antidepressants: Current Issues and New Drugs", Harvard Medical School/Massachussetts General Hospital Conference of Psychopharmacy, 17-19 October 1997.

24. Elliot S. Valenstein, *Blaming the Brain: The Truth About Drugs and Mental Health,* New York: The Free Press, 1998.

25. Elliot S. Valenstein, *Blaming the Brain: The Truth About Drugs and Mental Health,* New York: The Free Press, 1998, pps. 3, 241, 3 and 5.

26. Thomas Moore, *Prescription for Disaster: The Hidden Dangers in your Medicine Cabinet,* Dell, 1998, http://www.bible.ca/psychiatry/psychiatry-mental-illness-myths-chemical-imbalances.htm, accessed 27 February 2014.

27. Edward Shorter, *How Everyone Became Depressed,* 2013, Oxford: Oxford University Press, p. 157, from Ross Baldessarini interview in Ban, Oral History of NeuroPsychopharmacology, Vol. 5, 25.

28. Edward Shorter, *How Everyone Became Depressed,* 2013, Oxford: Oxford University Press, p. 157, from Ross Baldessarini interview in Ban, Oral History of NeuroPsychopharmacology, Vol. 5, 25.

29. David D. Burns, *The Feeling Good Handbook,* New York: Plume, 1999.

30. Stephen M., Stahl, *Essential Psychopharmacology: Neuroscientific Basis and Practical Applications,* Cambridge: Cambridge University Press, 2000, p. 601.

31. Steven E. Hyman, "The genetics of mental illness: implications for practice", Bulletin of the World Health Organization, 2000, 78 (4), p. 455.

32. Joseph Glenmullen, *Prozac Backlash: Overcoming the Dangers of Prozac, Zoloft, Paxil and Other Antidepressants with Safe, Effective Alternatives,* 2001, Simon & Shuster.

33. Ty Colbert, *The Rape of the Soul: How the Chemical Imbalance Model of Psychiatry has Failed its Patients,* California: Kevco Publishing, 2001, p. 79.

34. Tony Humphreys, in foreword to *Beyond Prozac: Healing Mental Suffering Without Drugs,* Dublin: Marino Books, 2001, p. 11.

35. Thomas Szasz, in "Psychiatric Hoax: The Subversion of Medicine", Citizen's Commission on Human Rights, 2002.

36. http://www.cmaj.ca/content/174/6/754.2, accessed 26 February 2014.

37. Bruce Levine, *Commonsense Rebellion: Taking Back your Life from Drugs, Shrinks, Corporations, and a World Gone Crazy,* Bloomsbury Academic 2003.

38. Psychiatrist David Burns, when asked about the scientific status of the serotonin theory in 2003, in J. R. Lacasse and T. Gomory, "Is graduate social work education promoting a critical approach to mental health practice?" *J Soc Work Educ* 2003, 39: 383–408.

39. Jonathan Leo, "The Biology of Mental Illness" *Society,* July/August 2004, Volume 41, Issue 5, pp. 45-53, http://link.springer.com/article/10.1007%2FBF02688217#page-1, accessed 19 August 2014.

40. Jonathan Leo, "The Biology of Mental Illness" *Society,* July/August 2004, Volume 41, Issue 5, pp. 45-53, http://link.springer.com/article/10.1007%2FBF02688217#page-1, accessed 19 August 2014.

41. Ron Leifer, http://www.anxietycentre.com/downloads/Chemical-Imbalance-Theory-is-False. pdf, accessed 28 February 2014.

42. Darshak Sanghavi, "Health Care System leaves Mentally Ill Children Behind", *Boston Globe,* 27 April 2004.

43. Kenneth S. Kendler, M.D., "Towards a Philosophical Structure for Psychiatry", *American Journal of Psychiatry,* 01 March 2005, 162:433-440. Doi:1176/appi.ajp.162.3.433, accessed 18 February 2014.

44. Joanna Moncrieff, quoted in "Advertisements for SSRIs May Be Misleading", by Laurie Barclay, MD, *Medscape,* 08 November 2005, http://www.medscape.com/viewarticle/516262, accessed 02 June 2014.

45. Gordon McCarter, quoted in "Advertisements for SSRIs May Be Misleading", by Laurie Barclay, MD, *Medscape,* 08 November 2005, http://www.medscape.com/viewarticle/516262, accessed 02 June 2014.

46. J.R. Lacasse & J. Leo, "Serotonin and depression: A Disconnect between the Advertisements and the Scientific Literature", *PLoS Med:* 2(12) e392, 08 November 2005, accessed 18 February 2014.

47. Sharon Begley, "Some Drugs Work to Treat depression, But It Isn't Clear How", *Wall Street Journal,* 18 November 2005, http://online.wsj.com/news/articles/SB113226807554400588, accessed 11 August 2014.

48. Vera Hassner Sharav, "Depression-serotonin: How did so many smart people get it so wrong", The Alliance for Human Research Protection, http://www.ahrp.org/cms/content/view/67/55/, 19 November 2005, accessed 31 December 2013.

49. David Healy, *Let them Eat Prozac: The Unhealthy Relationship between the Pharmaceutical Industry and Depression,* New York: New York University Press, 2006.

50. David Burns, *When Panic Attacks: The New Drug-Free Anxiety Therapy that can Change your Life,* Harmony, 2006.

51. Joanna Moncrieff & David Cohen, "Do Antidepressants Cure or Create Abnormal Brain States?", *PLoS Med.* 2006 July; 3(7): e240, http://www.ncbi.nlm.nih.gov/pmc/articles/ PMC1-472553/, accessed 30 December 2013.

52. Thomas Insel, quoted by Julie Scelfo in "Men and Depression: New Treatments", *Newsweek,* 25 February 2007, http://www.newsweek.com/men-and-depression-new-treatments-105091, accessed 20 May 2014.

53. Peter Breggin, Centre for the Study of Psychiatry and Psychology, http://www.alex-sk.de/mirror /braindis.html, 2007, accessed 27 November 2013.

54. Dorothy Rowe, "Real causes of depression", *Saga,* February 2007, http://dorothyrowe. com.au/articles/item/192-the-real-causes-of-depression-february-2007, accessed 24 November 2013.

55. Ivor Browne, *Music and Madness,* Cork: Cork University Press: Cork, 2008, p. 121.

56. Irving Kirsch, *The Emperor's New Drugs: Exploding the Antidepressant Myth,* London; Random House, 2009, pps.90-93.

57. Joanna Moncrieff, *The Myth of the Chemical Cure: A Critique of Psychiatric Drug Treatment,* Basingstoke: Palgrave Macmillan, 2009.

58. Marcia Angell, "Drug Companies and Doctors: A Story of Corruption", *New York Review of Books,* 15 January 2009.

59. Michael Corry, http://wellbeingfoundation.com/news2.html, accessed 19 May 2014.

60. Daniel Carlat, *Unhinged: The Trouble with Psychiatry—a Doctor's Revelations about a Profession in Crisis,* London: Free Press, 2010, p. 13.

61. Jonathan Rottenberg, "The Serotonin Theory of Depression is Collapsing", *Psychology Today,* 23 July 2010, accessed 03 January 2014.

62. Niall McLaren, http://biopsychiatry.ca/category/radio-show/dr-niall-mclaren/, 9 August 2010, accessed 11 May 2014.
63. Niall McLaren, http://biopsychiatry.ca/category/radio-show/dr-niall-mclaren/, 9 August 2010, accessed 11 May 2014.
64. Kirsten Weir, "The Roots of Mental Illness", *American Psychological Association*, June 2012, Vol. 43, No. 6, http://www.apa.org/monitor/2012/06/roots.aspx, accessed 26 March 2014.
65. Vivek Datta, "Chemical Imbalances and Other Black Unicorns", Mad in America website, 25 June 2012, http://www.madinamerica.com/ 2012/06/chemical-imbalances-and-other-black-unicorns /, accessed 27 February 2014.
66. Steven Reidbord, "Chemical imbalance—Sloppy thinking in psychiatry 1", in "Reidbord's Reflections", 29 April 2012, http://blog.stevenreidbordmd.com/?p=561, accessed 25 May 2014.
67. J.P. Jacobsen et al, "The 5-HT deficiency theory of depression: perspectives from a naturalistic 5-HT deficiency model, the tryptophan hydroxylase 2Aeg439Hisknockin mouse", *Philosophical transactions of the Royal Society of London. Series B, Biological Sciences.* 2012 Sep 5:367(1601):2444-59. doi: 10. 1089/rstb.2012.0109.
68. Edward Shorter, *How Everyone Became Depressed,* Oxford: Oxford University Press, 2013, pps. ix and 154.
69. Mary Maddock, in "The Mindfreedom Documentary", 07 May 2014, https://www.you-tube.com /watch?v=zeHaYUd9rXA accessed 25 May 2014.
70. J.J. Schildkraut, "The Catecholamine Hypothesis of Affective Disorders: a review of supporting evidence", *American Journal of Psychiatry,* 1965, 122: 509-22.
71. A. Coppen, (1967) "The Biochemistry of Affective Disorders", *British Journal of Psychiatry,* 1967, 113: pps. 1237-64.
72. Eugene Paykel, in discussion in 1985, in Ruth Porter, ed., *Antidepressants and Receptor Function,* Chichester: Wiley, 1986, p. 164.
73. B.K. Puri & I.T. Treaseden, *Textbook of Psychiatry,* Third Edition, Elsevier, 2011, p. 161.
74. John Grohol, "Low serotonin levels don't cause depression", Psych Central website, 13 September 2014, http://psychcentral.com/blog/archives/2014/09/13/low-serotonin-levels-dont-cause-depression/accessed 06 October 2014.
75. Pedro Delgado & Francisco Morena, "The role of Norepinephrine in depression" *Journal of Clinical Psychiatry,* 2000;61 Suppl 1:5-12.
76. Peter Kramer, in a letter to the *New York Times* in 2002, in "Serotonin and Depression: A Disconnect between the Advertisements and the Scientific Literature", by Jeffrey Lacasse and Jonathan Leo, *PLoS Medicine,* December 2005, Volume 2 Issue 12, e392, accessed 17 February 2014.
77. Irving Kirsch, *The Emperor's New Drugs: Exploding the Antidepressant Myth,* London: Random House, 2009, p. 80.
78. Daniel Carlat, *Unhinged: The Trouble with Psychiatry—a Doctor's Revelations about a Profession in Crisis,* London: Free Press, 2010, p. 76.
79. J.R. Lacasse & J. Leo, "Serotonin and depression: A Disconnect between the Advertisements and the Scientific Literature". *PLoS Med:* 2(12) e392, 2005, accessed 18 February 2014.
80. James Whitney Hicks, *50 Signs of Mental Illness: A Guide to Understanding Mental Health,* Yale: Yale University Press, 2005, p. 3.
81. Richard Bentall, *Doctoring the Mind: Why Psychiatric Treatments Fail,* London: Penguin Books Ltd, 2009, p. 77.
82. Daniel Carlat, *Unhinged: The Trouble with Psychiatry—a Doctor's Revelations about a Profession in Crisis,* London: Free Press, 2010, p. 76-77.
83. Daniel Carlat, *Unhinged: The Trouble with Psychiatry—a Doctor's Revelations about a Profession in Crisis,* London: Free Press, 2010.
84. Irving Kirsch, Thomas J. Moore & colleagues, "The Emperor's New Drugs: An Analysis of Antidepressant Medication Date Submitted to the U.S. Food and Drug Administration", *Prevention & Treatment,* Volume 5, Article 23, 2002, http://alphachoices.com/repository/assets/pdf/EmperorsNewDrugs.pdf. Kirsch and colleagues found that 80% of the benefits attributed to antidepressants were due to the placebo effect.
85. Irving Kirsch, *The Emperor's New Drugs: Exploding the Antidepressant Myth,* London; Random House, 2009, pps.90-93.

86. Such research has focused on areas such as the levels of tryptophan (a precursor of serotonin) in blood, urine and cerebrospinal fluid; the effects of depleting tryptophan levels and the levels of noradrenaline precursors; uptake patterns of serotonin and noradrenaline in platelets; the response of prolactin to fenfluramine, a drug thought to stimulate serotonin release into the synapses; growth hormone response to clonidine, a drug thought to increase noradrenaline levels in nerve synapses; serotonin and noradrenaline receptor density in the brains of people who have taken their own lives; serotonin and noradrenaline binding in living subjects using imaging and arterial assays of the metabolites of serotonin and noradrenaline. As described by Moncrieff, Joanna, in *The Myth of the Chemical Cure: A Critique of Psychiatric Drug Treatment*, Basingstoke: Palgrave Macmillan, 2009, p. 154. Clearly there is immense potential for inaccuracy and misinterpretation, given the level of indirectness that researchers have had to resort to in their efforts to identify brain chemical imbalance problems in depression.

87. Elliot S. Valenstein, *Blaming the Brain: The Truth About Drugs and Mental Health*, New York: The Free Press, 1998, p. 101.

88. Daniel Carlat, *Unhinged: The Trouble with Psychiatry—a Doctor's Revelations about a Profession in Crisis*, London: Free Press, 2010, p. 77.

89. Robert Whitaker, *Anatomy of an Epidemic: Magic Bullets, Psychiatric Drugs and the Astonishing Rise of Mental Illness in America*, New York: Crown Publishers, 2010, p. 70.

90. Daniel Carlat, *Unhinged: The Trouble with Psychiatry—a Doctor's Revelations about a Profession in Crisis*, London: Free Press, 2010, p. 77.

91. R.H. Belmaker & Galila Agam, "Major Depressive Disorder", *New England Journal of Medicine*, 358 2008, pps 55-68.

92. Philip Cowen, Paul Harrison & Tom Burns, *The Shorter Oxford Textbook of Psychiatry*, Oxford: Oxford University Press, 2012, p. 238.

93. http://www.merriam-webster.com/dictionary/biochemistry, accessed 28 December 2013.

94. L.G. Whitby, A.F. Smith & G.J. Beckett, *Lecture Notes on Clinical Chemistry*, 4th edition, Oxford: Blackwell Scientific Publications, 1988, p. 336.

95. L.G. Whitby, A.F. Smith & G.J. Beckett, *Lecture Notes on Clinical Chemistry*, 4th edition, Oxford: Blackwell Scientific Publications, 1988, p. 419.

96. Jocelyn Dow, Gordon Lindsey & Jim Morrison, *Biochemistry: Molecules, Cells and the Body*, Harrow: Addison-Wesley, 1995.

97. Michael L. Bishop, Janet L. Duben-Engelkirk & Edward P. Fody, *Clinical Chemistry: Principles, Procedures and Correlations*, 3rd edition, Philadelphia: Lippincott, 1996.

98. Michael L. Bishop, Janet L. Duben-Engelkirk & Edward P. Fody, *Clinical Chemistry: Principles, Procedures and Correlations*, 3rd edition, Philadelphia: Lippincott, 1996, p. 426.

99. N. V. Bhagavan, *Medical Biochemistry*, 4th edition, San Diego, Harcourt Academic Press, 2002.

100. John W. Baynes & Marek H. Dominiczak, *Medical Biochemistry*, Elsevier Mosby, Philadelphia, 2005.

101. Allan D. Marks, Michael Lieberman & Coleen Smith, *Mark's Basic Medical Biochemistry: A Clinical Approach*, 2nd edition, Lippincott, Baltimore: Williams & Wilkins, 2005.

102. Thomas M. Devlin, *The Textbook of Biochemistry with Clinical Correlations*, 6th edition, Hoboken, N.J.: Wiley-Liss, John Wiley & Sons, 2006.

103. Geoffrey Beckett, Simon Walker, Peter Rae, Peter Ashby, *Lecture Notes: Clinical Biochemistry*, 7th edition, Oxford: Blackwell Publishing Ltd, 2006.

104. Abraham L. Kierszenbaum and Laura L. Tres, *Histology and Cell Biology: An Introduction to Pathology*, 3rd edition, Philadelphia: Elsevier Saunders, 2012.

105. Michael Conn, ed., *Neuroscience in Medicine*, E-book, Totowa, NJ: Humana Press, 2008.

106. Jeffrey T. Joseph & David L. Cardozo, *Functional Neuroanatomy: An Interactive Text and Manual*, New Jersey: John Wiley & Sons, Inc., 2004, p. 284.

107. Gerard J. Tortora & Bryan Derrickson, *Principles of Anatomy and Physiology*, 11th edition, New Jersey: John Wiley & Sons, Inc, 2006, p. 267.

108. Gerard J. Tortora & Bryan Derrickson, *Principles of Anatomy and Physiology*, 11th edition, New Jersey: John Wiley & Sons, Inc, 2006, p. 429.

109. Paul Bentley, *Memorising Medicine: A Revision Guide*, London: Royal Society of Medicine Press Ltd, 2007.

110. Jeannette Naish, Patricia Revest & Denise Syndercombe Court, eds., *Medical Sciences*, Saunders: Elsevier, 2009, p. 390.

111. Alan F. Schatzberg & Charles B. Nemeroff, eds., *The American Psychiatric Publishing Textbook of Psychopharmacology,* Arlington, Va.: American Psychiatric Publishing Inc, 2009.
112. J.A. Muir Gray & Godfrey Fowler, *Essentials of Preventive Medicine,* Oxford: Blackwell Scientific Publications, 1984, p. 159.
113. John Nolte, *The Human Brain: An Introduction to its Functional Anatomy,* 6th edition, Elsevier: Philadelphia, 2009, p. 289.
114. John Nolte, *The Human Brain: An Introduction to its Functional Anatomy,* 6th edition, Elsevier: Philadelphia, 2009, p. 289.
115. According to the Fallacy Files website, a Wishful Thinking logical fallacy "usually takes the form of a bias towards the belief in P (in this case P being the belief that chemical imbalances occur in depression), which leads to the overestimating of the weight of evidence in favour of P, as well as the underestimating of the weight against. It can lead to ignoring the evidence against a cherished belief, which is a case of one-sidedness" http://www.fallacyfiles.org/wishthnk.html, accessed 02 January 2014.
116. Cynthia Chernecky, Professor of Physiological and Technological Nursing, Georgia Regents University, Augusta, & Barbara J. Berger, Director of Clinic Management, Summacare, Inc., Akron, Ohio, eds., *Laboratory Tests and Diagnostic Procedures,* 6th edition, St. Louis: Elsevier, 2013, p. 1010.
117. John Crocker & David Burnett, Eds, *The Science of Laboratory Diagnosis,* 2005, Chichester: John Wiley & Sons Ltd, p. 432: "Serotonin is synthesized from tryptophan and metabolized to 5-hydroxyindole acetic acid (5-HIAA) by monoamine oxidases. Carcinoid tumours secrete abnormal amounts of serotonin and measurement of blood/urine serotonin concentrations or urinary 5-HIAA excretion is useful in the detection of tumours and in monitoring therapy".
118. MedlinePlus, "Serum serotonin level", http://www.nlm.nih.gov/medlineplus/ency/article/003 562.htm, accessed 16 November 2014.

3. A HYPOTHESIS DISCREDITED A LONG TIME AGO

The notion that depression is caused by brain chemical abnormalities has long been discredited for a whole host of reasons. From the beginning, the idea that biochemical abnormalities caused depression was weak and far-fetched. Neuroscience professor Elliot Valenstein wrote in his 1998 book *Blaming the Brain: The Truth About Drugs and Mental Health*:

> Although it is often stated with great confidence that depressed people have a serotonin or norepinephrine deficiency, the actual evidence contradicts these claims ... The evidence is clear that none of the proposed biogenic amine theories of depression can possibly be correct. [1]

In this chapter, I discuss how the brain chemical imbalances notion in depression has long been discredited.

THE EXTRAORDINARY COMPLEXITY OF THE BRAIN

The human brain is one of the most extraordinary phenomena on this planet. Its complexity greatly surpasses that of all other human organs. Brain cells are called neurons. There are an estimated 100 billion neurons in the brain. It has been estimated that there may be one hundred trillion interconnections within the human brain. This demonstrates the currently unfathomable complexity and mystery of this remarkable organ. Our understanding of the human brain is still very primitive, but enough is known to create serious doubts regarding the simplistic brain chemical imbalance notion in depression. To conclude that the cause of depression is simply the unproven notion that brain synapse serotonin levels are low is an extraordinary oversimplification of this complexity.

In a 2000 World Health Organization Bulletin, psychiatry professor Steven Hyman, then Director of the National Institute of Mental Health, wrote an article titled "The genetics of mental illness: implications for practice". This bulletin concerned genetics in mental health, but Professor Hyman's comments apply equally to notions of biochemical brain abnormalities:

> The brain is the most complex object of investigation in the history of biological science. Its development depends on complex, often non-linear ... interactions ... associated with the interconnection of 100,000 million or more neurons. ... This complexity, however, has made progress in the neuroscience and genetics of mental illness exceedingly difficult. Each neuron in the brain makes thousands of connections or synapses with neighboring and distant neurons; there are probably more than 100 trillion such connections, and across them each neuron may utilize several of more than 100 chemical neurotransmitters ... The crowning

complexity of the brain, however, is that it is not static. Every time something new is learnt, whether a new name, a new skill or a new emotional reaction, the active neurons alter the synaptic architecture of the circuit in which the learning has occurred. This process is termed "plasticity"; new synapses may be formed and old ones may be pruned; existing synapses may be strengthened or weakened. As a result, information is processed differently. [2]

The vast complexity of the human brain was clearly recognized in a 1998 American Medical Association publication, *Essential Guide to Depression* (brackets mine):

Your brain contains between 10 billion and 100 billion neurons . . . The messages travel in the form of electrical impulses at incredible speed—taking less than 1/5,000 of a second to zip from one neuron to another . . . Each neuron has numerous dendrites (branches) to pick up messages and each has as many as 1,000 branches at the end of its axon to forward messages . . . Scientists once thought that the connections between neurons were fixed at birth and never affected by experience. Today, scientists have learned that events in our lives—the amount of nurturing we do or do not receive as infants, for example—have a great impact on how many of these connections are created. As you master new skills and feel new emotions, your network of neurons constantly forms new connections. For that reason, the connections between the neurons in your brain are unique. [3]

In other words, while psychiatry has consistently played down the importance of life experiences because they may cast doubt on the supposed primacy of biology, the American Medical Association recognised almost twenty years ago that "events in our lives . . . have a great impact" on brain structure and function. This passage portrays the brain as a dynamic and responsive organ rather than always being the director, the drive centre it is generally assumed to be. If the American Medical Association's assertion that the connections in the brain are unique to each person is correct, then a generalised lowering of serotonin as a general cause of depression becomes even more untenable. Professor Steven Hyman's 2000 World Health Organization Bulletin article just mentioned above contains a similar message; the human brain may be far more responsive to life experiences and external events than is generally assumed.

Neuroscientist Elliot Valenstein made similar comments regarding the extraordinary complexity of the brain in 1998. His comments reflect a healthy humility and considerable respect for the brain that contrasts with the hubris of many claims by doctors regarding how well they and their colleagues understand the brain:

The number of different brain changes that can occur over a three-week period of drug treatment is huge, as each change produces a cascade of other changes until the changes become unfathomable. [4]

Psychiatrist and historian Edward Shorter wrote in 2013 about the complexity of the brain relative to our understanding and our assumptions. In the following passage, he questioned the widespread importance placed on neurotransmission—how messages are passed between nerve cells:

> Neurotransmission is only a small part of the vast world—a world of hitherto unknowable size—of neurochemistry and neurophysiology. And it is not necessarily the central chemical mechanism in psychiatric illness. Nor has any psychiatric illness been convincingly attributed to a shortage of any particular transmitter. [5]

Shorter's point is important. Mainstream psychiatry makes extraordinary assumptions, assuming that the answers lie in the tiny proportion of brain activity of which we have become aware, and that to such a primitive degree. So much of brain function and its relation to experience remains a mystery that it is inappropriate at this time to make the remarkable presumption that the answers lie in the tiny bit we know. It is a classic example of the adage "a little knowledge can be a dangerous thing". Not nearly enough is known about the brain for anyone to claim with any degree of confidence that neurotransmitter function is a central mechanism in any psychiatric illness.

American psychotherapist and author Gary Greenberg wrote in a 2013 *New Yorker* article that rather than clarify how drugs might work within the brain:

> Research has mostly yielded more evidence that the brain, which has more neurons that the Milky Way has stars and is perhaps one of the most complex objects in the universe, is an elusive target for drugs. [6]

Despite the obvious complexity of the brain, some psychiatrists and GPs profess an understanding of this organ that is highly inconsistent with current scientific knowledge. Their comments smack of a level of arrogance that in my opinion is downright dangerous. In 1985 Nancy Andreasen, one of the world's leading psychiatrists and spokespersons for psychiatry of the past thirty years, was prepared to inform the public that:

> The mind and brain are in fact inseparable. The word *mind* refers to those functions of the body that reside in the brain. [7]

This remarkable and unsubstantiated claim reveals psychiatry's blind faith in biology in addition to its limited and distorted understanding of the human mind and of human beings. To describe the human mind as merely "those functions of the body that reside in the brain" is to present an alarmingly limited view of the human mind as merely some functions of the body. Such comments are often a reflection of the commonly held assumption within medicine that the mind is the servant of the brain. It is at least equally plausible that the brain is the servant of the mind, but for reasons of self-interest discussed in chapters twelve, thirteen and fourteen, psychiatry is largely blind to that possibility. Neither the mind nor the brain are understood to any significant degree, therefore claims such as Andreasen's made with certainty and authority are entirely inappropriate.

In his 2010 book, *Anatomy of an Epidemic: Magic Bullets, Psychiatric Drugs and the Astonishing Rise of Mental Illness in America*, journalist Robert Whitaker wrote:

> All of this physiology—the 100 billion neurons, the 150 trillion synapses, the various neurotransmitter pathways—tell of a brain that is almost infinitely complex. Yet the chemical imbalance theory of mental disorders boiled this complexity down to a simple disease mechanism, one easy to grasp. In depression, the problem was that the serotonergic neurons released too little serotonin into the synaptic gap, and thus the serotonergic pathways in the brain were "underactive". Antidepressants brought serotonin levels in the synaptic gap up to normal, and that allowed these pathways to transmit messages at the proper pace.[8]

Psychiatrist Daniel Carlat's 2010 commentary on the brain is accurate (brackets mine):

> The brain is extraordinarily complex, unfathomable really to current knowledge and technology. The brain contains approximately one hundred billion nerve cells, each of which interfaces through with up to ten thousand other nerve cells. This means that at any one time a quadrillion (that's one million billion) interface points or synapses are active at any given time—unfathomable—we should be in awe of its majesty rather than arrogantly and very prematurely assuming we understand it—the equivalent of 150,000 times the number of humans on earth, at any given moment. Almost incomputable. It is therefore no surprise that we know almost nothing definitive about the pathophysiology of mental illness. [9]

Only a handful of the estimated more than 100 neurotransmitters that have been identified have been researched to date, with new ones regularly coming to light. These test tube experiments typically check the effect of medication on up to just six of the many other neurotransmitters. Even within the narrow confines of the test tube, the effects of antidepressants on the many other known neurotransmitters have not been measured. It is akin to proclaiming to understand the mysteries of the galaxies because one has found a primitive telescope.

If brain chemical changes occur during and reflect our complex moment-to-moment thinking, feeling, behaviour and activities, these changes are likely to be remarkably fast-moving and complex, as our thoughts, feelings, behaviours and actions are. To conclude that patterns of thinking, feeling and experiencing can be simplistically explained as a persistent yet unidentified deficiency of one or two brain chemicals is counter-intuitive when the complexity of all this and of the brain itself is taken into account. Medical science has virtually no understanding of the extremely complex, interconnected and nuanced brain actions that occur hundreds of times per second each day of our lives. The interplay between our mind, thoughts and feelings and the brain remain largely a mystery. Given the extraordinary complexity of the brain and the virtually unfathomable degree of interconnectedness between brain cells, the suggestion that in depression there is a constant, unchanging biochemical imbalance so straightforward that it can be corrected by a pill is bordering on the absurd.

In my opinion, the remarkable level of hubris that exists within some quarters of psychiatry and general practice regarding depression, the brain and currently unknown future research outcomes is illustrated by Irish general practitioner Harry Barry's comment in his 2012 book *Flagging Depression: A Practical Guide* (italics mine):

> As this century, with its emphasis on the "mystery of the brain", advances, we *will* put to bed once and for all misconceptions about this illness. [10]

SEROTONIN DEPLETION DOES NOT CAUSE DEPRESSION

If low levels of brain chemicals such as serotonin caused depression, then reducing brain serotonin should cause people to become depressed. Research published in 2003 was designed to address this. Researchers developed drinks that were thought to deplete levels of serotonin or noradrenaline levels, in the case of serotonin by reducing levels of tryptophan, a precursor of serotonin. They hypothesised that if depression is caused by a deficiency in these neurotransmitters, these drinks should cause depression by depleting their levels.

That is not what happened. When people who were not diagnosed as being depressed ingested these substances, their mood remained unchanged and they did not become depressed. People diagnosed with depression and on treatment did not become more depressed upon taking these drinks. Some people deemed to have recovered from depression developed what the researchers called "transient depressive symptoms" without developing major depression. [11] As psychiatrist Daniel Carlat wrote subsequently, these results strongly imply that neurotransmitter deficiency is unlikely to cause depression. [12]

Neurotransmitter depletion has been attempted in at least 90 studies. The aim of these studies was to test the hypothesis that depression was caused by reduced levels of serotonin and noradrenaline. If this were true, then reducing brain levels of both should trigger depression. An evaluation of these studies was published in 2007. [13] In fact, such attempts to reduce serotonin, epinephrine and dopamine in people who had never been depressed did not affect their mood even to a slight degree. From these 90 studies, only one group of people were found in whom assumed depletion of serotonin sometimes resulted in clinical depression; depressed patients in remission who continued to take SSRIs. Approximately 50 per cent of this group experienced depression symptoms, which were transient and only occurred in those still taking SSRI antidepressants. [14]

Erroneous conclusions regarding the effects of the drug reserpine for over forty years have frequently been referred to as evidence that depression must be caused by a brain chemical abnormality. The importance of reserpine to the medical model of depression is reflected in neuroscientist Elliot Valenstein's comment:

> It was the neuropharmacological studies of reserpine that proved critical for the development of the biochemical theories of depression. [15]

Reserpine, used for decades to treat high blood pressure and on occasion to treat severe agitation, had been long thought to cause a depression-like state in some people. This drug was thought to reduce levels of serotonin and noradrenaline in the brain. [16] These two ideas were joined in the creation of a theory that concurred with the monoamine hypothesis and were wrongly taken as evidence supporting it. Since reserpine appeared to cause a depression-like state in some people and reserpine was thought to reduce brain levels of serotonin and noradrenaline, it was assumed that depression is likely caused by a depletion of brain levels of these chemicals. For several decades, many medical and psychiatric textbooks have referred to these assumed effects as evidence for the biochemical brain abnormality-depression hypothesis, misinforming their readers in the process. This has been commonly asserted as an established fact by psychiatrists, and as persuasive evidence that brain chemical deficiencies cause depression. But as neuroscientist Elliot Valenstein wrote in 1998:

> Contrary to the impression conveyed in a number of influential review articles, reserpine does not precipitate a clinical depression in most people. [17]

Research published in 1974 found that only six per cent of people taking even high doses of reserpine for several months developed symptoms that were even suggestive of depression. All of this six percent turned out to have a previous history of depression. The researchers concluded that rather than reserpine frequently causing depression, reserpine may reinstate depression in a relatively small number of susceptible patients. [18] This research, published in 1974 in the *Archives of General Psychiatry* fourteen years before Prozac's launch, found that drugs thought to deplete noradrenaline, serotonin and dopamine did not cause depression in humans. Commenting on this research in 1988, neuroscientist Elliot Valenstein wrote:

> Their summary of these articles should have delivered a crippling blow to any theory that assumed that either a serotonin or norepinephrine deficiency was the cause of depression, but actually it was ignored. [19]

Similar findings of just six percent of people taking reserpine becoming depressed had been found in research published three years previously. [20] The long-held belief in reserpine's supportive evidence of the model was built on very shaky grounds indeed.

Many drugs have been found to alleviate depression that have no action whatsoever on any of these neurotransmitters. In his 1993 book *Toxic Psychiatry* American psychiatrist Peter Breggin wrote:

> Eventually the theory was punched full of holes by contradictory evidence. For example, some drugs that mimicked these biochemical effects did not alleviate depression, and others that are thought to sometimes alleviate depression have a wholly different biochemical mechanism. [21]

The notion that deficiencies of brain chemicals such as serotonin are a regular feature of depression was dealt a further blow since the introduction of the drug tianeptine as an antidepressant (brand names include Stablon, Coaxil and Tatinol). In contrast to the SSRI antidepressants which are thought to increase serotonin levels in the spaces between brain cells, tianeptine is thought to have precisely the opposite effect, *decreasing* serotonin levels in these spaces. Yet tianeptine has a similar rate of success in treating depression as the SSRIs. The remarkably similar effectiveness rate for all types of antidepressants has led some researchers to conclude that these substances share a common mode of action—that of an active placebo—rather than any specific corrective action on brain chemicals. [22]

SELECTIVE SEROTONIN REUPTAKE INHIBITION DISCREDITED YEARS BEFORE PROZAC

Prozac was launched in 1988 as a breakthrough antidepressant drug, the first of a long line of selective serotonin reuptake inhibitors, the SSRIs. A major selling point for the SSRIs was the much-heralded selectivity of these drugs compared to their predecessors. It was claimed that these substances acted only on serotonin without interfering with any other aspect of brain chemical function. This claimed selectivity was considered such a key characteristic of SSRI antidepressants that serotonin selectivity became an intrinsic part of the name of this group of drugs. It turns out that years before Prozac was launched, major question-marks hung over these claims.

In 1978, ten years before the launch of Prozac, Seymour Kety, head of biological psychiatry at the Mailman Research Center at McLean Hospital in Belmont, Massachusetts wrote:

The simplistic notion of "one transmitter-one function" is no longer tenable. [23]

Similar major doubts were expressed in Britain in the 1970s. At a London conference in 1979 Laurent Maitre, a research scientist with Ciba-Geigy, stated:

It is very doubtful that there is a correlation between 5-HT (serotonin) uptake inhibition and clinical effects. [24]

At a 1979 conference in Monte Carlo, nine years before the launch of Prozac, Parisian pharmacist Alain Puech outlined the absurdity of the idea of selectively affecting one neurotransmitter while having no effect on others or on other aspects of brain function (brackets mine):

It is inconceivable that modifying one monoaminergic system (such as serotonin, dopamine or noradrenaline) can be done independently, because all the circuits are linked in a chain. Thus, every time there is a change in one neurotransmitter system, there is very probably at least one other neurotransmitter system than is modified. [25]

According to neuroscientist S.H. Snyder, in a 1980 *Science* article published eight years before the launch of Prozac:

> There may be over a hundred neurotransmitters rather than just a handful. Most drugs affect many more neurotransmitters than initially thought. [26]

The drug industry responded forcefully in 1988 with the launch of Prozac. Despite major concerns expressed by these and other experts regarding this drug's claimed serotonin selectivity, in an advertisement in the *Journal of the American Medical Association* in June 1988, the makers of Prozac championed this substance as:

> The first highly specific . . . highly potent blocker of serotonin uptake. [27]

Psychiatrist and historian of psychiatry Edward Shorter has been highly critical of this strategy:

> Using a model of drug action that had largely been discredited, Lilly and the other SSRI manufacturers went on to promote a drug class—and reap billions of dollars in profit—that captured the imagination of the public and the medical profession not just in the United States but in the whole world. [28]

In a 1991 *Journal of Clinical Psychiatry* article, neuroscientist Efrain C. Azmitia and his colleagues expressed major reservations about claims that SSRI antidepressants worked as selectively as was widely claimed:

> Even if these substances did selectively effect serotonin without affecting other chemicals, the situation remains extraordinarily complex in comparison to the simplistic picture that is presented by those with vested interests. There are hundreds of thousands of brain cells that involve serotonin, cells that extend to virtually every area of the brain. Each serotonin brain cell branches over 500,000 times as it makes contact with vast numbers of other brain cells. Through this extraordinarily complex brain circuitry, brain cells are in a continuous process of inter-communication involving delicate balances and feedback loops of such complexity that are currently so far from our current levels of understanding. This reality alone should engender modesty, humility and a reluctance among those who should know better, who are frequently given to making pronouncements regarding brain function that they simply cannot confirm through scientific means. The interconnectivity of the brain just referred to, where one cell connects with at least 500,000 others, renders blenderized rat brain test tube experiments irrelevant and inappropriate, since the interconnectivity of cells is destroyed in the blending and killing process. [29]

In 1998 neuroscientist Elliot Valenstein wrote that research suggested that the different brain neurotransmitters are interlinked through complex interconnected brain circuitry. Interfering with one affects the functioning of the others. In response to the artificially-created chemical imbalance created by the drugs, many secondary, tertiary and even more remote compensatory changes take place in the brain, and many of these changes do not involve serotonin or noradrenaline. [30] Psychiatrist Joseph Glenmullen wrote in 2001:

> To talk about "selectivity" in smashed brains in test tubes where fragments of brain cells no longer influence one another is irrelevant; to talk about it in regard to living humans is simply folly . . . The Prozac group were hailed as a breakthrough because they were "selective" for serotonin. This selectivity gives the impression that serotonin is localized in a depression center in the brain. If a depressed person's serotonin is low, the impression is given that the drugs top it up in a safe, targeted manner. This impression does not match reality, however . . . while pharmaceutical companies have marketed Prozac, Zoloft, Paxil and Luvox as "selective" for serotonin, serotonin is anything but selective in its widespread effects. [31]

In 2005, American psychiatrist Grace Jackson wrote in her book *Rethinking Psychiatric Drugs: A Guide for Informed Consent*:

> The very concept that an antidepressant might be specific for one type of chemical (serotonin) has fallen by the wayside, as researchers have demonstrated the complex interactions which exist between and among the neurotransmitter systems in the brain. [32]

THE TIMING OF DRUG EFFECTS

An awkward conundrum for proponents of the biochemical deficiency theory of depression is that it generally takes at least two-three weeks for antidepressants to kick in. Common sense would suggest that treatment for a chemical imbalance should have a more rapid effect, particularly since research suggests that noradrenaline and serotonin reach their maximum levels within one-two days of drug commencement. [33] As psychiatrist Daniel Carlat wrote in 2010:

> Another challenge to the chemical imbalance theory is the well-known delay in the effect of antidepressants—in most patients, these drugs take at least two weeks to work. Yet, the drugs begin altering levels of serotonin and norepinephrine immediately. In order to explain this, authorities have created increasingly elaborate theories about "downstream" effects of antidepressants . . . Again, the theories are ingenious but unproven. [34]

Several theories have been put forward in an attempt to square this circle, none of which has reliable corroborating scientific evidence. One of the theories most referred to is that antidepressants may increase the number of neurotransmitter receptors in the brain. According to this theory, bringing the number of receptors up to the required level takes time, and this is the likely reason for the delay in action of antidepressants. This theory has serious limitations. There is no reliable scientific supportive evidence for this notion, which smacks of wishful thinking. The assumption that these substances would know precisely how many new receptors are necessary and create just this amount is fanciful in the extreme. There is no clarity regarding what the required level of receptors is, and there is no evidence of a reduced number of neurotransmitter receptors in the brain prior to the initiation of treatment.

"AN ASTONISHING BETRAYAL OF TRUST"

In a 2012 *Spectator* interview, psychologist and Nobel Prize winner in economics Daniel Kahneman described the strong link between trust and credibility:

> People aren't convinced by arguments, they don't believe conclusions because they believe in the arguments they read in favour of them. They're convinced because they read or hear the conclusions from people they trust. You trust someone and you believe what they say. That's how ideas are communicated. The arguments come later. [35]

The trust that people place in doctors has contributed greatly to the widespread delusion that brain chemical imbalances are a known feature of depression. Having heard such claims from doctors over many years, in the media and in the doctor's office, the public have come to assume that chemical abnormalities in depression are established facts. The possibility that so many doctors would consistently tell untruths is one that few people would consider.

In a *Truthout* 2014 article titled "Psychiatry Now Admits It's Been Wrong in Big Ways—But Can It Change?" psychologist and author Bruce Levine interviewed award-winning journalist Robert Whitaker, author of the 2010 *Anatomy of an Epidemic: Magic Bullets, Psychiatric Drugs and the Astonishing Rise of Mental Illness in America*. Here are some extracts from that article:

> B.L. In *Anatomy of an Epidemic*, you also discussed the pseudoscience behind the "chemical imbalance" theories of mental illness—theories that made it easy to sell psychiatric drugs. In the last few years, I've noticed establishment psychiatry figures doing some major backpedaling on these chemical imbalance theories. For example, Ronald Pies, editor-in-chief of the *Psychiatric Times* stated in 2011, "in truth, the 'chemical imbalance' notion was always a kind of urban legend—never a theory serious propounded by well-informed psychiatrists". What's your take on this?
>
> R.W. This is quite interesting and revealing, I would say. In a sense, Ronald Pies is right. Those psychiatrists who were "well informed" about investigations into the chemical imbalance theory of mental disorders knew it hadn't really panned out, with such findings dating back to the late 1970s and early 1980s. But why, then, did we as a society come to believe that mental disorders were due to

chemical imbalances, which were then fixed by the drugs? Dr. Pies puts the blame on the drug companies. But if you track the rise of this belief, it is easy to see that the American Psychiatric Association promoted it in some of their promotional materials to the public and that "well informed" psychiatrists often spoke of this metaphor in their interviews with the media. So what you find in this statement by Dr. Pies is a remarkable confession; psychiatry, all along, knew that the evidence wasn't really there to support the chemical imbalance notion, that it was a hypothesis that hadn't panned out, and yet psychiatry failed to inform the public of this crucial fact. By doing so, psychiatry allowed a "little white lie" to take hold in the public mind, which helps sell drugs and, of course, made it seem that psychiatry had magic bullets for psychiatric disorders. That is an astonishing betrayal of trust that the public puts in a medical discipline; we don't expect to be misled in such a basic way.

B.L. But why now? Why are we hearing these admissions from Dr. Pies and others now?

R.W. I am not sure, but I think there are two reasons. One, the low-serotonin theory of depression has been so completely discredited by leading researchers that maintaining the story with the public has just become untenable. It is too easy for critics to point to the scientific findings that contradict it.

The second reason Whitaker mentioned was the fact that, as I discussed in chapter one, drug companies are moving away from psychiatric research and from the chemical imbalance theory, a major development that will accelerate "the public collapse" of the "fabrication" that is the brain chemical imbalance notion. [36]

In her 2010 book *Why we Lie*, psychologist and author Dorothy Rowe wrote:

Lying words are used in great abundance in the professions. Because professionals are supposed to be experts, non-professionals assume that the words used by professionals must be truthful, when in fact professionals use them to deceive. Often the professionals themselves do not realize they are doing this. To them, they are using the language of their profession, and, since the theories they have learnt must be true, so the words they use must be true . . . To become a member of a profession you have to pass qualifying examinations where you are tested on your knowledge of the theory, practice, and language of the profession. Completing this can take many years and a great deal of hard work. We all hate the feeling of having wasted our time, and so, many professionals are very reluctant to let themselves see when they use their professional language to deceive. Among themselves, they argue the finer points of theory or the value of a particular type of research, but they cannot bear to allow themselves to see the untruths in what they do. Thus, they deceive others, and they deceive themselves. [37]

It is said that watching what people do provides greater insight into people than listening to or believing what they say, and this is certainly true regarding the brain chemical imbalance notion. There is no practical hands-on application of this theory at any level within the medical approach to depression. Observing the medical approach to depression and its treatment reveals the true situation in relation to serotonin, a scenario very different from the one so vigorously promoted for the past five decades.

NOTES TO CHAPTER THREE

1. Elliot S. Valenstein, *Blaming the Brain: The Truth About Drugs and Mental Health*, New York: The Free Press, 1998, p. 100-102.
2. Stephen E. Hyman, "The genetics of mental illness: implications for practice", Bulletin of the World Health Organization, 2000, 78 (4).
3. American Medical Association, *Essential Guide to Depression,* New York: Simon & Schuster, 1998, pps. 60-61.
4. Elliot S. Valenstein, *Blaming the Brain: The Truth About Drugs and Mental Health*, 1998, New York: The Free Press, p. 99.
5. Edward Shorter, *How Everyone Became Depressed,* Oxford: Oxford University Press, 2013, p. 154.
6. Gary Greenberg, "The Psychiatric Drug Crisis", September 3, 2013, http://www.newyorker.com /online/blogs/elements/2013/09/psychiatry-prozac-ssri-mental-health-theory-discredited. html, accessed 28 February 2014.
7. Nancy Andreasen, *The Broken Brain: The Biological Revolution in Psychiatry,* New York: Harper & Row, 1985, p. 219
8. Robert Whitaker, *Anatomy of an Epidemic: Magic Bullets, Psychiatric Drugs and the Astonishing Rise of Mental Illness in America,* New York: Random House, 2010, p. 70.
9. Daniel Carlat, *Unhinged: The Trouble with Psychiatry—a Doctor's Revelations about a Profession in Crisis,* London: Free Press, 2010, p. 6.
10. Harry Barry, *Flagging Depression: A Practical Guide*, Dublin: Liberties Press, 2012.
11. Linda Booij et al., "Monoamine Depletion in Psychiatric and Health Populations: Review", *Molecular Psychiatry* 8 (2003): pps. 951-973.
12. Daniel Carlat, *Unhinged: The Trouble with Psychiatry—a Doctor's Revelations about a Profession in Crisis,* London: Free Press, 2010, p. 78.
13. H.G. Ruhe et al, "Mood is Indirectly Related to Serotonin, Norepinephrine and Dopamine Levels in Humans: a Meta-analysis of Monoamine Depletion Studies", *Molecular Psychiatry,* 12, 2007.
14. Irving Kirsch, *The Emperor's New Drugs: Exploding the Antidepressant Myth,* London; Random House, 2009, pps. 91-2.
15. Elliot S. Valenstein, *Blaming the Brain: The Truth About Drugs and Mental Health*, New York: The Free Press, 1998, pps. 71, 98-9.
16. Joanna Moncrieff, *The Myth of the Chemical Cure: A Critique of Psychiatric Drug Treatment,* Basingstoke: Palgrave Macmillan, 2009.
17. Elliot S. Valenstein, *Blaming the Brain: The Truth About Drugs and Mental Health*, New York: The Free Press, 1998, p. 97.
18. Joseph Mendels and Alan Frazer, 'Brain Biogenic Amine Depletion and Mood', *Archives of General Psychiatry* 30, no. 4 (1974): 447-51.
19. Elliot S. Valenstein, *Blaming the Brain: The Truth About Drugs and Mental Health*, New York: The Free Press, 1998.
20. Goodwin & Bunney Jr., "Depressions following reserpine: a reevaluation", *Semin.Psychiatry*, vol. 3, no. 4, 1971, pps 435-448.
21. Peter Breggin, *Toxic Psychiatry,* London: HarperCollins, 1993, pps. 173-5.
22. An active placebo is a substance used in research that has no effect on the condition being researched but does produce noticeable side effects, often similar to those of the drug to which it is being compared. Compared to an inactive placebo—such as a sugar pill—which produces no effects whatsoever, a person who experiences the effects of an active placebo may be more open to the possibility that this substance is an active drug for their condition. This expectation may then give rise to an enhanced placebo response.

23. Seymour Kety, in Morris A. Lipton et al., eds., *Psychopharmacology: A Generation in Progress*, 1978, New York: Raven Press, 1978, 7-11, p. 10.

24. From: Laurent Maitre, discussion, in 'Biogenic Amines and Affective Disorders: Proceedings of a Symposium held in London 18-21 January 1979", in T.H. Svensson and A. Carlsson, Eds., *Acta Psychiatrica Scandinavica*, 61 (Suppl. 280) (1980), 19, in Shorter, Edward, (2013), *How Everyone Became Depressed,* Oxford: Oxford University Press, p. 159.

25. A.J. Puech, discussion, in 'Colloque international sur l'approche modern des desordres de l'humeur, Monte-Carlo, 3-5 Mai 1979', in P. Deniker, Ed., *L'Encephale* ns 5 (1979), Suppl. 581.

26. S.H. Snyder, "Brain Peptides as Neurotransmitters", *Science*, 1980, 209, pps. 976-83.

27. Prozac advertisement, *Journal of the American Medical Association*, 259, 03 June 1988, 3092 a-c.

28. Edward Shorter, *How Everyone Became Depressed*, Oxford: Oxford University Press, 2013, p. 161.

29. E.C. Azmitia, E.C. & P.M. Whitaker-Azmitia, "Awakening the Sleeping Giant: Anatomy and Plasticity of the Brain Serotonergic System", *Journal of Clinical Psychiatry* 52, 1991, [12, suppl]: 4-16.

30. Elliot S. Valenstein, *Blaming the Brain: The Truth About Drugs and Mental Health*, New York: The Free Press, 1998, p. 99.

31. Joseph Glenmullen, *Prozac Backlash: Overcoming the Dangers of Prozac, Zoloft, Paxil and Other Antidepressants with Safe, Effective Alternatives,* Simon & Shuster, 2001, pp. 202 and 16-17.

32. Grace Jackson, *Rethinking Psychiatric Drugs: A Guide for Informed Consent,* Bloomington: Authorhouse, 2005, p. 72.

33. Elliot S. Valenstein, *Blaming the Brain: The Truth About Drugs and Mental Health,* New York: The Free Press, 1998, p. 100.

34. Daniel Carlat, *Unhinged: The Trouble with Psychiatry—a Doctor's Revelations about a Profession in Crisis,* London: Free Press, 2010, p. 78.

35. Daniel Kahneman, in Alisdair Palmer, "Mad Money", *Spectator,* 28 July 2012, http:// planet 3.org /2012/08/27/the-way-scientists-try-to-convince-people-is-hopeless/, accessed 17 May 2014.

36. Bruce Levine, "Psychiatry Now Admits It's Been Wrong in Big Ways—But Can It Change?", *Truthout,* 05 March 2014, http://truth-out.org/news/item/22266-psychiatry-now-admits-its-been - wrong-in-big-ways-but-can-it-change-a-conversation-with-investigative-reporter-robert-whitaker, accessed 12 March 2014.

37. Dorothy Rowe, *Why We Lie*, 2010, London: Fourth Estate, 2010, pps. 115-6.

4. THERE IS A BETTER WAY

The brain chemical imbalance delusion has dominated medical, psychological and public thinking about depression for the past fifty years. Parties with a vested interest see nothing wrong with this. Nor do the vast majority of the general public, for whom the depression brain chemical imbalance idea feels as familiar and logical as raised blood sugar in diabetes. There are two main reasons why psychiatrists and GPs have embraced the biochemical imbalance delusion with such enthusiasm. This notion portrays doctors and their drug treatment in a positive light, as real doctors treating biological abnormalities consistent with the treatment of diseases generally in medicine. Secondly, having observed for thirty years how my medical colleagues in psychiatry and general practice work, I do not believe they know any other way of understanding or responding to depression other than as an assumed biological abnormality. I remain unconvinced that there is sufficient breadth of vision within mainstream psychiatry or medicine to see or to move beyond the rigidly held belief that depression is primarily a biological disorder. Yet, the majority of the experiences categorized as depression are primarily emotional and psychological or have a significant emotional input.

THE DEPRESSION DELUSION AND THE REPACKAGING OF EMOTIONAL DISTRESS

The medical view of depression is an interpretation and a repackaging of people's experiences, done primarily on the assumption that doctors know best. Doctors are presumed to have the necessary expertise and scientific objectivity in addition to having the public interest at heart. Human experiences are filtered through and interpreted within the radar and value system of psychiatry, which values certain things and discounts many others in accordance with the degree to which they appear to concur with the psychiatric system of interpretation. People's experiences of distress are reinterpreted as symptoms of illness. The medical interpretation is then given precedence over the person's experiences.

In the current medical climate where depression is so commonly diagnosed, a wide range of human experiences are interpreted under the guise of depression. Many understandable human experiences consequently become lost, missed, inaccessible and unnecessarily pathologized under the umbrella term, "depression". Once diagnosed, depression becomes the primary focus. Everything is explained, justified and understood under the guise of the person's biological illness, their chemical imbalance, their depression. "I am hurting", "I feel numb and don't feel anything" becomes repackaged as "I am suffering from an illness called 'depression'". The person's behaviours, habits and patterns are not acknowledged or addressed in their own right, but as part of an illness. The experiences themselves all make sense and can be understood from an emotional and psychological perspective. [1] When they are jumbled up in the melting pot of depression they become inaccessible and apparently incomprehensible, other than as a claimed consequence of abnormal brain function.

Their meaning and significance is often lost. The waters become muddied. The depression brain chemical imbalance delusion, with proclaimed biochemical abnormality at its heart, has legitimized this practice of reinterpretation.

Existence is complicated and experienced differently by different individuals. Yet existence can be understood and understood deeply, but this is not what psychiatry sets out to do, except within the narrow context of human biology. This is a very limited way of seeking to understand people, humanity, life and existence. There is so much more to us human beings, to life, humanity and existence than our biology. The medical approach does not do justice to the reality that the various components of experience and behaviour that become labeled as depression are closely related to existence and to the realities of life. In most countries, guidance on how to live and deal effectively with life, existence and challenge is provided not by psychiatrists but by either psychologists or psychotherapists. This further points to the lack of ability of psychiatrists to provide people with a deep understanding of themselves and of life, and their inability or unwillingness to help people with the many challenges that may confront human beings in life.

Life in the twenty-first century can be very challenging. There are many potential pitfalls and curved balls. Life is not always fair. I have worked with many people diagnosed with depression who through no fault of their own have encountered far more than their fair share of bad luck and wounding. I am repeatedly stuck by the failure of many doctors to adequately consider their patients' distress in the context of their life and existence, choosing instead to reframe distress in terms of mental illness. That they can do this and consider this acceptable is testament to the degree of molding into the psychiatric ideology that occurs within medical education and training.

While there is a lot of good, kindness and generosity in the world, there is also considerable selfishness, carelessness and lack of humanity. There can be a dog-eat-dog attitude out there in the world with which many people find difficult to cope. It is no coincidence that people who have experienced sexual, emotional or physical abuse and neglect are more likely to have experiences and exhibit behaviours that doctors diagnose as depression. These experiences can leave scars on our hearts and minds. Many others who do not appear to have experienced such abuses are nevertheless at an increased risk of being diagnosed with depression if for them engaging with the world has become something to be feared.

Unable or unwilling to fit into society's limited pathways of how to progress and get ahead in life, it is not difficult to fall between the cracks. Some people may drop out of education. Some struggle with the challenges involved in seeking and maintaining employment. Many become psychiatric patients with a psychiatric diagnosis such as depression. Some became embroiled in the psychiatric system, often for much of their life. Many feel ostracized by society and may increasingly feel the need to ostracize themselves. Preoccupied with their fixed beliefs linking human distress to illness, many doctors fail to sufficiently consider and appreciate these realities.

Believing that they are real doctors treating real illnesses like other medical specialists, psychiatrists tend to approach things in similar fashion to other medical specialists. Many are somewhat distant and clinical and do not spend the degree of quality time with their patients that is necessary to build up levels of trust and rapport that might encourage the person to really open up. Many of their patients already have trust issues relating to situations and relationships. For them, building up trust will take time and effort on the doctor's part, more time and attention than many doctors realize. Many doctors don't seem to rate their patients really opening up to them as particularly important. Even when people do open up to their psychiatrists, what they say is generally filtered through the psychiatric diagnostic system. Opportunities to work through deeply-held emotional and psychological distress and unfinished business are thus regularly missed.

THE CORE COMPONENTS OF DEPRESSION ARE *NOT* BIOLOGICAL

I do not work as most of my GP or psychiatric colleagues do. Having obtained a master's degree in psychotherapy in addition to twelve years previously working as a general practitioner, for the past thirteen years I have provided a recovery-oriented mental health service. I do not need to resort to fictitious notions of brain chemical imbalances to explain depression either to myself or to people who attend me. I find depression and its components to be eminently understandable. My critique of the depression brain chemical imbalance delusion stems as much from my experience that there is a much more accurate and effective way to understand and respond to depression as from my knowledge that there is no scientific basis to the brain chemical imbalance idea.

I will discuss depression and its components in detail in a future book, already largely written. It is appropriate to discuss what depression is briefly here. The core aspects of people's experiences that subsequently become labelled as depression are emotional and psychological rather than physical. Some of these experiences have physical components, but this does make these experiences fundamentally biological in nature, as many GPs and psychiatrists would have you believe. Core components of depression include emotional and psychological woundedness; shock; emotional and psychological distress in many forms, and increasing reliance on defense mechanisms such as selfhood reduction, [2] avoidance, shutdown and withdrawal.

Unlike notions of chemical imbalances that cannot be verified in any of the millions of people worldwide who have been diagnosed with depression during the past fifty years, these core components of depression are always there to varying degrees. They are always a part of the person's story, experiences and behaviour. Many doctors do not possess the skills to identify these components. When they do identify them, many doctors underestimate their significance, preferring to interpret the person's situation through their familiar lenses of illness and brain chemistry.

Don't be fooled into thinking that doctors are totally objective about all this. As I discuss in detail in chapter twelve, it is very difficult for most doctors involved in mental health to be truly impartial. Their identity and status is intricately tied up with depression being seen as a fundamentally biological illness. The possibility that they might be wrong is not a possibility to which many doctors are willing to give much consideration.

NINE CASES OF DEPRESSION

I now present brief summaries of the stories and experiences of nine people who have attended me. Each received a diagnosis of depression from a GP, psychiatrist or both. Each was prescribed or recommended antidepressants by a doctor prior to attending me. Most were severe cases of depression. They were all told by their doctors that they had a brain chemical imbalance that needed long-term correction with antidepressants.

In each of these cases, the person either never took medication for depression or gradually came off medication fully and successfully during the course of our work together. I fully respect the fact that some people choose to take antidepressant substances because they feel helped by them. I do prescribe medication, though a great deal less than the majority of my medical colleagues. As I discuss in more detail under the "Misinformed and manufactured consent" heading in chapter sixteen, the ethical rules and guidelines regarding informed consent in medical care apply to the information provided to people by doctors regarding depression and how antidepressants work. Only then can people make informed choices. Any doctor or health professional who tells their patients that depression is characterized by brain chemical imbalances and that antidepressants correct these imbalances is misinforming their patients. I will address in detail how antidepressants act in a future book.

In 2009, a fifteen-year-old girl attended me, accompanied by her parents. She had been attending the psychiatric services for eighteen months. Her situation had deteriorated considerably since she attended the child and adolescent mental health services. Her parents were distraught and had lost hope, despairing at the deterioration and apparent hopelessness of the situation despite eighteen months of attending the experts. She had been diagnosed with depression and was taking both Prozac 20 mgs and Xanax 0. 25 mgs daily, a benzodiazepine tranquillizer. She and her family had been told that she had a brain chemical imbalance that needed treatment with Prozac. Her life was in turmoil. She had felt unable to attend school, and had missed the majority of school during the past nine months.

Within our first few meetings, I was able to identify that emotional and psychological wounding, shock, great emotional distress and many defense mechanisms including the reduction of her sense of self were the key issues for her, not imagined and unidentifiable biochemical imbalances. We worked together, meeting every week or two for the next eighteen months, less frequently after that. Gradually she improved. Her school accommodated her situation as best they could, and gradually her attendance at school improved. She managed to complete her final school examinations and enter a third level course. On completion of this course she obtained employment relating to the course she had just completed. She has not needed to attend me for over three years. Two months ago I happened to meet her mother on the street, who told me that her daughter is happy, confident and fulfilled in her life. She has been off all medication for five years.

A fifteen-year-old boy had been attending the Child and Adolescent Mental Health Services accompanied by his parents for two months prior to attending me. His parents felt that these services were not getting to grips with the boy's problems and that if anything they were compounding his already difficult situation. His parents contacted me following a recommendation by a friend. In his mother's first email to me, she said that she and her husband felt that these services "were only making matters worse".

Having met with the boy and his parents on two occasions, the family decided that they wanted their son to continue attending me. I suggested they continue attending the psychiatrist, for the moment at least. Initially the psychiatrist wanted the boy to attend one of his team for counselling rather than me. When the parents insisted that he attend me, the psychiatrist eventually agreed to this.

In a letter to me, the boy's psychiatrist listed the "working diagnoses". It was quite a list. There were seven in total, including "Depression with psychomotor retardation". [3] The boy's parents were informed by the psychiatrist that their son needed medication because his situation was most likely caused by a brain chemical imbalance.

The boy and his parents experienced their visits to the psychiatric services as very stressful. His parents felt that they were being questioned as parents and were coming under considerable scrutiny by the psychiatrist, and to a degree this was confirmed in the psychiatrist's communications to me. According to his parents, in the initial stages the psychiatrist was very forceful, strongly encouraging the parents to virtually force-feed their son. A psychiatric in-patient admission to a unit more than sixty miles from his home was being recommended, as was a formal psychological autism assessment.

I understood the psychiatrist's concerns. The first and most immediate priority was to get this young man to gain some weight so that his life would not be in any danger from malnutrition. But from the perspective of the boy and his parents, the psychiatrist lost their trust in the process. The boy felt very unsafe in the offices of the psychiatrist and his team. He therefore communicated little of his inner experiential world to them. His parents also felt unsafe. They did not trust the psychiatrist or the system. They came to see this doctor as a threat rather an ally, as someone with great power who could make recommendations about their son against their will.

Creating high quality relationships and a safe space for people to talk freely about themselves and their life is one of my greatest priorities, even more so when I am in the company of a very frightened, unsure and overwhelmed fifteen-year-old. Within the first few sessions it was clear that the boy and his parents felt good about attending me. He gradually opened up to me. I helped the boy and his parents make sense of his experiences and behaviours. I listened carefully and respectfully to everything he and his parents said. In return, they listened well to me and took my suggestions on board.

He made great progress during the following six months. He gradually increased his food intake. Three months after he first attended me, his weight was just a pound or two short of his ideal weight. Through our work, he came to better understand himself. He found the courage to begin to express himself; for years he had remained very quiet. Pleasantly surprised by the encouraging responses he received from those around him when he did express himself, he risked going gradually further down the road of self-expression, self-honouring and self-worth.

As a result of his parents' obvious love for their son and their commitment to do anything that would help, the boy's relationships with his parents improved exponentially. He had become so quiet for such a long time, his parents had been trying to read his mind and he theirs. Such mind-reading can lead to very erroneous conclusions. I encouraged all three to be more expressive to each other. This helped the boy enormously.

For six months, he continued to attend the psychiatrist. He has been fully discharged from the psychiatric services for nine months now. Neither the inpatient psychiatric admission, the formal psychological assessment nor medication turned out to be necessary. He is back in school fulltime. He is risking to express himself more to his peers in school. As at home, he has been delighted to find that many fellow teenagers are actually quite happy to listen to what he has to say.

As is generally the case in my work with clients, I paid no attention whatsoever to the boy's supposed brain chemical imbalance. I find this notion of no practical help in my work with people, and I am not prepared to inform people of something that I know is not true.

This young man's major improvement in a relatively short time is very obvious. He looks so much better. His eyes are bright. He is more spontaneous. The psychomotor retardation the psychiatrist spoke of—a general and obvious physical and mental slowing down—has disappeared, without ever taking the medication that the vast majority of psychiatrists and GPs erroneously consider to be essential in all such cases.

A sixteen-year-old girl began attending me eight years ago. She had been diagnosed with depression three years previously. She and her parents had been told that she had a brain chemical imbalance, for which she was taking 300 mgs Effexor. Despite this high dose of a treatment that was supposed to help her greatly by correcting her so-called chemical imbalance, the girl was in crisis. She had already had three psychiatric hospital admissions in her young life and was facing a fourth. Her psychiatrist was now recommending electroconvulsive therapy, which prompted her parents to bring her to me. Her life story was filled with emotional wounding and distress. None of these realities of her life experience received much attention from the mental health services she attended. Her sense of self was on the floor. She had experienced bullying from other girls since she was seven years old, to such a degree that she changed schools twice. On each occasion she quickly found herself in familiar territory, again being bullied and isolated by other girls. Always a "yes" girl, terrified of saying "no" to people in case they would disapprove of her, she had largely lost her sense of self from her early childhood. [4] She told me that from age seven onwards for several years, she would cry every day in front of the television after school. She hated her time in school, especially what she experienced as her shame of the aloneness she experienced in school. She had taken a drug overdose two years previously, which sounded like a serious attempt to end her life. She described her most recent summer school holidays as "horrible", staying in bed until 6 or 7 pm, getting up for a few hours, rarely getting out of her pyjamas or leaving the house.

Her habits and patterns of living were already entrenched by the time she began attending me. Over the years she had become a perfectionist, and regularly felt devastated when she did not achieve her own very high expectations. Having few comforts in life, she regularly used food as a way of comforting herself. Very easily hurt, engaging with the world was for her like going into a major battle every time with no suit of armour to protect her. Her academic ability had always been one of the few things about herself in which she trusted. That too had taken a severe blow in recent years as she had felt unable to sit any formal exams in school. By the time she attended me, she had already missed out on sitting two sets of state examinations.

She attended me for about four years, very regularly for the first three. Getting her life back on track was a major challenge for her, but gradually she managed to do so. In summary, our work focused on creating a very good relationship, raising her sense of self, releasing the considerable well of distress and grief that had accumulated within her, and gradually getting back into mainstream life at a pace that could work for her. I felt that her high dose of medication was interfering with her ability to think and feel, therefore I worked with her to gradually reduce her medication over the initial eighteen month period.

She never did have electroconvulsive therapy or any further psychiatric admissions. Her journey of recovery took several years. This is to be expected. The duration and intensity of the journey of recovery are generally proportional to the degree of distress experienced and accumulated over the years. Other factors are also relevant including the degree to which the person has come to rely on defense mechanisms to get by; the degree to which they have removed themselves from everyday life and experience; the level of support they have; the degree to which they have become disempowered and lost their sense of self; and whether or not there are aspects of themselves and their life that can be utilized as stepping stones on the journey. I address the reduction of selfhood in my 2011 book *Selfhood: A Key to the Recovery of Emotional Wellbeing, Mental Health and the Prevention of Mental Health Problems*.

Through our work, she gradually developed a deep understanding of herself. Within six months, of her own volition, she had stopped attending the psychiatric services and never returned to them. Her progress during the first two years was slow. This too was to be expected. Her degree of accumulated emotional wounding and reliance on defense mechanisms was enormous, as was her loss of self. Making gradual changes terrified her. The pace of change needed to honour her terror of change.

She did make a very good recovery. She last attended me about three years ago. By then her need to attend me had become occasional and sporadic. She was then in college, had friends, a boyfriend, and was generally pretty happy with life. She had been off all medication for the previous three years. This was by far the best period of her life. She still struggled somewhat with stress around exam time. She still needed to be mindful of old habits and patterns such as avoidance, procrastination and withdrawal, which surfaced from time to time. Coincidentally I saw her twice recently in local shops. On both occasions she was with a male companion and she looked happy. The first time I saw her in a shop, she flashed me a big smile and quickly looked away. My hunch was that she may not have told this young man about this painful part of her past. Meeting me in his company may therefore have been something she would prefer not to happen.

A thirty-five-year-old man began attending me nine years ago. He had been attending a psychiatrist for the previous three years. The psychiatrist he attended had diagnosed depression and prescribed antidepressants. He was told by the psychiatrist that antidepressants work by balancing brain chemical levels that have become deficient in depression. He felt that he was getting nowhere, and he was referred to me by his GP. He was taking 75 mgs of Effexor daily when he attended me, a moderate dose compared to the 225 mgs he was being prescribed by the psychiatrist six months previously. In consultation with his GP, he had gradually reduced the dose from 225 mgs to 75 mgs. Neither he nor his GP knew what to do next, hence the referral to me.

As is so often the case in my experience, it emerged that many key emotional and psychological contributing factors to this man's distress had been either missed completely or their importance underestimated by his psychiatrist. This is one of the unfortunate consequences of the depression brain chemical imbalance delusion. Most treating doctors focus on the imagined chemical imbalances and their treatment, failing to see the crucial importance of factors such as emotional and psychological woundedness, unresolved shock, emotional distress, the many defense mechanisms people employ such as shutdown and avoidance, and great loss of sense of self, what I refer to as loss of selfhood. [5]

This man had accumulated a great deal of emotional wounding, loss and grief in his life, which had gone unrecognized and unresolved despite attending doctors for several years. Circumstances in his childhood had not been easy. His father had major alcohol problems. The eldest of four children, even as a child he saw it as his duty to protect and mind his mother as much as possible. He became a great carer for others, finding it very difficult to let others care for him or to care for himself. He lived like an adult while still a young boy, missing out on much of his childhood, experiencing aspects of the adult world at an age when he was ill prepared for the uncertainties and challenges of adult life. His way of operating in the world was shaped in his childhood. Habits and patterns he had developed in response to the relationships and environments of his younger life as ways of coping and surviving were now coming back to haunt him. Addressing these was a key aspect of our work together, including him recognizing, honouring and expressing his own needs, building up his sense of self, releasing the grief he had held within for many years, and giving himself permission to feel and express the wide range of human feelings.

Aspects of his current life needed addressing too. Some of these problems were in part created by the habits and patterns shaped within him during his childhood. Excellent at his work, his inability to say "no" contributed to him being expected to work under very difficult conditions and extremely long hours. Unfortunately he appeared to work for people who were prepared to take advantage of his high quality work ethic and his willingness to do the work of three men. When he did eventually question his working conditions, his employers were apparently less than sympathetic to his situation. Aspects of his long-term relationship also needed attention. He brought his highly skilled caring nature and his hesitancy to meet and to express his own needs that he developed in his childhood into this relationship. I helped him balance the importance of his partner's needs with his own equally legitimate needs.

Within a year of attending me he was off all medication. The months after stopping the antidepressant were difficult. He cried a great deal during this time. Most doctors would have seen this as a recurrence of his depression. I saw this as the expression of long-held pent-up emotion that was better released than held within, in addition to withdrawal effects from the drug. This went on for many weeks. With my support and reassurance he came through this, reaching a point of inner peace, self-empowerment and contentment that he had never previously known.

In 2012, a woman in her early 20s was told by a psychiatrist with stated psychotherapy training that she had endogenous depression. The psychiatrist told her that endogenous depression was a long-term biological illness involving brain chemical deficiencies for which she would need long-term medication. She attended me for a second opinion. It did not take long for me to identify that her current state was largely a reaction to life as she experienced it. For more than a year this young woman had many experiences of emotional wounding, distress and defense mechanisms including shock, anxiety, withdrawal, avoidance patterns, tearfulness, sadness, unexpressed grief, fear of change, fear of both failure and success, and selfhood reduction. Despite having stated expertise in psychotherapy, the psychiatrist was unable to identify sufficient reason for these changes and therefore diagnosed endogenous depression due to a brain chemical imbalance that the doctor claimed required long-term medication. I was able to make sense of her experiences. I picked up many things that the psychiatrist had missed. Her story made perfect sense to me, and this formed the platform for full recovery without medication. We met regularly over six months. She has returned successfully to work, without ever taking the medication that her psychiatrist told her was so essential.

A man in his late 40s attended me six years ago. He had been diagnosed with depression by his GP, who had tried him on several antidepressant drugs with little improvement. His GP had told him that he had a deficiency of serotonin in his brain for which he needed antidepressants, but he wasn't convinced. He had read my book *Beyond Prozac* and he wanted another opinion regarding his situation. When he first attended me he was taking 75 mgs of the antidepressant Effexor and 15 mgs of Dalmane, a sleeping tablet. Within two or three meetings I formed the opinion that rather than depression being his problem, his main issues were largely emotional and psychological. Since his early life he had put great emphasis on pleasing others, always putting on a brave face, disowning and disconnecting from his own emotions. He was very conscientious, to a fault. He was very sensitive, hating anything that even vaguely resembled a criticism. Having little self-confidence, he did not feel he could deal with people on an equal footing. He therefore spent a great deal of energy and time trying to anticipate what people wanted, trying to keep one step ahead.

Over a six-month period I weaned him off both drugs. He went through major withdrawal reactions in the weeks after coming off Effexor. Misinterpreting this as a recurrence of the person's supposed depression, the medical trend in this situation has been for doctors to encourage the person to go back on their medication. Knowing that Effexor is one of the worst offenders regarding withdrawal reactions from antidepressants, I supported him during this withdrawal period. He came through it, and has not needed to recommence antidepressants since then.

During one of our meetings, he told me some of the things his GP had previously said to him. His GP had advised him that he had a brain chemical imbalance, which was why he prescribed the antidepressant for him. His GP had strongly advised him against coming off Effexor. To justify this advice, the GP told him that coming off the antidepressant was comparable to removing arm-bands in the swimming pool. In a subsequent letter to his GP, I referred to this dubious analogy:

> This man said to me that on one occasion you expressed considerable concern regarding his desire to come off Effexor. He mentioned that you compared this to removing armbands in the swimming pool. Carrying this analogy a stage further, the purpose of armbands in the swimming pool is to keep the person safe until they have learned how to swim. Few people would aspire to relying long-term on armbands in the swimming pool.

I knew that, with the right approach and support, this man was well capable of living without arm-bands, and so he has. That was five years ago. Since then he has attended me about six times. He has not been depressed during this time. He has been well able to work, maintain important relationships and remain effective in his everyday life. His few attendances in recent years have been with the purpose of resolving underlying emotional unfinished business from the past, which he has successfully managed to do. He attended me rather than his GP as he felt sure that his GP would simply recommend antidepressants again. In my letter to the GP I also wrote:

> I formed the opinion that his underlying problem was not depression. Rather, it was primarily anxiety related to the uncertainty and fear created by certain changes in his life over the preceding months, not least major changes in his work situation. We worked together on his self-esteem, and on helping him understand precisely what had happened to him. He made steady progress . . . Please bear this letter in mind for future situations such as insurance policies he might take out.

I included the last sentence because a diagnosis of depression can affect a person's life in many ways including their ability to obtain life insurance cover.

This man's GP knew me. Before I gave up working as a GP to work full-time in mental health thirteen years ago, I had intermittent contact with him. A pleasant gregarious man, I bumped into him at a social event about five years after my book *Beyond Prozac* was published. He greeted me with "How is the most courageous doctor in Ireland?". He was familiar with what I was doing and how I worked. His patient began attending me about two years after our paths crossed at that social occasion. This man had clearly had a far better outcome working with me than with his own doctor. GPs tend to be pragmatic people. When they come across professionals who can help some of their patients, most GPs tend to refer more of their patients to that person. Although we live and work in the same city, in the five and a half years since I wrote that letter, that GP has not referred any patients to me. This is a situation I have encountered on many occasions. I have come to the conclusion that with a few exceptions, doctors do not refer patients to me because my way of working often runs counter to theirs. And for many doctors, that is more important than the possibility that I might be able to help some their patients.

A fifty-year-old woman attended me several years ago. She took antidepressants for ten years, having been diagnosed with depression. On three occasions she tried to stop the antidepressants. On each occasion she developed intense emotions including anxiety, sadness and much crying. Finding these emotions too much to handle, on each occasion she went back on antidepressants within weeks. She was encouraged to do so by her doctor, who informed her that her experiences upon stopping antidepressants proved that she was ill with depression and that she needed long-term medication. Within a few meetings, I came to understand her. What her doctor had diagnosed as a brain chemical imbalance, as depression, was in fact a combination of psychological and emotional features such as a very low sense of self and much unfinished emotional business that had accumulated during her life. On lower doses of antidepressants and off them, she experienced obsessive thoughts regarding the passage of time, ageing, guilt, panic, feeling out in control of her life. Her doctors interpreted these as the recurrence of depression, recommenced or increased antidepressants and did little else. I helped her understand and work through these experiences, many of which were in the background of her life since her childhood. In this work she grieved considerably, something that is often necessary. I also worked with her to raise her sense of self and to feel, express and honour her feelings of sadness and loss rather than run from them or numb them with drugs. She worked through her feelings, came out the other side, and for the first time in twenty years, lived well without antidepressants. A changed person, more in touch with herself and her needs, more expressive of herself, she felt better than she had all those years on medication.

A man in his early fifties began attending me three years ago. His GP had diagnosed him with depression and prescribed Lexapro to treat his brain chemical imbalance several months previously. He was in great distress—agitated, highly anxious and overwhelmed. He exhibited several features consistent with what doctors diagnose as depression. He stayed in bed for much of the day and avoided contact with reality as much as possible.

His distress was triggered by major financial difficulties that had arisen in recent years. Like many people in Ireland, he had become financially over-extended at the peak of the Irish economic and property boom of the early and mid-2000s. Having always been financially comfortable, for the first time in his life he suddenly found himself out of his depth, in real financial trouble when the property bust and the accompanying Irish economic crisis hit hard in the late 2000s. His business collapsed. He owed the bank several million euros, and now looked like having no way of paying this back.

During this time he also attended a psychiatrist. His GP and psychiatrist focused primarily on treating his "mental illness" called "depression", on treating his "chemical imbalance" with drugs. I focused primarily on him, his life, the major challenges he faced, and how he might gradually address these and regain some sense of empowerment during this process. Over a period of six months, he went from spending most of the day under the duvet, in terror and great distress to increasingly taking action. As I generally suggest, this began with little things that he was neglecting, such as cutting the grass, general financial house-keeping, and getting more clarity on the precise level of his financial situation. Initially reluctant to do anything, gradually he noticed that he was feeling a little better and slightly more empowered as a result of doing and completing tasks. Excellent at looking after others, I also encouraged him to take better care of himself and his own needs.

Once he experienced that he felt somewhat better by taking charge in this way, he really got into the practice of taking action, small steps, completing small tasks and seeing them as little victories. Within six months he had taken whatever action he could to deal with the financial pressures he faced. He engaged fully with his banks.

He attends me about twice a year now. Although the facts of his financial situation have not changed, his approach to it has vastly changed, as has his general wellbeing. He feels empowered and ready for whatever stresses and challenges come his way. I have repeatedly been very impressed with his emotional and mental strength, and I have told his so on many occasions. More than once in his company I have wondered out loud whether I would have handled such immense stress so well. He has not taken an antidepressant for eighteen months.

A woman in her seventies began attending me in 2008. A member of a religious community, she had felt very depressed for many years. She was taking antidepressants prescribed by her GP, who wanted to refer her to a psychiatrist since she was not getting any better. Her GP told her that the antidepressants were to treat her brain chemical imbalance. She decided not to attend a psychiatrist, and attended me instead.

There had been many changes in her life over the preceding years. Always an active member of her religious and local community, she felt that she had been sidelined considerably. Other people were taking over roles she had happily fulfilled for many years. The previous year she had been quite ill, spending several months recuperating in a nursing home. She felt bullied and badly treated there. She spoke of a black cloud that followed her everywhere. She hated that cloud, and frequently became very angry with it. I suggested that she dialogue with the black cloud rather than continuously fight with it. She documented this dialogue in a journal. At my suggestion she asked the cloud many questions, and was frequently surprised at the answers that surfaced within her. Through this process she realized that rather than being an enemy, "black cloud" knew she was hurting and was trying to protect her from further hurt. Through this process of dialogue she cried many times, releasing the pent-up emotion that had accumulated within her in recent years. She gradually made peace and made friends with "black cloud", which gradually lost its heaviness and blackness in proportion to her progressively feeling better. Within twelve months, she was off medication and felt that our work together was complete. I wrote a letter to her GP summing up our work together and filling him in on her current situation. In the letter I wrote:

> This woman attended me because she was depressed. I understand you were sufficiently worried about her to recommend that she attend a psychiatrist. Her depression might be more accurately described as a protective reaction to a great deal of hurt and emotional pain she had experienced in the year prior to attending me. We worked together on these matters. She reports a considerable improvement in her situation. She has reconnected with her community, and has begun becoming more involved in many activities which used to mean so much to her.

I am not suggesting that everyone who attends me makes such a wonderful recovery. Several factors affect outcomes, including the brain chemical imbalance culture. The public perception that depression is a chronic illness caused by a brain chemical imbalance has created the expectation that recovery and living without medication is rarely a viable option. Many people do not have sufficient supports to embark successfully on the process involved in recovery. Some people have such a degree of self-doubt that they find the process too difficult and do not persist. Others have such a degree of emotional distress within them that the process seems to be endless and they lose hope. Still others find it extremely difficult to allow themselves to fully feel their woundedness and distress and to grieve for as long as they need to. If the ubiquitous nature of emotional woundedness, shock, distress, and defense mechanism creation were accepted as they are; if they were seen as part of a person's life journey, a difficult but often transformative experience when worked through rather than suppressed, and not transmuted into invented brain chemical imbalance notions; then people in distress would feel far more accepted within communities and society. Education about emotions, emotional and psychological distress, and the creation and maintenance of a strong sense of selfhood should be *the* most important subject in schools. Young people would then be familiar with these crucially important issues and have a language with which to express and address them. Recovery rates from depression would be much higher in such a society, in my opinion.

NOTES TO CHAPTER FOUR

1. In a future book on depression, largely already written, I set out and explain the experiences and behaviours that become diagnosed as depression, how they make sense, and how they can be worked with emotionally and psychologically.
2. I refer to selfhood as a global sense of self. The commonly used term "self-esteem" is insufficient to encapsulate a global sense of self, since it is just one aspect of selfhood. Selfhood reduction is a common response to actual or perceived threat. I describe selfhood and its relationship to emotional and mental health in my book *Selfhood: A Key to the Recovery of Emotional Wellbeing, Mental Health and the Prevention of Mental Health Problems*, Limerick: Mental Health Publishing, 2011.
3. Psychomotor retardation means a slowing-down and reduction of thought and physical movements. It is generally considered by doctors as evidence of severity.
4. For information on selfhood see note 2 in this chapter.
5. For information on selfhood see note 2 in this chapter.

5. DOCTORS PROMOTING DEPRESSION AS A BRAIN CHEMICAL IMBALANCE

Despite the absence of any direct evidence confirming the existence of brain chemical abnormalities in depression, the promotion of the chemical abnormality notion as a fact or so-near-a-fact-as-makes-makes-no-difference has come from many sources, but primarily from the medical profession and the pharmaceutical industry. Following their lead, the idea has been picked up and promoted widely by other mental health care professions such as psychology, mental health organizations, the media and many members of the public.

Doctors rarely state publicly or to their patients that there is no reliable scientific evidence to support this notion or that the hypothesis has been largely discredited. They state or imply it as a proven fact or as so close to proven as makes no difference, or as a strongly held belief by a reliable scientific profession, held with sufficient conviction to persuade the majority of the public to believe in it too.

Psychologist and researcher Irving Kirsch wrote about this in his 2009 book *The Emperor's New Drugs: Exploding the Antidepressant Myth:*

> If the evidence for a chemical imbalance as a cause of depression is so weak, why was the theory so widely accepted and why do people still cling to it? Certainly the serotonin story was a good one—everyone could grasp it. Serotonin was good; lack of serotonin was bad. The evidence did not really fit the story, but few doctors had the time to carefully sift through the data. They see drug-company advertising in their professional journals, and they read the labelling information approved by the FDA and other regulatory agencies. At medical conferences they meet drug-company representatives, who present the company's interpretation of the evidence, an interpretation that is consistent with the simple chemical imbalance theory. [1]

The widespread diagnosing of depression and prescribing of antidepressants sits easily within the medical mindset, the medical way of seeing the world. As far as doctors are concerned, the ideal is to develop magic bullet treatments, drugs that specifically target an identified deficiency or problem in the body. In the case of depression, the supposed abnormality is assumed. As Dr. Marcia Angell wrote in a 2009 *New York Review of Books* article:

> Physicians learn to practice a very drug-intensive style of medicine. [2]

The climate of medical training is such that when they qualify, young doctors are already cultured into the understanding that the prescribing of medication is the norm for most medical conditions. Doctors are trained into that way of thinking. The chemical imbalance notion has been central to persuading doctors and the public that depression is a disease like any other. Once convinced that depression is an illness, prescribing for it becomes accepted medical practice. Any sense of questioning of this idea they may have had upon entering medical school has usually been eradicated long before they graduate.

The medical profession has been enthusiastic in promoting imagined biochemical abnormalities as central to the cause of depression. This is particularly true of both psychiatry and general practice, the two areas of medicine most involved in depression. Informing people that depression is caused by a brain chemical deficiency has been a consistent pattern of doctors over the past thirty years. Psychiatrists and GPs have enthusiastically and at times forcefully promoted this message in their consultations, writings and public interviews. Here are some examples of this practice.

PSYCHIATRY

The American Psychiatric Association places biochemistry firmly at the top of their list of causes of depression. According to this association's website:

> Biochemistry . . . can play a role in the onset of depression . . . abnormalities in two chemicals in the brain, serotonin and noradrenaline, might contribute to symptoms of depression. [3]

They add that other brain networks are "undoubtedly" involved as well. An American Psychiatric Association information leaflet on depression titled "Let's Talk facts About Depression" claimed:

> Antidepressants may be prescribed to correct imbalances in the levels of chemicals in the brain. [4]

These are false claims. That they are made by the one of the foremost mental health organizations in the world makes them all the more outrageous. The American Psychiatric Association is well aware that biochemistry has never been found to "play a role in depression"; that "abnormalities in two chemicals in the brain" have never been found; and that it cannot be claimed that "antidepressants may be prescribed to correct imbalances in the levels of chemicals in the brain" when no such imbalances have even been identified to exist.

The Royal College of Psychiatrists' 2006 public information sheet claimed that:

> Upwards of 100 different chemicals are active in different areas of the brain. It is thought that in depression, two of these neurotransmitters are particularly affected—serotonin, sometimes referred to as 5HT, and noradrenaline. Antidepressants increase concentrations of these two chemicals at nerve endings and so seem to boost the function of those parts of the brain that use serotonin and noradrenaline. [5]

As psychologist Dorothy Rowe has written, the Royal College of Psychiatrists have removed most of their references to chemical abnormalities from their website since 2006. [6] Their website still contains subtle messages that demonstrate the continuing leanings of the medical profession toward biological causation. For example, according to the Royal College of Psychiatrists' website, physical illnesses cause depression because:

> Some physical illnesses . . . can affect the way the brain works. They cause anxiety and depression directly. [7]

The clear implication of this sentence is that it is because of brain changes that occur in people with physical illnesses that they may become depressed. This has never been established. A further example appears on the Royal College of Psychiatrists' "Antidepressant" webpage:

> We don't know for certain, but we think that antidepressants work by increasing the activity of certain chemicals in our brain called neurotransmitters. They pass signals from one cell to another. The chemicals most involved in depression are thought to be serotonin and noradrenaline. [8]

This passage is problematic. Claiming that they don't know *for certain* is misleading. The truth is that they don't know this *at all*. The Royal College of Psychiatrists has neglected to mention that there is not a shred of scientific evidence confirming that there is any neurotransmitter deficiency that needs correcting.

In 1970 psychiatrist Morris Lipton PhD was Professor and Chair of Psychiatry at the University of North Carolina when he wrote in a psychiatry journal:

> Since the pharmacological agents that ameliorate depression and mania appear to act upon and alter the concentration and metabolism of the biogenic amines in what are presumably corrective directions, it may be inferred that in the affective disorders there exists a chemical pathology related to these compounds . . . positive evidence is slowly accumulating and negative evidence is thus far lacking.[9]

It is quite a leap of faith to infer the existence of brain chemical abnormalities without any direct supportive scientific evidence. No evidence has been "slowly accumulating", not in 1970 when this professor of psychiatry wrote this nor since then.

The following comment in their 1973 book *Psychiatry* by British professors of psychiatry E. Anderson and W. Trethowen appears innocuous:

> The state of mental depression may well be the result of some biochemical cause which affects whatever homeostatic process that normally controls mood. This at least can be regarded as a working hypothesis. [10]

This position is reasonable, as long as the other half of this premise is given due regard; while depression may be the result of some biochemical or biological cause, it is equally possible that depression may not be fundamentally biological at all. This latter position generally receives little consideration within psychiatry. Focusing on "some biochemical cause" that "may well" be causing depression is problematic. This book was written over forty years ago. With repetition, people including doctors and medical students have become familiar with such ideas. Hearing the same ideas repeatedly often results in people gradually believing them to be facts. Many trusted authority figures such as doctors consistently mention chemical abnormalities as by far the most likely cause of depression. It is hardly surprising that in the eyes of the media and general public, the line between theory and established fact has become blurred. Public acceptance of this theory as fact has many benefits for the groups who promote these notions including the medical profession and the pharmaceutical industry.

The Mayo Clinic is one of the most prestigious and respected medical centres in America and beyond. According to its website, the Mayo Clinic has four "major campuses" in America and "the Mayo Clinic Health System has dozens of locations in several states". [11] Their website contains clear misinformation about depression and brain chemicals.

On the Mayo Clinic website, depression is stated to be a "medical illness", a "chronic illness that usually needs long-term treatment, like diabetes or high blood pressure". A video titled "Antidepressants—How they help relieve depression" appears on their "Diseases and conditions" webpage. The video and the accompanying transcript contain the following claims:

> If you have depression, you may have a serotonin imbalance. Your overall level of serotonin may be low, and some of it may be reabsorbed too soon. As a result, communication between the brain cells is impaired. An SSRI, or selective serotonin reuptake inhibitor, is a medication designed to help increase the amount of serotonin in the synapse by blocking its reabsorption. As serotonin builds up, normal communication between cells can resume and your symptoms of depression may improve. [12]

This passage, from a highly respected source, contains several examples of false information and flawed logic. The word "may" appears three times in the first two sentences, illustrating a distinct lack of definiteness regarding what is being presented. You *may* have a chemical imbalance; your serotonin *may* be low and *may* be reabsorbed too soon. Then again, perhaps you don't have any of these postulated actions going on within you. The very next sentence involves a miraculous transformation from possibility to fact: "As a result, communication between the brain cells *is* impaired". Such a seismic shift from "may" to "is" should never occur in any properly reasoned argument. The final sentence contains false information. The claim that "normal communication between cells can resume" implies that communication between these cells is known to have been abnormal, and there is absolutely no evidence of any such abnormality. No wonder the public have become mistakenly convinced that chemical imbalances are a known feature of depression, when so many authoritative sources wrongly tell them so.

American psychiatrist Nancy Andreasen has been an eminent psychiatrist on the world mental health stage for thirty years. She is currently Chair of Psychiatry at the University of Iowa. She was a member of the Task Forces of both the *DSM-3* and *DSM-4*. In her influential 1984 book *The Broken Brain*, Andreasen referred to the biology of mental illnesses as a known certainty, including abnormalities in the levels of brain chemicals:

> The various forms of mental illnesses are due to the many different types of brain abnormalities, including the loss of nerve cells and excesses and deficits in chemical transmission between neurons. [13]

When considering why people may respond differently to different antidepressants, Andreasen unequivocally claimed:

> One suffers from a serotonin deficiency in the brain, while the other suffers from a norepinephrine deficiency. [14]

These assertions by a highly respected psychiatrist had no basis in fact, but the reader could not have known this. These claims therefore were and continue to be grossly misleading. In the same book Andreasen contradicted this attractive scenario of certainty. She wrote that there were many:

> Hints that mental illness is due to chemical imbalances in the brain and that treatment involves correcting these imbalances. [15]

If the biology of depression were indeed a certainty, one would expect psychiatry to rely on evidence rather than "hints". In common with the views of many of her colleagues to this day, Andreasen regulated the role of psychotherapy to secondary importance compared to underlying chemical imbalances, although the latter have never been identified to exist. According to Andreasen, the main role of psychotherapy is to help the person cope with their brain chemical disorder and its consequences:

> While the patient may require a somatic therapy to correct the underlying chemical imbalance, he may also need psychotherapy to deal with the personal and social consequences of his illness. He may need help with his marriage, with learning to find a new type of work, or simply with learning to live with the fact that he has had an episode of mental illness. [16]

Many psychiatrists responded enthusiastically to Andreasen's book, perhaps because her book made psychiatry appear a great deal more scientific than it actually is. Andreasen and her writings have impacted widely on mental health worldwide. She is regularly referred to by other psychiatrists and writers on mental health. For example, referring to Andreasen's 1985 book title *The Broken Brain* in his book *Depression: The Mood Disease* published eleven years later, Johns Hopkins University psychiatrist Francis Mondimore wrote:

The title makes the point that psychiatric illnesses like major depressive disorder, bipolar disorder and schizophrenia are caused in large part by biological and chemical malfunctions in the brain. [17]

Mondimore's unequivocal claim that "psychiatric illnesses are caused in large part by biological and chemical malfunctions in the brain" has no basis in fact. He followed this statement with:

> Although we still don't know exactly what these malfunctions are, we are getting very close to understanding some of the biological mechanisms that might be involved . . . what scientists think might be broken. [18]

This passage oozes flawed logic, misinformation and exaggeration. Since it is not known "exactly what these malfunctions are", assuming (a) that they exist and (b) that if they exist, they are the cause of psychiatric illness, is highly inappropriate both logically and scientifically. Mondimore either knows or should know that claiming "we are getting very close to understanding some of the biological mechanisms that might be involved" is a gross misrepresentation of the facts. Mondimore might have served his readers better if he had exhibited some of the humility and realness of his fellow American psychiatrist Daniel Carlat who as mentioned earlier, wrote the following, four years *after* Mondimore's book:

> The shocking truth is that psychiatry has yet to develop a convincing explanation for the pathophysiology of any illness at all. [19]

As I mentioned earlier, pathophysiology is the study of functional changes in the body that occur in response to disease or injury. The enthusiasm for the notion of biochemical abnormalities was enormous in the early days of Prozac and the other SSRI antidepressants, far outstripping the scientific evidence. This was not surprising in a profession searching for a role and identity, a profession that largely became intoxicated by an idea they really wanted and needed to be true, their reason and judgement being correspondingly compromised. The majority of psychiatrists and GPs became convinced by their own rhetoric. The biological basis of depression and antidepressant action soon became a belief beyond questioning, akin to a religious dogma.

In her book *Prozac Diary* Lauren Slater described how in 1988 her doctor, whom she referred to as her "Prozac doctor", explained the action of Prozac. She was one of the first tranche of people to receive the new wonder-drug. Her doctor enthused that:

> Prozac marked a revolution in psychopharmacology because of its selectivity on the serotonin system; it was a drug with the precision of a Scud missile, launched miles away from its target only to land, with a proud flare, right on the enemy's roof. [20]

This colourful description was certainly exciting and persuasive, but it had no basis in fact.

In a 1995 book a University of Washington psychiatrist described a "world-wide epidemic of depression" caused by the "serotonin depleting times" people were then living in. According to psychiatrist Michael J. Norden, perhaps we are all serotonin-deficient. The first chapter of Norden's book *Beyond Prozac: Brain Toxic Lifestyles, Natural Antidotes and New Generation Antidepressants* is titled "Is nearly everyone serotonin deficient?" [21] Having sown this seed in the reader's mind, the reader may not notice that Norden failed to answer his own question satisfactorily. Norden wrote:

> The way we sleep, the way we eat, even the air we breathe draw on the same account, weakening the specific neurochemical "stress shield" that Prozac is designed to bolster—the vital neurochemical known as serotonin. In a certain sense, our lifestyles have made us "Prozac deficient", or more accurately, serotonin deficient. [22]

Norden provided no scientific evidence for this remarkable conclusion of global serotonin deficiency. His only reference is to a questionnaire he came up with himself:

> Your answers to the questionnaire in Chapter 1 will give you an idea of your biochemical vulnerability. [23]

Final-year medical students know that real "biochemical vulnerability" is identified not by a questionnaire but by biochemical tests. Undaunted, Norden continued:

> An optimal level exists for just about every chemical inside us . . . We do not know the desired level of serotonin because we have no conclusive way to measure it. A number of tests exist at a research level, but none is reliable enough to justify widespread use. We can, however, roughly measure the *function* of brain serotonin by various indirect means. It is this I refer to in discussions of laboratory assessments of brain serotonin levels. [24]

In this passage, Norden admitted that psychiatrists do not even know what the desirable level of serotonin should be. He acknowledged that psychiatry has no way of measuring serotonin. His assertion that the function of brain serotonin can be measured fairly reliably by various indirect means is untrue, as discussed in chapter two and elsewhere in this book. Norden valued serotonin so highly that he referred to it as a "surrogate parent". [25] Yet after all that enthusiasm, Norden acknowledged:

> There is little direct evidence to correlate changes in a person's mood with serotonin fluctuation. [26]

In fact, there is *no* such evidence. Norden's acknowledgement that brain serotonin levels cannot even be measured does not prevent him from concluding that a mass serotonin deficiency has somehow descended upon humanity:

Why should our brains have suddenly become deficient in serotonin? The short answer is that while our physical evolution fitted us well for life in the plains of Africa, our cultural evolution demands far more of us, especially in the last century ... Have you fallen prey to the onslaught of our serotonin-depleting times? The following questionnaire is designed to help determine that. However, until the test is standardized in large populations, your answers can serve only as an initial guide to identifying a relative deficiency ... even one yes may indicate relative weakness in your serotonin system. [27]

The following are examples of the general and non-specific nature of these questions:

"I do not handle stress well".
"I have a close relative who is alcohol/drug addicted".
"I have been in at least one fight since age 18".
"I have a low tolerance for heat".
"I smoke cigarettes." [28]

Assuming that the answers to these and similar questions provide reliable evidence of brain serotonin levels is about as real as fantasy fiction material, but the lay reader may assume it is trustworthy since it is written by a psychiatrist. Perhaps seduced by his own ideas, Norden pushed the boat out even further:

It's intriguing to speculate whether the general decline in serotonin function has contributed to the withering of behavior traditionally known as "virtuous". [29]

This is a classic Begging the Question logical fallacy, [30] since the premise upon which it is built—"the general decline in serotonin function"—has not been established as a reality in even one person, never mind the general population. Many of Norden's readers may not be aware that this is utter conjecture and may have been persuaded to believe him, given his credentials as a psychiatrist. Many of his readers may also be unaware of neuroscientist Elliot Valenstein's direct response to Norden's views:

Actually, there is not a shred of evidence of any worldwide decrease in brain serotonin. [31]

According to then professor of psychiatry Dr. C. Thompson at the University of Southampton in 1997:

For more than 30 years the dominant hypotheses of the biological basis for depression have been related to noradrenaline and serotonin. [32]

This statement is a Begging the Question logical fallacy. [33] Dr. Thompson presented the unsubstantiated premise that there is a biological basis for depression as a fact, which strengthened the apparent legitimacy of the hypotheses to which he referred. It is also a Proof of Tradition logical fallacy. [34] The notion that there is an underlying biological depression has no scientific basis; it has become widely accepted within psychiatry and general practice largely through familiarity and repetition.

I fully accept that there is no conscious malicious intent to deceive or misinform on the part of the vast majority of doctors. It is very likely that Dr. Thompson did conscientiously believe that there is a fundamental biological basis for depression. But belief without evidence is just that—a faith-based belief rather than an evidence-based established fact. Many doctors have mistakenly become convinced that their unproven beliefs are established facts. They are not aware that when they present their beliefs as though they were either established facts—or so close to being established facts as makes no difference—they are in effect misinforming those who hear or read their words. Regardless of the intent or bona fides of the speaker, misinformation is misinformation.

Daniel Amen is a well-known American psychiatrist. He has written over 30 books, five of which have been on the *New York Times* bestsellers list. Dr. Amen has contributed to the depression brain chemical imbalance delusion with unequivocal claims like the following, from his highly successful 1998 book *Change Your Brain, Change Your Life*:

> Depression is known to be caused by a deficit of certain neurochemicals or neurotransmitters, especially norepinephrine and serotonin. [35]

Dr. Amen and his methods have many critics, including some psychiatrists. Criticism from mainstream psychiatrists has not extended to Amen's unsubstantiated chemical imbalance claims. [36] Psychiatrist Richard Harding, then president of the American Psychiatric Association, wrote in 2001:

> In the last decade, neuroscience and psychiatric research has begun to unlock the brain's secrets. We now know that mental illnesses—such as depression or schizophrenia—are not "moral weaknesses" or "imagined", but real diseases caused by abnormalities of brain structure and imbalances of chemicals in the brain. [37]

This passage contains serious errors of fact and logic by a senior member of the psychiatry fraternity. It was not "known" in 2001 nor since that date that "mental illnesses" were "real diseases caused by abnormalities of brain structure and imbalances of chemicals in the brain." This eminent psychiatrist resorts to a logical fallacy frequently employed by promoters of the brain chemical imbalance delusion in favour of their position; the False Dilemma logical fallacy. [38] In this passage, the only other possible explanations considered for depression and other psychiatric diagnoses are "moral weaknesses" or "imagined" problems. Both are quite unpalatable to the reader, rendering the acceptance of the preferred position of the writer more likely, in this case, the acceptance by the public that depression is a disease caused by brain chemical imbalances. As I discussed in chapter four, there are other ways of understanding depression that are not so unpalatable. However, acknowledging these might reduce the likelihood of this psychiatrist's preferred position being widely accepted.

Also in 2001, Dr. Nada L. Stotland was professor at the Departments of Psychiatry and Obstetrics and Gynaecology, Rush Medical College in Chicago. In 2001 she wrote:

Antidepressants are not "uppers" and they have no effect on normal mood. They restore brain chemistry to normal. [39]

This psychiatrist should not have unequivocally asserted that antidepressants "return brain chemistry to normal" since there is no evidence that brain chemistry was abnormal to begin with or that these substances normalize brain function. Her claim that antidepressants "have no effect on normal mood" is very questionable, given that Prozac and similar drugs quickly earned a reputation for making people feel better than well. I believe that this claim is an example of the common human tendency to assert as a fact what one wants to be a fact but isn't.

In their 2002 book *Getting Your Life Back: The Complete Guide to Recovery from Depression*, psychiatrist Jesse Wright and psychologist Monica Ramirez claimed:

All of these (SSRI antidepressant) drugs work by increasing serotonin, a chemical in your brain. [40]

This sentence conveys the unequivocal message that these substances work by correcting a serotonin imbalance. Since no brain serotonin imbalance has ever been identified in people diagnosed with depression, this assertion is a Begging the Question logical fallacy. [41] It is also a classic False Cause logical fallacy. [42] It does not follow that because antidepressants increase serotonin levels and some people taking these substances feel better, one causes the other. Indeed, many researchers claim that the brain quickly attempts to adjust to the interference caused by these drugs in an attempt to return to the state of equilibrium present prior to the ingestion of the substance.

In her 2003 book *Depression: What You Really Need to Know*, Canadian psychiatrist Virginia Edwards presented the following impressive piece of fiction to her readers:

Since the brain has too few neurotransmitters in the gap (between nerve cells), the number of receptors on the wall of the receiving cell greatly increases, so these receptors can grab the scarce neurotransmitters going by. Once antidepressants increase the supply of neurotransmitters in the gap, the receiving cell can "relax" and the number of receptors can decrease. At this point the depression improves. This is the current theory of depression, and how antidepressants help. [43]

Science has not verified any of Dr. Edwards' assertions. It has never been scientifically established that supplies of neurotransmitters are "scarce" in depression. In the final sentence, she does acknowledge that this is the current *theory* of depression. However, like many of her colleagues, Dr. Edwards presents the above passage with such detail and definiteness that the line between fact and theory easily becomes blurred in the eyes of the reader. Virginia Edwards finished this paragraph with:

Keep in mind, though, that scientists are constantly making new discoveries, and adjusting the theory. [44]

This sentence conveys quite a misleading impression of reality to the reader. Since the brain chemical deficiency theory was first proposed almost fifty years ago, no "new discoveries" have conferred any scientific validity upon this theory. There have been few adjustments to the theory during the past half-century. Those that have been made were generally done to provide a rationale for new medication use that appeared credible. The recent exodus of several drug companies from psychiatric research as discussed in chapter one does not support this claim either. If scientists were indeed "constantly making new discoveries", drug companies would be increasing their involvement rather than decreasing it.

James Whitney Hicks is a New York psychiatrist. A graduate of Yale University where he also completed his psychiatrist residency, Hicks is board-certified in general psychiatry and forensic psychiatry. In his 2005 book *50 Signs of Mental Illness*, Hicks provided another example of the tendency exhibited by Dr. Thompson as I discussed three pages ago; the tendency to question aspects of depression that do not threaten the medical view and to remain silent regarding more fundamental questions, the examination of which might be quite threatening to psychiatric beliefs and practices (italics mine):

> Scientists are uncertain about *which* physical changes in the brain lead to psychiatric symptoms. They have studied brain volume, hormone levels, blood flow, and other physiological data without finding conclusive answers. We know that abnormal proteins cause plaques in the brains of people who suffer from Alzheimer's dementia, but no smoking gun has been found for depression, schizophrenia, or other major (psychiatric) illnesses. [45]

While Hicks did acknowledge how little real progress has been made in spite of great effort, his comments are logically flawed, a Begging the Question logical fallacy. [46] His words portray an unquestioning acceptance that there are physical changes in the brain that lead to psychiatric problems, but no scientific evidence confirms this to be the case. Since this fundamental aspect of his argument is logically flawed, so is the remainder of his assertion, though his readers are unlikely to have enough information to identify these fundamental flaws. Given the extraordinary complexity of the brain, Dr. Hicks' scientifically unsubstantiated claims are a grossly misleading and erroneous simplification of brain function. His introduction of dementia is interesting. Dementia is fundamentally a known neurological rather than psychiatric illness, diagnosed principally by neurologists, not psychiatrists. I discuss this in detail in chapter twelve. The following also appears in Hicks' 2005 book:

> Psychiatrists believe that depression is ultimately the expression of a chemical imbalance. Abnormal levels of neurotransmitters have been detected in depression. [47]

Hicks' assertion that many psychiatrists believe that depression is ultimately an expression of a chemical imbalance is certainly true. As I outlined in chapter two, this is merely a belief, for which there is no reliable scientific evidence that supports it and plenty that contradicts it. Hicks' claim that "abnormal levels of neurotransmitters have been detected in depression" is false. Hicks either knew that or should have known that at the time he wrote this untruth. As I described in detail in chapter two, abnormal levels of neurotransmitters have never been reliably scientifically detected in depression. Readers of this passage are very likely to erroneously conclude that abnormal levels of neurotransmitters are an established fact in depression.

Dr. Sabina Dosani is a psychiatrist at the Maudsley Hospital, London. In her 2005 book *Defeat Depression: Tips and Techniques for Healing a Troubled Mind*, she wrote:

> Low levels of the neurotransmitter serotonin lead to depression . . . Serotonin drives our sleep and wake cycles . . . You might have heard that levels of serotonin are low in people with depression. Instead of spreading communication in the synapse between adjacent brain cells, serotonin is reabsorbed, so communications about mood, sleep, appetite and sex are lost. [48]

While it is widely *believed* that serotonin drives sleep and wake cycles, the current primitive understanding of the brain does not permit us to make such statements as fact. Here is yet another psychiatrist making untrue assertions about serotonin and depression. No reliable scientific evidence has established that communications about mood, sleep, appetite and sex are lost because serotonin is reabsorbed. There is no evidence that serotonin absorption is faulty at all, let alone that serotonin problems cause depression. If "communications about sex" are "lost" due to serotonin deficiency, how come up to sixty per cent of people taking antidepressants experience sex-related problems? The misinformation in psychiatrist Dosani's book does not end there. She continued:

> Noradrenaline is like a party planner, controlling brain activity. But when you're depressed, noradrenaline is released from brain cells at a snail's pace, so activity levels plummet. [49]

This is yet another falsehood misrepresented as truth by a respected mental health professional. As with serotonin, the current primitive understanding of brain function does not permit extravagant and unsubstantiated claims that noradrenaline controls brain activity or that "noradrenaline is released from brain cells at a snail's pace, so activity levels plummet". To assert as a fact that activity levels plummet because of noradrenaline deficiency when a noradrenaline deficiency has not even been established is wrong and misleading. Coming from a person identified in society as an expert on mental health, the reader will likely conclude these to be facts and end up grossly misinformed.

According to the 2005 book *A Simple Guide to Depression*, written by neuro-chemistry Ph.D. Rebecca Fox-Spencer and edited by psychiatry professor Allan Young, under the heading "Causes of depression" the author stated that "a number of factors

. . . are thought to cause or worsen depression". She included the sub-heading "Biological factors", of which she mentioned two. The first was genetics, which I will address in my next book. The second was the statement, "depleted levels of neurotransmitters in your brain. [50] The author did not inform the reader that there is no scientific evidence whatsoever to support this "thought".

Research published by psychiatrist G.S. Malhi in 2005 asserted that the chemical imbalance theory of depression is supported by "the indisputable therapeutic efficacy of these (antidepressant) drugs", [51] which according to these researchers:

> Suggests that serotonergic and/or noradrenergic underactivity is the key to the pathophysiology of clinical depression. [52]

In fact, the effectiveness of antidepressants is highly disputed, particularly the often-exaggerated claims of their effectiveness. [53] Reliable and replicated research indicates that antidepressants are little more effective than active placebos. [54] To conclude that exaggerated claims of drug effectiveness are "the key" to understanding the biological processes that may be involved in depression is highly questionable. Brain underactivity of either serotonin or noradrenaline has never been established to exist. From a scientific perspective, it seems cavalier in the extreme to assume that something that has never been established to exist is likely to be the key to understanding depression.

According to Johns Hopkins University psychiatrist Francis Mondimore in his 2006 book *Depression: The Mood Disease:*

> In mood disorders, the alterations in functioning in the brain are just beginning to be measured. It is quite clear that the changes in the actual structure of the brain are extremely subtle; almost no changes in the structure of the brain can be seen with a CT scan or MRI scan or under a microscope. Very subtle changes in the size of certain brain structures have been demonstrated in depression. However, the changes are not enough to be useful for diagnosing the illness in individuals. Because the amounts of brain chemicals involved are so small and difficult to measure, chemical analysis has not been much help either. [55]

These comments require some analysis. Mondimore's assertion that "the alterations in functioning in the brain are just beginning to be measured" is rather dubious. Researchers have been intensively trying to find alterations in brain functioning for over fifty years and have not come up with any scientifically valid evidence of altered brain function in depression. His statements suggest that alterations in brain functioning are now being measured. This was as untrue in 2006 when he wrote this as it is now. This psychiatrist's statement that "Because the amounts of brain chemicals involved are so small and difficult to measure, chemical analysis has not been much help either" is also highly suspect, though the reader is not likely to realize this. It is certainly true that chemical analysis has not been much help. Indeed it is no help whatsoever, apart from its role in ruling out known physical illnesses that might cause a person to become depressed. Mondimore's assertion that this is because the amounts of chemicals are so small is highly problematic. This claim conveys the misleading message to the reader that slight alterations of brain chemical levels or function are known to occur in depression. The problem is set out to be the minute levels of brain chemical abnormality being "difficult to measure". The truth is quite different; no such abnormalities have been identified at all, small or otherwise. This claim is therefore false and misleading.

Psychiatrist Siobhan Barry has been a leading figure in Irish psychiatry for many years. According to Dr. Barry in 2006:

> Irregularities in brain chemistry can involve substances called neurotransmitters and electrolytes. Many of the commonly effective antidepressants act to increase levels of the neurotransmitter serotonin, which suggests that irregularities in this neurotransmitter may be involved in depression. There is also evidence that abnormalities in the neurotransmitter noradrenaline are involved in other types of depression. [56]

Several issues arise in the above passage. The reader may understandably but erroneously conclude that "irregularities in brain chemistry can involve substances called neurotransmitters and electrolytes" in depression means that such irregularities have been identified and are therefore demonstrated to exist. Siobhan Barry summarised the rationale behind the belief in chemical abnormalities; because antidepressants increase neurotransmitter levels, and antidepressants help depression, perhaps irregularities in neurotransmitter levels are involved in depression. As a hypothesis, this is reasonable. When presented as an established fact, as it is by many doctors, drug companies and others, it becomes a False Cause logical fallacy. [57] Since one half of the supposed correlation has not even been established, such claims are also examples of the Begging the Question logical fallacy. [58] Dr. Barry's claim that "there is also evidence that abnormalities in the neurotransmitter noradrenaline are involved in other types of depression" is not supported by any reliable scientific evidence.

A 2007 *New York Times* article contained serious misinformation regarding brain biochemicals and depression. In a generally far-fetched article, psychiatry professor Richard M. Friedman, director of the psychopharmacology clinic at the Weill Cornell Medical College, wrote:

> Some depressed patients who have abnormally low levels of serotonin respond to SSRIs, which relieve depression, in part, by flooding the brain with serotonin. [59]

This is utter misinformation, since "abnormally low levels of serotonin" have not been reliably linked to depression, or indeed reliably identified at all. Nor is there any reliable scientific evidence to support the claim that "flooding the brain with serotonin" "relieves depression". This is both a False Cause logical fallacy [60] and a Begging the Question logical fallacy. [61] Friedman was requested to provide evidence to substantiate this claim by neuroanatomy professor Jonathan Leo and social work professor Jeffrey Lacasse. Lacasse and Leo subsequently wrote that the supporting "evidence" Friedman produced was not even a research paper on serotonin at all. They wrote that Friedman:

Supplied a 2000 paper by Nestler titled "Neurobiology of depression", which focuses on the hypothalamic-pituitary system, but not on serotonin". [62]

Psychiatrist Daniel Carlat was interviewed in 2010 on the Fresh Air programme on NPR radio. During the interview Dr. Carlat talked about how antidepressants work:

> What we think these medications do is they prevent the neurons of the brain from sort of vacuuming up the excess chemicals and neurotransmitters that the neurons generate so that if the depression or anxiety disorder is due to a deficiency of a chemical, a reuptake would act by pumping out or allowing the neuron to pump out more neurotransmitter, thereby famously balancing the chemicals. [63]

The following observations increase the accuracy of Dr. Carlat's statements. For "what we think", read "what we think, hope, wish and want to be true". There is absolutely no evidence of any "excess" of brain chemicals. His total lack of certainty is revealed by his comment "*if* the depression or anxiety disorder is due to a deficiency of a chemical" (italics mine). His hope that "a reuptake" would result in "famously balancing the chemicals" represents fantastical wishful thinking, given the extraordinary complexity of the brain, our primitive understanding of this organ, and the complete lack of any supporting scientific evidence.

In his 2010 book *Unhinged: The Trouble with Psychiatry—a Doctor's Revelations about a Profession in Crisis*, psychiatrist Daniel Carlat wrote:

> Patients often view psychiatrists as wizards of neurotransmitters, who can choose just the right medication for whatever chemical imbalance is at play. This exaggerated conception of our abilities has been encouraged by drug companies, by psychiatrists ourselves, and by our patients' understandable hopes for cures. [64]

Not for the first time, Carlat's candidness is welcome. Psychiatrists have indeed played a major part in creating and fostering the growth of the depression delusion, including the widespread mistaken belief that biochemical brain abnormalities have been established as a scientific reality in depression. While Carlat's comment that this misperception of psychiatrists has been encouraged by drug companies who stood to gain enormously is true, blaming "our patients' understandable hopes for cures" is not credible. Patients with advanced cancer also have understandable hopes for cures, but their doctors do not generally depart from their solemn duty not to misinform, even in such difficult circumstances. Irrespective of the wishes of people to be cured of any ailment, it behoves all members of the medical profession to refrain from misinforming their patients. This is a fundamental ethical principle of medical practice. Patients' belief that psychiatrists are neurotransmitter experts and wizards is there because they have been led to believe this, primarily by psychiatrists.

Leading American psychiatrist Jeffrey Lieberman participated in a 2012 video produced by the University Hospital of Columbia and Cornwall titled "Causes of Depression". Dr. Lieberman was then Psychiatrist-in-Chief at the New York

Presbyterian/Columbia University Medical Center and President-elect of the American Psychiatric Association. On this video Dr. Lieberman stated unequivocally:

> Major psychiatric disorders in general involve a disturbance in a specific area of the brain that is involved in regulating mood or mediating mental functions like cognition or perception . . . frequently the disturbance is of a neurochemical nature, meaning that the way nerves talk to one another, and communicate, is through the secretion of a chemical called a neurotransmitter, which stimulates the circuit to be activated. And when this regulation of chemical neurotransmission is disturbed, you have the alterations in the functions that those brain area are supposed to mediate. So in a condition like depression, or mania, which occurs in bipolar disorder, you have a disturbance in the neurochemistry in the part of the brain that regulates emotion. [65]

This prominent psychiatrist apparently saw no wrong in grossly misinforming the many viewers of this video which in the eyes of the viewer originates from a highly authoritative and reliable source. He wrongly portrayed disturbance in the regulation of chemical neurotransmitters as a known fact. He further asserted that this supposed disturbance causes depression and bipolar disorder. Since there is no scientific evidence that this is the case, this is both a Begging the Question logical fallacy [66] and a False Cause logical fallacy. [67]

Dr. Lieberman went even further. He informed his viewers that brain "disturbances" in psychiatric disorders including depression were known organic or functional disturbances, similar to the biological abnormalities that occur in a stroke:

> It's like, if you have a little stroke or seizure, if your stroke is in an area of the brain that affects your motor function, you'll have weakness in one arm or one leg, if it affects your sensory perception, you won't be able to feel things, if it affects your speech area you won't be able to talk or understand. In psychiatric disorders, the disturbance is in an area that regulates emotion or affects mental functions like cognition, perception, thinking. [68]

Dr. Lieberman either knows or should know that this is gross misinformation. A stroke is a known biological event in the brain that results in physical damage to brain tissue. The brain damage caused by a stroke is reliably identified by investigations like a CT or an MRI scan. A seizure is known to be characterised by abnormal brain wave patterns. An electroencephalogram (EEG) reading of the brain of a person during a seizure will show abnormal brain wave patterns characteristic of a seizure. In complete contrast, no such abnormalities have been identified to exist in psychiatric disorders including depression. Therefore no test is used to identify the so-called "disturbances" in psychiatric disorders. It is rather difficult to test for something that has not been identified to exist. Dr. Lieberman's inappropriate comparison between a stroke, a seizure and major psychiatric disorders is therefore a Weak Analogy logical fallacy. [69] That such basic inaccuracies of fact and logic would emanate from a leading psychiatrist in a public educational video—Jeffrey Lieberman was president of the

American Psychiatric Association from May 2013 to May 2014—is extremely worrying though regrettably not uncommon.

In an article that formed part of *The Guardian's* special report on depression in November 2013, psychiatrist Tim Cantopher of the Priory Hospitals Group in Britain wrote:

> Antidepressants do work, but only for real clinical depression, the type involving a chemical imbalance in the brain, with a full range of characteristic physical symptoms. [70]

This sentence clearly implies that brain chemical imbalances have been demonstrated to occur in "real clinical depression". Since no such brain chemical imbalances have ever been demonstrated to exist, this claim is a falsehood, one likely to lead the reader to erroneously conclude that brain chemical imbalances are an established scientific fact in clinical depression. Dr. Cantopher either knows or should know that since this unequivocally-made claim is not supported by any direct scientific evidence, he is in effect misinforming the many readers of the *Guardian.*

Currently a prominent Irish health care website, irishhealth.com is designed to provide the public with accurate health care information. The site had 157,840 registered users at the end of August 2014, and probably hundreds of thousands more visitors to the site. According to the site, irishhealth.com is:

> Ireland's most visited health website and has been ranked in the world's top 10 "Health News & Media" websites. [71]

Two of the eight named Expert Video Panel members are prominent Irish professors of psychiatry. [72] While the authors of many of their articles are not identified, a clear editorial policy is applied to all contents on the site:

> Articles on the site have been reviewed by our panel of healthcare professionals. The medical content has been developed in Ireland by medical writers in conjunction with medical professionals. [73]

One might reasonably assume that all of the content on irishhealth.com is accurate and trustworthy. In the case of depression, this is certainly not the case. The following false information appears:

> Whatever the cause, it has been found that people with depression have an imbalance of certain chemicals in their brain, which affect mood. [74]

This is a blatant falsehood, and the authors either know or should know that. No imbalance of any brain chemical "has been found". It shocks me that such false information regularly appears from sources purporting to be expert and trustworthy. The authors even went so far as to claim that these "chemical imbalances" are "found" "whatever the cause", that is, in every case of depression. I am not sure whether this represents arrogance, audacity or ignorance on the part of the authors and the site. The pervasive nature of the depression chemical imbalance delusion within society facilitates the acceptance of such misinformation from supposedly trustworthy sources such as irishhealth.com. People are so familiar with the idea that chemical imbalances occur in depression that they do not blink an eye upon seeing such assertions, having heard such claims on many previous occasions. Also according to irishhealth.com:

> Antidepressant drugs work to restore the imbalance of certain chemicals in the brain, which occurs in depression. [75]

This is another false claim. Since chemical imbalances have never been identified in depression, claims that these substances correct a chemical imbalance that has not been demonstrated to exist are untenable, a Begging the Question logical fallacy. [76] The misinformation does not stop there. According to this site:

> There are many different types of antidepressant drugs, and there have been major improvements over the past 20 years, with newer classes of drugs proving to be very effective with less side effects that the older drugs. [77]

In fact, it has been long accepted within the medical profession that newer antidepressants are no more effective than the older antidepressants that have been around for fifty years and more. Further misinformation occurs on the "Depression Clinic: How antidepressants work" webpage on the irishhealth.com website:

> It is believed that depression is linked to an imbalance of chemicals within the brain. Different antidepressants have been designed to deal with these imbalances but they do so in slightly different ways. Within the brain there are a number of chemical messengers. These are called neurotransmitters. Key neurotransmitters are serotonin and noradrenaline. When these behave normally, mood is regulated. However, if these neurotransmitters are not moving freely as they should, depression occurs. In different ways, antidepressants act on the brain to keep these neurotransmitters working properly. [78]

Let's go through this passage sentence by sentence. The first sentence is correct. Depression is widely *believed* to be linked to an imbalance of brain chemicals, although there is not a shred of reliable verifying evidence to validate this belief. The authors either know or should know that their assertions that antidepressants "deal with these imbalances" are false claims. No such claims can be correctly made when no such imbalances have even been identified. The next three sentences are red herrings. Descriptions of brain neurotransmitters have no relevance here, since no pre-existing imbalances have been identified. The reader is not likely to know this, and may be impressed and tempted to believe that this is relevant.

The final three sentences each contain some serious misinformation. Here they are again:

When these behave normally, mood is regulated. However, if these neurotransmitters are not moving freely as they should, depression occurs. In different ways, antidepressants act on the brain to keep these neurotransmitters working properly.

In my opinion, the first sentence is disingenuous. The authors either know or should know that brain chemicals have never been identified as behaving abnormally to begin with. The authors speak confidently about neurotransmitters "not moving freely as they should", as if this is a known phenomenon, which it is not. They further claim that depression occurs when the as yet unidentified phenomenon of "not moving freely as they should" occurs. And since neurotransmitters have never been found not to be "working properly", these claims are patent nonsense.

That is quite a collection of false information and inaccuracies on one website, a site that describes itself as:

Ireland's independent health site, designed to offer users a comprehensive yet easy to use online source of medical and healthcare information and up-to-the-minute health news. [79]

It is no coincidence that the misinformation emanating from this and so many other sources all have one thing in common; they make the medical profession and its approach to depression look far more scientific and credible than it is in reality.

THE BRITISH MEDICAL ASSOCIATION ENDORSES THE DEPRESSION DELUSION

As I was researching for this book, I came across two current books that were published in association with the British Medical Association that contain blatant misinformation regarding depression and brain chemicals. The fact that these falsehoods were not identified by the British Medical Association—either before or since publication—is further evidence of the pervasive nature of the depression delusion.

Understanding Depression is a 2006 book written by psychiatrist Kwame McKenzie. It is stated on the cover of the copy I read that this book is published in association with the British Medical Association, and therefore has this important Association's explicit blessing. Over 175,000 copies had been sold prior to the printing of the copy I read. Dr. McKenzie is professor of psychiatry at the University of Toronto and Senior Psychiatrist at the Center for Addictions and Mental Health. Dr. McKenzie informed his readers that:

In depression there are physical changes to the way in which your body works and antidepressants can help put things back to normal . . . the levels of these neurotransmitters are low in depression—it's as if the baton were being dropped. [80]

This assertion is utterly unproven scientifically, yet this psychiatrist and the British Medical Association have seen fit to misrepresent this notion to the public as an unequivocally established fact. I fail to see how readers cannot but be misinformed upon reading this. In this book McKenzie asserted the following sentences as facts, whereas in truth they are blatant falsehoods:

> Studies have shown that three important neurotransmitters, dopamine, serotonin and noradrenaline, are in short supply in depression. The levels are low in synapses, and this leads to faulty brain communication and message passing which may be the cause of depressive symptoms. [81]

This psychiatrist either knew or should have known that these statements are not true. He continued:

> Nobody knows what causes these low levels of chemicals. Scientists do not know whether they cause the depressed mood or they are caused by the depressed mood. [82]

At first glance this appears a reasonable statement. One might be initially impressed by this psychiatrist's openness to both possibilities; that low neurotransmitter levels might either cause depression or be caused by depression. The reader cannot be expected to know that his fundamental premise itself is groundless. There is no reliable scientific evidence of any lowering of brain neurotransmitter levels to begin with. It is noteworthy that the psychiatrist did not share this information with the reader. Scientific ignorance is therefore at a far more fundamental level than that acknowledged by this psychiatrist, since scientists have no evidence of any abnormalities in brain chemicals to begin with. Many of his medical colleagues make the further error of assuming that one is caused by the other, an assumption which at least McKenzie has not made. The question of whether chemical imbalances are caused by or cause depression is a Red Herring logical fallacy. It distracts the reader from the deeper reality that no brain chemical imbalances have ever been demonstrated to exist. The fact that these falsehoods are endorsed by support from the British Medical Association only adds to the degree of concern such assertions create.

This psychiatrist asserted a further false statement as a truth, this time at the head of an impressive-looking colour diagram outlining how antidepressants are thought to act:

> In depression, the levels of neurotransmitters are low. [83]

Currently in its eighth edition, The British Medical Association's 2011 *New Guide to Medicines and Drugs: The Complete Home Reference to over 2,500 Medicines* is this important medical association's official guide for the general public about medications. This book contains several falsehoods regarding depression and brain chemicals. According to the authors:

Depression is thought to be caused by a reduction in the level of certain chemicals in the brain called neurotransmitters. [84]

The authors followed this statement of theory with a statement presented as fact that is actually an utter falsehood:

Normally, the brain cells release sufficient quantities of excitatory chemicals known as neurotransmitters to stimulate neighbouring cells . . . In depression, fewer neurotransmitters are released. [85]

This statement is accompanied by a diagram depicting this, with the caption:

The brain cells release fewer neurotransmitters than normal, leading to reduced stimulation. [86]

Informing the public that "in depression, fewer neurotransmitters are released" and that "the brain cells release fewer neurotransmitters than normal, leading to reduced stimulation" when no scientific evidence exists that backs up such claims is clearly worrying. That such false information is communicated with the explicit support of the British Medical Association only adds to the inappropriateness of such assertions.

FAMILY PHYSICIANS (GPS)

GPs—also referred to as general practitioners, family doctors, family practitioners and family physicians—are an integral part of the medical approach to depression. The majority of diagnoses of and treatment for depression are initiated and managed by GPs. Only a minority of people diagnosed with depression are referred to psychiatrists. For this reason, and because of their status in society as trusted medical physicians, what GPs believe and say about depression and brain biochemistry has considerable significance and influence.

THE DEPRESSION DELUSION, AS SEEN ON BRITISH TV

As a general rule, when a mass delusion is discussed in public, virtually everyone who is involved in the conversation takes for granted that the subject matter is an established fact. Few people notice the delusion. An example of this occurred in ITV's *This Morning* show on 18 March 2014. This ITV programme is regularly watched by up to one-and-a-half million viewers per programme. [87]

A phone-in discussion about depression took place on the show, during which Dr. Chris Steele provided expert medical advice. Chris Steele is one of Britain's best known doctors. A general practitioner, he has been awarded a Member of the Most Excellent Order of the British Empire (MBE). Steele has been a resident doctor on ITV's *This Morning* daytime magazine show since 1988. Chris Steele's comments, including assertions about depression and chemical imbalances, were typical of what doctors have been saying about depression for over thirty years. It is therefore not surprising that his words would be accepted as facts by the programme's very large audience, and by the presenters and producers of this programme. [88]

On two occasions during this programme, Dr. Chris Steele misinformed both the people to whom he was directly talking on the show and the large television audience regarding brain chemicals and depression. In each case, the misinformation concerned claims made by Dr. Steele as established facts, when no scientific evidence verifies any such claims. In conversation with and about Dee Kelly, Dr. Steele stated unequivocally:

> She had a lot of stress. It drained her brain of natural chemicals and she got depression. The antidepressants basically elevate those chemicals back to normal and you start feeling better. And you will get better with depression if you take the medical treatment and the medical advice. [89]

On the same *This Morning* show, within 80 seconds of caller "Nicola" beginning to tell her story, shaking his head and smiling knowingly, Dr. Steele said:

> Straight away, this is the frustration of depression. Look, if you had a hormone problem due to low hormones, you'd be given hormone therapy to take those levels up to normal to help you to feel normal. With depression, something has caused the chemicals in your brain to be drained down, and antidepressants help these chemicals to come back up to normal, to put you on an even keel. [90]

Dr. Steele either knows or should know that notions of brain chemical abnormalities associated with depression are unproven and discredited hypotheses. It is entirely inappropriate and misleading that Dr. Steele would present such notions on two occasions in this programme as established facts to an audience likely to accept his words as truth. This is a Begging the Question logical fallacy. [91] By claiming that being "drained" of brain chemicals causes depression, he committed a False Cause logical fallacy. [92]

Dr. Chris Steele uploaded a video on depression to YouTube on 14 June 2011. The explanation of depression he provided on this video is similar to the claims he made on the aforementioned ITV's *This Morning* show:

> Let me just simply explain depression. Basically, your brain is drained of the chemicals that keep you in a sort of a level mood, and one of those chemicals is called serotonin, and when you drain your brain of serotonin, then depression can creep upon you. And the antidepressants that we use now boost the levels of serotonin in your brain, and put you back to normal. It's not unlike hormone replacement therapy; your body's running short of hormones so you take hormone replacement therapy to boost those levels. So, think of depression as a condition where you are replacing substances that your brain has actually become very low in, and that makes it easier to accept. [93]

On both ITV's *This Morning* programme and his YouTube video, Dr. Steele compared depression to hormone replacement therapy. On neither forum did Dr. Steele allude to an obvious major difference between the two. I am sure that like any conscientious doctor, Dr. Steele would not diagnose a hormonal imbalance or deficiency without laboratory investigations that confirm the diagnosis. I am also certain that since there are no tests for brain serotonin levels, he has never confirmed a single case of "drained brain chemicals" in depression by any laboratory test in even one of the possibly thousands of people he has treated for depression during his long medical career. As was the case in the ITV *This Morning* programme, Dr. Chris Steele's YouTube claims of reduced serotonin levels in depression are a Begging the Question logical fallacy. [94] His assertion that serotonin deficiency causes depression is a False Cause logical fallacy. [95]

Such misinformation may not have been identified as such by the ITV programme's editors and producers. This is understandable. Like the vast majority of the public, they too are likely to mistakenly believe that doctors would only make such claims of serotonin deficiency in depression if these findings had been reliably identified by solid scientific evidence. This public espousing of the depression delusion by a respected medical expert was noticed by Julie Leonovs, a mental health activist and holder of a Master of Science degree in Psychological Research Methods. With contributions from Nick Redman of the Bristol Hearing Voices network, Julie Leonovs wrote an open letter dated 15 April 2014 to ITV regarding this programme which was subsequently published on the Mad in America website. [96] Since the falsehoods about depression and brain chemical deficiencies espoused on the programme were made by Dr. Chris Steele, Julie Leonovs addressed her letter directly to him. Here are some extracts from that letter:

> We would like to express our grave concern over the information and advice you gave several of your participants on the programme including Dee, and then Nicola and Dan specifically, during the phone-in. On the majority of occasions whilst imparting your medical knowledge (and personal experience) on depression, you clearly stated that this condition was due to a "chemical imbalance" in the brain caused through a depletion of serotonin . . . It was clear that Dee has major social difficulties and this is having an impact on her ability to manage and cope. Although you stated Dee's circumstances caused a depletion in serotonin in her brain and the drugs would correct this, there is no scientific evidence to support your assertion that Dee actually has a depletion or chemical imbalance and that antidepressants correct any imbalance. What is the proper level of serotonin? What medically established, peer reviewed test, measures serotonin in the brain? . . . The notion of a "chemical imbalance" is now a fairly outdated view, and it is irresponsible and unethical to continue to indicate to the public that they suffer from an imbalance where none has ever been consistently found and replicated within peer reviewed professional journals . . . Dr. Steele, bearing in mind the findings from the research we have highlighted above and the ever growing publication of research on this subject matter, we trust you will take our concerns on board and refrain from using information that cannot be substantiated

scientifically. To continue to do so is not only misleading but also grossly unethical. Making claims via the media that cannot be proven scientifically we feel actually has serious implications for the health and wellbeing of *This Morning's* viewing audience and therefore the programme could be an infringement of broadcasting legislation. [97]

Is Julie Leonovs right to be concerned that this experienced and respected medical doctor has been "irresponsible and unethical"? If she is, how can it be that such an experienced and caring doctor could and would behave in this way on British television, in front of potentially millions of viewers?

The answers to these questions become clearer when due consideration of the mass depression brain chemical imbalance delusion is taken into account. I imagine that Dr. Chris Steele did not wilfully intend to misinform or to behave unethically or irresponsibly. I am also pretty certain that if a major public controversy had arisen regarding his comments, he would have received a great deal of support from his medical colleagues. This is what happens in a collective delusion; fellow believers generally row in to support one of their own. Presumably Dr. Steele made assertions about brain biochemical levels and depression because like most of his colleagues he believed this to be true. But as Julie Leonovs correctly pointed out, these assertions are not true. They are not established facts at all. They are an integral part of the depression brain chemical imbalance delusion. Doctors have become so familiar with their own rhetoric that they have come to perceive these fanciful notions as incontrovertible established facts. It seems to me that misinforming the large audience of this ITV programme, including the several people whose depression he discussed and advised upon, can hardly be described as responsible and ethical behaviour. Given his role as a television expert, I believe that Chris Steele has a solemn duty to familiarize himself with the facts prior to speaking with authority in the media on any subject, including depression and brain chemical imbalances. Ironically, the collective depression delusion may be Dr. Steele's best defense. He was articulating a conviction that is widely held as a fact within the medical profession and the general public. Perhaps he and many of his medical colleagues believe what he said to be true. Whether or not Chris Steele knowingly misinformed ITV's *This Morning* audience does not affect the degree to which the audience were misinformed by his words.

An unfortunate consequence of the medical domination of mental health is that people perceived as experts are frequently far less expert than others who have a perceived lesser status. Based on their expressed familiarity with the facts, in my opinion Julie Leonovs and Nick Redman know far more about the facts regarding depression and biochemical abnormalities than Dr. Chris Steele. But the possession of a medical degree results in doctors being generally perceived as *the* experts. What they say goes. What they espouse is believed. When a highly respected doctor asserts a delusional idea as if it was an established fact, the listeners can hardly be blamed for believing him.

On 19 April 2014, British psychiatrist Joanna Moncrieff posted the following response to Julie Leonovs' letter to Dr. Chris Steele and ITV on the Mad in America website:

Excellent letter, thank you to all involved for sharing it. I gave a lecture to some university academics the other day (from arts and humanities faculty), and they were shocked to hear that the chemical imbalance theory of depression has no scientific grounding. I just mention this to illustrate how successful the marketing of the chemical imbalance has been. The general public just have no access to information debunking it, and as you point out, the media continue to propagate it. Leading psychiatrists know that the chemical imbalance theory of depression and justification for antidepressant use is unproven and "metaphorical". They do not want to challenge it publicly though because it helps to support disease-based theories of depression, which psychiatry is so fearful of losing. [98]

Joanna Moncrieff's experience of university academics being shocked that there is no scientific basis to the biochemical deficiency depression notion illustrates just how pervasive the depression delusion has become. These academics had unwittingly succumbed to the collective depression delusion that has infiltrated virtually every area of modern life. Hence their shock at being informed that there is no scientific basis to this notion. Elsewhere in this book I refer to similar comments made by Joanna Moncrieff regarding a group of journalists she spoke to being similarly shocked to hear that the chemical imbalance notion has no scientific foundation. [99]

Six people wrote comments in response to Dr. Steele's YouTube video from which the above quote is taken. Four out of the six comments refer directly to Dr. Steele's error in regard to depression and brain chemical imbalances. It is both clear and worrying that all four—psychologist Dr. Toby Watson and mental health activists Leonie Fennell, Bob Fiddaman and Julie Leonovs—appear to have a far greater grasp of the facts than Dr. Steele. The comments appear in the order just listed: [100]

The chemical imbalance theory of the subjective idea of "depression" has been discredited decades ago Dr. Chris. You have got to be kidding that you are still allowing this misleading information on the internet.

Seriously, Dr. Chris seems like a nice guy but the chemical imbalance theory has been well and truly debunked. There is no such thing Dr Chris—please stop misinforming the public!

Where on earth did you read that people become depressed because their brains are drained of serotonin? If you are going to issue statements like this then could you please back it up with science. You reach out to many people, the information in this video is very misleading. The chemical imbalance theory was a marketing tool to convince people they had a brain disease. It's no longer used . . . really surprised that you haven't done your homework on this Dr. Steele.

Where is the proof for a "chemical imbalance" Dr. Steele? This is not like hormone depletion at all. Have you read Dr. Joanna Moncrieff and *The Myth of the Chemical Cure*, amongst other books on this subject matter? Your "expert" opinion is very misleading here.

The last comment above was written by Julie Leonovs, the author of the letter to ITV's *This Morning* programme discussed earlier. The authors of these four comments are correct. Dr. Chris Steele's assertions regarding serotonin and depression are grossly incorrect and therefore seriously misleading. There is not a shred of scientific evidence that verifies any of Dr. Steele's assertions which are misrepresented to his audience as established facts.

As outlined, on three occasions Dr. Chris Steele's asserted unequivocally that brain chemicals are "drained down" in depression, twice on ITV's *This Morning* programme and again on his YouTube video on depression. You may have noticed that "drained down" could hardly be described as a scientifically precise statement. Such imprecise language is not surprising given the utter lack of any corroborating scientific evidence for Dr. Steele's claims.

On 12 August 2014, the day after actor Robin Williams' suicide, ITV's *This Morning* programme again focused on depression. Well known British GP Dr. Dawn Harper regularly appears on this programme as a medical expert. On this occasion, Dr. Harper misinformed the programme's viewers with unequivocal but utterly unproven claims about depression and brain chemicals:

It is very much a chemical illness . . . The reason that antidepressants work is that we know that they alter the chemicals in the brain and rebalance them. [101]

Dr. Dawn Harper's assertion that depression "is very much a chemical illness" is a Begging the Question logical fallacy. [102] This claim is totally unsubstantiated scientifically, as is her statement that antidepressants "rebalance" brain chemicals. This too is a Begging the Question logical fallacy. [103] Her claim that antidepressants work by altering brain chemical levels is a False Cause logical fallacy; [104] it does not follow that because antidepressants interfere with brain chemicals, and because some people taking these substances feel better, antidepressants work because they interfere with brain chemistry. [105] I discuss claims made by Dawn Harper on this programme regarding depression and diabetes in chapter ten.

GPs: Behind Closed Doors is a popular British Channel 5 television show in which actual patient consultations are a regular feature. The episode screened on 29 April 2014 featured a GP's consultation with a woman named as Laura that culminated in a prescription for antidepressants. Here is how the consultation went:

Dr. Opong: "Tell me more about your mood".
Laura: "I've been feeling really depressed lately because of a lot of personal issues. Everything that pretty much could possibly go wrong in my life, has. I've been feeling suicidal at points as well, I cry every night and not feeling sociable and don't really go out, I just feel really down.
Dr. Opong: "What's specifically happened? You said there have been some things that happened, what's happened?"
Laura: "My granddad died."
Dr. Opong: "I'm sorry to hear that".

Laura: "My brother was stabbed. My mum and my stepdad are getting divorced. I've lost my boyfriend also, he's in prison, as well, so that's quite stressful. I feel like I'm under a constant battle with my conditions (epilepsy and other conditions as well) and stuff, and I just feel so worried".

Dr. Opong: "You talked about feeling suicidal. What is it you thought about doing?"

Laura: "I just don't see the point of going on. I have no one, no one there for me at all, just to comfort me even. I'm not really much of a talker anyway, just to have that bit of comfort, just to have a hug and say that everything's gonna be alright kind of thing, intimate, really.

Dr. Opong: What is it you've thought of doing, to do that?"

Laura: "Slitting my wrists, chucking myself under a train".

Dr. Opong: "How's your sleep?"

Laura: "Not good. I've never been a good sleeper anyway, but there's not really a lot I can do about it because of the medication I take for my epilepsy."

Dr. Opong: "When you talked about feeling suicidal, would you ever act on these thoughts?"

Laura: "No, because I'm not a selfish person, and I'd cause a lot of hurt to a lot of people if I'd done that."

Dr. Opong: "It's important, if you are feeling suicidal, you need to let us know or let someone else know, because we don't want to see any harm coming to you."

Laura: "I wouldn't do that because I'm not a selfish person. I wouldn't do that to them."

Dr. Opong: "Have you suffered depression in the past?"

Laura: "Yeah, bad things in life going on but, not like I feel at the moment".

Dr. Opong: We can refer you for counselling here if you want."

Laura: "I've never been a great fan of counselling. I'm quite a private person and like I said I'm not really much of a talker. I can take everyone else's problems on board, I'm a great listener, and I could just sit there for hours for someone talking to me and listen, but I don't really like the idea of just talking to some random person."

Dr. Opong: "Have you thought about anything like antidepressants or medications? Is that something that you've thought about?"

Laura: "Yeah."

Dr. Opong: "So, one of the theories behind when people get low mood or depressed is that one of the chemicals in the brain is low. So, antidepressants help to boost that bad chemical. Quite often, you have to take these for at least a month before you might see any benefits of taking the antidepressant. You can get side-effects, a couple of side-effects with antidepressants, nausea, vomiting, stomach upsets, can cause problems with vision as well. Antidepressants, I wouldn't say that they are a long-term solution. I think they can be good to help get people out of a rut, in combination with other things as well, cos you've got to look at different life aspects, is there something that's making someone feel depressed, to deal with that as well."

Laura: "I guess it's something that I can try."

Dr. Opong: "You want to try them?"
Laura: "Yeah."
Dr. Opong: "Because of the other medications you are on I have to check about what I can give you".
Laura: "Okay".
Dr. Opong: "I'll get back to you at lunchtime today".
Laura "Okay".

Most GPs and patients are likely to consider this a fairly typical consultation in which Dr. Opong did a good job. Dr. Opong's compassion for Laura is obvious. A logical rationale for both understanding disease and treatment is commonplace in all areas of medicine. People expect doctors to know how the substances they prescribe work. Immediately after introducing antidepressants into the conversation, Dr. Opong offered a rationale for how they work:

So, one of the theories behind when people get low mood or depressed is that one of the chemicals in the brain is low. So, antidepressants help to boost that bad chemical.

This statement is problematic for several reasons. Dr. Opong either knew or should have known that this theory has no scientific basis and has been discredited for over twenty years, but he did not convey this to Laura. Like many of his colleagues, Dr. Opong slipped seamlessly from theory in the first sentence to fact in the second; from "one of the theories" to "antidepressants help to boost that bad chemical". The chemical is now referred to as "bad", without any evidence that there are any actual problems with Laura's or anyone else's brain chemicals. Dr. Opong said on air that:

You've got to look at different life aspects, is there something that's making someone feel depressed, to deal with that as well.

Laura told Dr. Opong of least five very significant current life aspects—her grandfather's recent death, her brother being stabbed, her mother and step-father getting divorced, losing her boyfriend who is now in prison, and a constant battle with her medical conditions including epilepsy. In addition, Laura alluded to great loneliness and hopelessness, and the pain of not having someone there with whom to share her life. Other than offering counselling once, Dr. Opong took no steps in this consultation to explore these major issues or to recommend counselling or other possible interventions and supports to help Laura deal with any of these major life issues.

While Dr. Opong mentioned and offered counselling, he mentioned it just once. He did not actually recommend counselling at all or explain what counselling is. He did not describe how counselling might work for or help her, as he did regarding antidepressants. Once Laura said that she was not a fan of counselling, the doctor quickly moved the conversation to medication. Yet, in addition to the five significant current life events in her life, Laura had provided other important information that suggested counselling might well be helpful for her. Dr. Opong did not appear to notice the potential significance of Laura's comment that she could listen to other people's problems for hours but does not talk about her own, because she is a "private person". Such people often benefit from counselling, which can provide a safe space to begin to express oneself and work through one's emotional pain. He did not reassure Laura that a counsellor is not a "random person", but one trained to work with people in distress.

Dr. Opong said that this consultation is typical of many such consultations that every GP has several times a day:

> A big proportion of our patients will come in either depressed, or in a low mood, anxious, or in a distressed state. On a daily basis I'd see maybe five or six patients that are going through some form of distress.

It is therefore entirely possible that the process of medicalization of human loss and distress that occurred during Laura's consultation is widespread within Dr. Opong's practice and within GP's surgeries generally. I am not criticizing Dr. Opong per se. He was caring and compassionate. He acted as most GPs would do, in accordance with his training and the prevailing medical approach to emotional and mental health, and that is the real problem. Doctors are trained to medicalize people's distress and problems of living. In order to do so, as psychiatrist Daniel Carlat has said, doctors must come up with some sort of rationale that persuades the public that they know what they are doing. [106] That is why doctors resort to the chemical imbalance notion in their consultations. Since there is no real basis to this notion, doctors generally end up distorting the truth in order to sound convincing. Dr. Opong either knows or should know that his statement regarding depression and brain chemicals was not grounded upon any established scientific evidence. He is not alone in providing such misinformation to patients. In 2014 the newly-formed Council for Evidence-Based Psychiatry carried out a survey of people reporting difficulties withdrawing from psychiatric medication prescribed by a GP or psychiatrist. Of 435 responses to the question, "Were you told by your doctor or psychiatrist that you have a 'chemical imbalance'?", just under half (47%) replied "yes", 14% couldn't recall, and 38% replied "no". [107]

DR. GREG'S NEUROTRANSMITTER NONSENSE

In June 2014 I came across a YouTube video published on 11 May 2013 titled "Depression, Anxiety, OCD and More: Serotonin the Master chemical" by American doctor Greg Castello. [108] Dr. Castello described himself as "board certified in Family Practice". [109] Since his video epitomized the understanding of depression and serotonin among many general practitioners, I include extracts of his video and my exchanges with Greg Castello. Dr. Castello included the following text on the video webpage:

> Many people suffer from depression and anxiety. They share a common condition with those that have Obsessive Compulsive Disorder (OCD), anorexia nervosa,

bulimia, Post Traumatic Stress Disorder (PTSD) and even insomnia. They are all due to a deficiency of serotonin, a neurotransmitter in the brain.

The brain communicates and functions with the help of three important neurotransmitters; serotonin, noradrenaline and dopamine. The ends of nerve cells release the neurotransmitter, it floats across the gap and is picked up by the next cell, which becomes activated, and it then carries a message to the next nerve cell, which becomes activated, and it then carries a message to the next nerve cell. If there is not enough neurotransmitter, the cells do not communicate effectively, and brain function can be affected.

The same serotonin deficiency can cause different problems in different people. One person may have depression, another may have insomnia or anorexia. Think about hypothyroid, one person may be tired, another dry skin and hair, and yet another may present with constipation. All have low thyroid, but have different symptoms. [110]

In his video, Dr. Greg Castello stated:

Today we're going to talk about depression, and anxiety, and obsessive compulsive disorder, and anorexia, and bulimia, and post-traumatic stress disorder, and insomnia. And you might ask, how the heck am I gonna do all that in four or five minutes. Well, I'm actually gonna talk about the cause of all of these problems. And although they are very different problems, they are actually all related to something called serotonin deficiency.

Your brain has three neurotransmitters or three chemicals it uses to communicate from cell to cell. When a cell wants to send an electrical impulse or message to another cell next to it, it releases a neurotransmitter into the little space in between the two cells called a synapse . . . When you have a serotonin deficiency in your brain, this neurotransmitter is either not present in sufficient quantities or it gets absorbed quicker than it should, and you don't have enough of this chemical for your cells to communicate from cell to cell, and then things kind of fall apart. The interesting thing is that in different people a low serotonin level will cause different symptoms. One person will come in with depressive symptoms, another person may come in with anxiety or panic. Many times there's a common combination of depression and anxiety. You might actually just come in (to the doctor's office) and have trouble sleeping. You can't stay asleep at night. You wake up frequently. That's serotonin related. There's different clues to serotonin deficiency and they are very very different constellations of symptoms.

When you come in (to the doctor's office), if the doctor puts you on an antidepressant medication, it may not be for depression. It may be for anxiety. It may be for body image issues. It may be because you got mugged and have Post Traumatic Stress Disorder, and you have a relative serotonin deficiency. Generically speaking we call these antidepressants but we have to understand that they are actually serotonin raising drugs. So, your Lexapro, Prozac, Paxil, Zoloft, these medications all raise serotonin levels in your body and fix the underlying problem. [111]

He then compared all of this to a thyroid deficiency problem:

> Your doctor does blood work and determines that you are hypothyroid . . . If you came in and you were hypothyroid, you wouldn't feel inadequate about yourself because it's a chemical abnormality and you don't really have control over that. If you came in with depression or anxiety, likewise that's a chemical issue. I don't have a blood test to show you on paper that your chemicals are low, but we do know this. So you really shouldn't feel bad if you have to go on one of these medications because it's not necessarily in your control. [112]

Dr. Castello spoke of what he described as a typical scenario, a woman in a nice home with children, who seems to have it all but is unhappy and depressed: "Her serotonin levels are low and she needs to go on medication". [113] Castello spoke of:

> Internal depression, strictly chemical-related, nothing you really did about it, and you probably need to be on medication . . . Think of depression as being a symptom not the disease. The disease is low serotonin and the depression or the anxiety or the OCD is just a manifestation of it, and you want to treat the problem, not the manifestations. [114]

This video had been watched by 5,508 people by the end of February 2015, many of whom wrote comments of appreciation for this "informative" video. I posted the following comment on Greg Castello's video webpage on 09 June 2014:

> Dr. Castello, this is nonsense. There are no identified serotonin deficiencies and you should know that. Stop misinforming people. What should a person's serotonin be? Have you ever checked a patient's serotonin? There are no tests. Please inform your viewers NOW regarding what the normal brain serotonin should be. There is not a single piece of reliable scientific evidence that has ever identified ANY serotonin imbalance or deficiency. [115]

Dr. Castello was none too pleased with my comments. Within 24 hours he replied:

> Terry, as I clearly stated, there is no serotonin test in humans, that animal brain biopsy studies were used. Do you suggest we start doing brain biopsies on humans? Maybe you could be the first volunteer. I have twenty years of experience treating people, please tell me your experience on the subject, other than reading the internet. [116]

My reply included the following:

> Hi Greg, thanks for your reply. Your irritation at my comments was pretty obvious. Your comments regarding my volunteering for a brain biopsy are comical, juvenile and quite unprofessional. They are not worthy of a response. [117]

I included seven of the many references in this book that confirm that no evidence of a serotonin deficiency has ever been found. I then continued:

> You may indeed have "20 years of experience treating people", but you have zero hands-on experience with serotonin in depression, unlike all real biochemical imbalance conditions you treat, e.g. diabetes and hypothyroidism, in which virtually all of what you do clinically is dictated by laboratory tests. You would likely be regularly sued for malpractice and complained to your professional regulatory body if you did not approach real biochemical deficiency conditions in this manner.
>
> Your unequivocal claims regarding serotonin deficiency as the cause of depression, anxiety, OCD, eating disorders, insomnia etc. etc. are scientifically unsubstantiated nonsense.
>
> I recognize that you are not deliberately seeking to misinform. You seem like a nice guy. Like many of our well-meaning medical colleagues, you have become seduced by the brain chemical imbalance-depression notion. You have come to believe something as a *fact* that is in truth a discredited *hypothesis*. By informing your viewers unequivocally that this is a *fact*, you are by definition misinforming your viewers, albeit unintentionally. A hypothesis should never be presented as a fact; in particular, a hypothesis with no direct supporting scientific evidence and a great deal of contradictory evidence.
>
> It may interest you to know that the collective brain chemical imbalance in depression notion (that most of society has erroneously subscribed to) meets the *DSM-5* criteria of a delusion. It would appear that you are a believer in the delusion and through your words, a promoter of it also. My hunch is that much of this is news to you. [118]

Dr. Castello responded within 24 hours. He apologized for his comments that I might become the first human volunteer for a brain biopsy. His reply included the following:

> I absolutely concede there is no direct human data to support the serotonin theory. It would require a brain biopsy. May I get you to agree that in animal studies, the mechanism of action of SSRIs is decreased degradation of serotonin and now with the newer agents, an increase in output of serotonin, resulting in more neurotransmitter in the synapses?
>
> You mention that I track lab tests on patients for other diseases, and that is true. Since I have no objective data to diagnose a depressed or OCD patient, what other than my clinical experience am I supposed to use?
>
> If not serotonin, then what causes one person to get these illnesses and not another? How come people feel better when they take these medications?
>
> I haven't figured out whether you are against the class of drugs, or just the concept of serotonin deficiency as an explanation. [119]

The following was part of my response:

Hi Greg,

Apology accepted.

You may not have noticed that on two occasions in your most recent reply to me, you directly contradicted your unequivocal video claims that serotonin deficiency is known to cause the list of psychiatric illnesses you mentioned including depression. In your reply, you refer to "the serotonin theory" and "the concept of serotonin deficiency as an explanation". In both your video and the text accompanying this video you proclaim serotonin deficiency to be a known *fact*, but when challenged you admit that it is just a *theory*, a *concept*. Something cannot simultaneously be both a fact and a theory/concept, yet according to you, serotonin deficiency in depression and many other conditions can be both. Is this contradiction not obvious to you? Using generally accepted principles of logic and reasoning, I cannot square this circle. Please explain how you manage to square this circle.

I'm glad you concede that "there is no direct human data to support the serotonin theory". This is a pretty important reality don't you think? I expect this will come as news to many of the viewers of this video. Do you not think your viewers might like and need to know this, and that you should therefore have stated this rather relevant fact in your video? Would the fact that there is no direct evidence whatsoever in humans (fifty years after such theories were first mooted) not make you even a little uncomfortable about assuming and unequivocally claiming in public that all the conditions you listed are definitely caused by a serotonin deficiency? Your conviction regarding serotonin deficiency and that of your many colleagues is clearly faith-based rather than evidence-based; it clearly is not based on any reliable direct scientific evidence, since no such evidence exists.

The hypothesis that problems with brain serotonin cause depression is largely based upon the observation that SSRIs raise serotonin in brain tissue of rats. Not living rats with fully functioning brains at the time of testing; in killed rats, whose brains are removed, smashed to bits and blenderized; fragments of dead rats' brains, assessed in a test tube. The level of credibility of claims that conclusions can be extrapolated from such experimentation that reliably apply to the living human brain is anyone's guess. In your reply, you seem to have missed the rather obvious fact that SSRIs increasing serotonin synapse levels does not mean that there is a serotonin deficiency there to begin with. Also there is considerable evidence that the body takes action over a period of weeks to rebalance the artificially raised serotonin secondary to SSRIs, so the situation is far more complex than just elevation of serotonin by SSRIs.

You are clearly well-intentioned, but in regard to serotonin, you are seriously misguided. As I said in my last message, you are far from alone in this. This has become a mass collective delusion within the medical profession and consequently within society, fuelled by the pharmaceutical industry that has reaped astonishing rewards as a consequence.

Your question, "Since I have no objective data to diagnose a depressed or OCD patient, what other than my clinical experience am I supposed to use?" is interesting on several levels. Think about that for a second. Does the reality that "you have no objective data" not raise even a slight degree of questioning of the "logic" of concluding that people have a serotonin deficiency that you cannot ever confirm through any test and that no doctor anywhere in the world has ever identified through any test or investigation?

In your most recent reply, you bring in a whole other set of questions and issues into the mix. While these are important, they are off topic, i.e. the topic of your video and my initial reason for responding, i.e. your unequivocal assertions that a string of psychiatric illnesses are caused by a serotonin deficiency. I have plenty to say about these issues elsewhere. I deal with many of these issues in a talk I gave in 2013 at the Athlone Literary Festival. [120] I am addressing some of these questions in my next book, in future books, and indeed in my two current books, *Beyond Prozac* and *Selfhood*. Here and now, I am going to stay on topic, the topic you chose as the subject for this video, i.e. serotonin deficiency.

You say in your reply that "it would require a brain biopsy" to "support the serotonin theory". To be accurate, you might have said that it would require brain biopsies that reliably established a brain serotonin deficiency, quite a different thing. Post mortem brain biopsies have been carried out for decades in people with depression and in people who have ended their lives. These biopsies and brain studies have been inconclusive, as have studies of cerebrospinal fluid and urine.

As a matter of interest; you say that you stop antidepressants as soon as you can, when the person is "feeling better"; how do you scientifically determine that the person's "serotonin deficiency" has returned to "normal" in these situations? What is the "normal" serotonin level that you want your patients to attain? Are you seriously saying that the person "feeling better" can be taken scientifically as the sole and reliable indicator of the rebalancing of serotonin within the extraordinarily complex and dynamic human brain, which contains approximately one hundred billion nerve cells, each of which interfaces with up to ten thousand other nerve cells at any given moment?

The facts of the matter remain: There is not a shred of direct scientific evidence of any serotonin deficiency in depression or any of the mental health problems in which you claim serotonin deficiency as the cause in your video. Please stick to the facts, or at least inform the public when you are theorizing. [121]

In my exchanges with Dr. Greg Castello, I went into considerable detail because I felt that such claims made by trusted doctors need to be comprehensively challenged. Although I requested that he address my questions, Greg Castello did not reply. His video remains on YouTube at the time of writing.

Many of Greg Castello's statements reveal a great deal about the real level of understanding of emotional and mental health that pertains within the medical profession, none more so than the following:

If not serotonin, then what causes one person to get these illnesses and not another?

In this sentence, this conscientious but misguided doctor unwittingly revealed that he had no other way of computing people's difficult experiences and behaviours other than through the lens of imagined abnormal brain biology such as chemical brain abnormalities. In his 2010 book *Unhinged: The Trouble with Psychiatry—a Doctor's Revelations about a Profession in Crisis*, psychiatrist Daniel Carlat made a similar observation:

> How could mental illness not be, ultimately, biological? All thoughts and emotions come from the brain, and so disordered thoughts and emotions must come from a disordered brain . . . Depression must be caused by something that has gone wrong in the brain. [122]

The comments of these two doctors illustrate the one-dimensional nature of the medical approach to depression; depression *must* be caused by "something that has gone wrong with the brain". Carlat's assertion that "All thoughts and emotions come from the brain, and so disordered thoughts and emotions must come from a disordered brain" is logically unsound. It discounts the very real possibility that thoughts and feelings originate in the mind and are then subsequently reflected in the brain. This position reveals a shocking truth, of which I have been aware for over ten years:

> *The subtleties of the emotional and psychological aspects of human beings, of emotional and mental health and distress are poorly understood by the majority of doctors.*

Many people naturally assume that the medical preference for biology over the emotional and psychological aspects of people's experiences and behaviours is grounded upon a comprehensive understanding of all of these aspects. People might understandably presume that psychiatrists and GPs know all the emotional and psychological stuff that therapists know, and in addition have a deep understanding of biology and medication which therapists do not possess. The actual position is that these doctors have far less understanding of the emotional and psychological aspects of mental health than many well-trained therapists. Their preoccupation with biology is based on their collective ignorance of emotionality and psychology in addition to their need for biology to be seen as *the* most important aspect of mental health in order for their position at the top of the mental health tree to be maintained. As demonstrated in this and in my next book, the medical understanding of the biology of depression is frequently exaggerated and distorted.

OTHER GPS PROMOTE THE BRAIN CHEMICAL IMBALANCE DELUSION

Dr. Caroline Shreeve is a GP with a special interest in mental health. She trained in psychiatry and has worked as a GP in Australia and in the United Kingdom. Caroline Shreeve has been a regular contributor to many medical journals, newspapers and magazines. She is the author of sixteen books including *Dealing with Depression: Understanding and Overcoming the Symptoms of Depression*. Originally published in 2005,

I read a copy of the 2010 edition. This book contains the following misinformation about depression and brain chemical imbalances:

> All these familiar stresses certainly can tip us over the edge into depressive illness if . . . we have naturally low levels of neurotransmitters (brain chemicals) serotonin, adrenaline and noradrenaline. [123]

> Dopamine, serotonin and noradrenaline . . . are known as the monoamines . . . Monoamine supplies are low in depression, which explains why our mood flattens and sinks, and why we lose interest and a sense of purpose, and suffer from insomnia and appetite disturbances when depressed. [124]

> Scientifically derived evidence of chemical changes in the brain may convince you—or someone close to you, perhaps, who is skeptical about depression as a whole—that the illness under discussion is not the product of a hypochondriac's fantasy. [125]

In the first two quotes above, Dr. Caroline Shreeve unequivocally asserted that low levels of brain chemicals are a known characteristic of depression. This is not true, and Dr. Shreeve either knows or should know this. Perhaps she too has fallen for the depression brain chemical imbalance delusion. The first two quotes above are both Begging the Question logical fallacies. [126] The premise in both quotes is that brain chemicals in depression are known to be low, and this deficiency causes the effects referred to. Since low levels of brain chemicals have never been established in depression, these claims are clearly wrong. The second quote is particularly noteworthy. This doctor is prepared to assert that the many listed features of depression are definitely caused by low brain chemical levels that have not even been established to exist. This is further evidence of the very limited medical understanding of mental health I referred to earlier in this chapter. Only in terms of brain chemicals and other unproven brain abnormalities can most doctors attempt to explain the experiences and behaviours that become labelled as depression.

Dr. Shreeve's claim in the third quote above of "scientifically derived evidence of chemical changes in the brain" in depression is also highly problematic. No scientifically derived evidence of any such chemical changes in the brain has been found. As many others including many doctors have done, in this passage Caroline Shreeve presents a False Dilemma logical fallacy in order to convince the reader. [127] She presented the reader with just two ways of interpreting the experiences and behaviours of depression. Either it is a brain chemical imbalance or "the product of a hypochondriac's fantasy". Faced with just these two options, which one would you pick?

As I discussed in chapter four and will discuss in more detail in a future book, there is a third way of understanding the experiences and behaviours of depression, a way which is far more accurate than those presented by Dr. Caroline Shreeve. Few doctors understand this way, for two main reasons. Their understanding of human emotionality and psychology is far more primitive than most people realize. Secondly, most medical doctors are seriously biased in favour of a biological understanding, since their identity, modus operandi and status in mental health and in society depends on maintaining this bias and convincing the public to be so biased also.

Irish GP Harry Barry has written several books on mental health. He has become a nationally respected commentator on mental health in Ireland. According to Dr. Barry (emphases his):

> Depression occurs essentially because of a lack of communication in the brain . . . our emotional and logical brains are connected by three mood cables, which operate like simple telephone lines between the two. There is the SEROTONIN cable, the NORADRENALINE cable and the DOPAMINE cable. When we develop Major Depression, these three mood cables become underactive . . . The three mood cables, which communicate using serotonin, noradrenaline and dopamine, are normally depleted in varying degrees during depression . . . There has been such a depletion of the three main mood neurotransmitters—serotonin, noradrenaline and dopamine—and such extensive damage to the mood departments that these drugs cannot block the re-uptake of neurotransmitters, as they are not being released in sufficient amounts into the synapses. [128]

There are numerous inaccuracies, falsehoods and logical fallacies in these passages. None of these claims are known to be facts. Depression being caused by a lack of communication within the brain is an utterly unsubstantiated assertion, as are Barry's claims of depleted mood cables and "extensive damage to the mood departments". His claim that this damage—which has never been found to exist—causes features of depression is a remarkable piece of creative writing, yet it is presented as an established fact. This is all misinformation, a series of Begging the Question logical fallacies. [129] In my opinion, such unsubstantiated unequivocal statements should not be made by a doctor. It is theorising and wishful thinking misrepresented as established facts, to a public who cannot be expected to know the difference.

Barry's remarkable claims of complete cable breakdown and total depletion of transmitters in severe depression are followed by the equally extraordinary and unsubstantiated assertion that suicide being "at the top of the agenda" in severe depression is due to "total depletion of the serotonin cable", [130] a remarkable False Cause logical fallacy. [131] The reader is likely to conclude from this passage that science has firmly established that suicide is caused by a "total depletion of the serotonin cable". There is no serotonin cable, and reliable links between serotonin and suicide have not been established. It is another example of grossly flawed logic, another Begging the Question logical fallacy, [132] since his claim of total depletion of serotonin is utterly unverified scientifically. Barry contradicted these assertions of certainty regarding brain function in depression later in this book (brackets mine):

> The causes of this illness (depression) and its exact neurological mechanisms will take some time for researchers to understand fully. Science is only beginning to understand the workings of the brain, and how an illness like depression operates. [133]

Barry also acknowledged that researchers are "struggling to answer" questions of causation of depression, an admission that runs contrary to his aforementioned unequivocal claims. [134] Yet on the same page, he referred to the "biological causes of depression", and the "biological underpinnings of depression", as if these were scientifically-established certainties. [135] These inferences are not appropriate, given his admission regarding how little the brain and its relation to depression is currently understood.

Dr. Harry Barry's assertion that "three mood cables"—serotonin, noradrenaline and dopamine—connect our "emotional and logical brains" and operate "like simple telephone lines between the two" is absurdly simplistic and erroneous. There are no such serotonin, noradrenaline or dopamine cables. Compare Barry's assertions to the factual descriptions of the brain as I discuss in chapter three, in which the vast and currently unfathomable complexity of the brain is repeatedly acknowledged by many leading world authorities.

Levels of serotonin, noradrenaline and dopamine are not "normally depleted to varying degrees in depression". As I discussed in chapter two, no scientific evidence exists that identifies levels of these neurotransmitters as being reduced to any degree in depression. Therefore all of Dr. Harry Barry's claims regarding neurotransmitter depletion and damage and "complete breakdown of mood cables and structures" are without foundation.

In his book *Flagging Depression: A Practical Guide* Dr. Harry Barry repeatedly referred to the Raggy Doll Club. This club is "mentioned so often in this book" because Barry believed that the Raggy Doll Club gets to the "real secret of good long-term mental health"; rating ourselves and others. He wrote:

> If we can learn to remove the whole idea of judging and rating ourselves and allow others to do so, we will have taken a crucial step towards staying well . . . we are too hard on ourselves and never learn to accept ourselves without conditions. As a result, we remain exposed to depression arriving back in our lives. If you can grasp this concept, you will stay well. I cannot guarantee that you will never again suffer a bout of depression, but you will have seriously reduced the chances of this occurring. [136]

His Raggy Doll Club is quite a useful concept, but there are major inherent contradictions here which Harry Barry does not appear to see. If the core problem in depression really was a brain chemical deficiency and "extensive damage" to "mood cables" as Barry claims, such fundamentally psychological advice and action is highly unlikely to prevent a relapse of a chemical imbalance problem. It is highly unlikely that such an idea would make a major difference or considered a "crucial step" in the treatment of diabetes or an underactive thyroid gland, conditions in which known chemical imbalances are at the core of the problem, which is why such comments as Harry Barry's would not be made regarding diabetes or other chemical imbalance conditions. If anything, these contradictions point away from biology, toward the importance of the emotional and psychological aspects in depression.

In 2001, the year in which he was named Irish Medical Journalist of the Year, Irish general practitioner and *Irish Times* medical correspondent Dr. Muiris Houston wrote:

> Depression, in my view, is no different from diabetes. In one you take insulin and in the other you take Prozac or some other antidepressant. Both substances are simply designed to replace natural chemicals missing from the body. [137]

This grossly simplistic view contained several inaccuracies. As outlined earlier, science has as yet failed to demonstrate any "natural chemicals missing from the body" in depression. This is not my opinion; it is a fact. No doctor should present something in a national newspaper as a fact which is not a fact but rather a wholly unproven theory. More about the often-used comparison of depression with diabetes in chapter ten.

Muiris Houston wrote this *Irish Times* article following a radio programme in which he, psychiatrist Professor Ivor Browne, I and others participated. He wrote that the programme consisted of a discussion regarding:

> Whether there was a biological basis for depression. Both Ivor Browne and Terry Lynch, the other two doctors who contributed, would tend towards a position which would be sceptical of demonstrable biochemical changes in people who suffer from depression. [138]

The clear inference of this passage is that both Professor Ivor Browne and I do not accept either that depression has a "biological basis" or the "demonstrable biochemical changes in people who suffer from depression". Whether intentional or not, these comments conveyed the impression that Ivor Browne and I were unreasonable and irrational doctors who stubbornly refused to accept the existence of demonstrable biochemical changes that were reliably identified to occur in people suffering from depression.

Readers of this article could not have known that Houston's assertion of "demonstrable biochemical changes in people who suffer from depression" is a falsehood. Perhaps Dr. Houston himself did not realize that either, since most general practitioners have come to believe the rhetoric they have heard from psychiatrists and drug companies over the past four decades. This falsehood was presented as an established fact in a reputable national Irish newspaper, written by a trusted and respected medical doctor. The many thousands of readers of this article were in effect misinformed. Readers would naturally presume that Dr. Muiris Houston had his facts right and that his words could be taken as true.

In 2015, fourteen years later, "demonstrable biochemical changes" have still not been identified in depression. Whether this misinformation was provided deliberately or not has no bearing on the fact that Dr. Muiris Houston's comments were untrue and therefore misleading.

When an idea has been widely accepted within society as a fact and regularly promoted as such by trusted medical doctors, it is not surprising that some people would be taken aback to hear this theory being challenged. The live radio program Muiris Houston referred to lasted just under an hour. Many calls and emails to the program were read out on line by presenter Vincent Browne. Some callers expressed surprise that depression as a biological illness was being questioned at all. Many callers welcomed the openness of the discussion, although you would not deduce this from reading Muiris Houston's article. In his *Irish Times* article, Houston focused primarily on one call supporting his position received in relation to the show, the "most striking reaction" that was received after the show. I believe this was an example of *confirmation bias*, described by author Rolf Dobelli as:

> The mother of all misconceptions. It is the tendency to interpret new information so that it becomes compatible with our existing theories, beliefs and convictions. [139]

Dobelli quoted international investor Warren Buffett:

> What the human being is best at doing, is interpreting all new information so that their prior conclusions remain intact. [140]

There were several other examples of flawed logic in Muiris Houston's article. On two occasions, he used "evangelistic" references. Having named both Ivor Browne and I as being in opposition to him on the radio programme, Houston wrote that he did "not have an evangelical view on these matters" and later, "my advice is to ignore all evangelical approaches to this subject". The clear inference was that both Professor Ivor Browne and I were "evangelical" in our approach. I think it is reasonable to conclude that Muiris Houston was not using this term in a complimentary fashion. Whatever about me, for this GP to describe or to imply that Professor Ivor Browne is "evangelical" was in my opinion a striking piece of arrogance. Now eighty-six years old, Ivor Browne has been one of Ireland's most loved and respected psychiatrists for half a century, described as a "towering and powerful influential figure in Irish psychiatry" by internationally renowned award-winning Irish author Colm Toibin. [141]

Implying that Ivor Browne and I were evangelists is an example of a Straw Man logical fallacy. [142] It could be argued that the term "evangelist" applies to any doctor who, convinced in their belief that biochemical abnormalities occur in depression, seeks to convince the public to believe in their version, claiming that their faith-based convictions are the fundamental truth, which in the case of claims of chemical brain abnormalities in depression, they most certainly are not.

OTHER PHYSICIANS AND BRAIN CHEMICAL IMBALANCES

The delusion that brain biochemical abnormalities occur in depression has spread well beyond the area of depression into other areas of medicine. The lack of basic logical reasoning regarding the brain and postulated chemical imbalances in high places is at times breath-taking, as the following passage from the American Medical Association 1998 book *Essential Guide to Depression* illustrates:

Researchers are uncertain exactly why changing levels of neurotransmitters can lead to depression. [143]

Given the authoritative origin of this book, most readers will likely take what they read in it to be factual. The reader is likely to interpret this passage to mean that changing levels of neurotransmitters have been scientifically identified, that these changing levels can lead to depression, and that all that remains to be identified is why changing levels of neurotransmitters leads to depression. Given its apparently reliable source, the reader is unlikely to question these statements.

Readers of that book are not likely to be aware that this short sentence contains two instances of misinformation. Changing levels of neurotransmitters—changes that are identified as abnormal—have never been scientifically identified to occur in depression. Therefore, there cannot be reliable scientific evidence that has established any direct connection between changing levels of neurotransmitters and depression. This assertion is therefore a classic example of the Begging the Question logical fallacy.[144] These flaws and inconsistencies becomes clearer in the sentences that follow:

Part of their uncertainty results from the difficulty they have in studying these substances. Each neurotransmitter occurs in minute quantities, is found only in specific parts of the brain, and is quickly removed once its job is done. Because the neurotransmitters disappear so quickly, there is no way to measure levels of them directly within the brain. Instead, scientists measure levels of substances that are left over after the brain uses a neurotransmitter. These substances, called metabolites, are found in such body fluids as urine, blood and cerebrospinal fluid. By measuring the changes in the level of serotonin metabolites in the body, scientists gauge the change in the levels of neurotransmitters in the brain. [145]

It is clear from this passage that scientists have had little success in deriving definitive information about serotonin by studying serotonin function in the brain. As I discussed in chapter two of this book, years of research into the by-products—metabolites—of serotonin has not yielded any reliable results. The implication that measuring these metabolites in urine, blood and cerebrospinal fluid provides an indication of brain neurotransmitters is therefore untrue, having no basis in scientific evidence. One might expect better from the American Medical Association. I encountered other pieces of misinformation regarding depression and neurotransmitters in this American Medical Association book including the following:

Researchers are also uncertain whether depressive illness results from or causes changes in the level of certain neurotransmitters. [146]

There is no evidence of any neurotransmitter abnormalities in depression to begin with. Questioning whether "changes in the levels of certain neurotransmitters" is the cause or the result of depressive illness is therefore a Red Herring logical fallacy. [147] As we have seen, many doctors are less humble than the American Medical Association, assuming and preaching that one causes the other, without the one even having been established. The authors wrote:

> The neurotransmitter serotonin is also involved in depression. Researchers have found low levels of serotonin in some severely depressed people, including some who were suicidal . . . Here again, however, the link between low levels of serotonin and depressive illness is unclear, as some depressed people have too much serotonin. [148]

There are several errors in this passage. It has never been established that "serotonin is also involved in depression". What is definitely established is that serotonin is very much involved in the medical imagination regarding what happens in depression. The assertion that "researchers have found low levels of serotonin in some severely depressed people, including some who were suicidal" is utter misinformation. Researchers have never reliably identified low levels of serotonin in depression, yet the American Medical Association presents this assertion as a known established fact. Nor has it ever been scientifically demonstrated that some people with depression have elevated levels of serotonin.

The authors also claimed that "Antidepressants improve your mood by interfering with this cleanup process", that is, the breaking down or reuptake of neurotransmitters from the synapses. [149] While their use of the word "interfering" is accurate, presuming that this interference "improves your mood" is a major assumption for which there is no evidence; rather, this is a Wishful Thinking logical fallacy. [150] No scientific evidence exists that confirms any problems with this "clean-up process" that require any form of interference.

Notice the apparent scientific nuance and certainty of the following passage from this American Medical Association book (italics mine):

> Doctors *believe* depression comes from having too much or too little of certain neurotransmitters—such as serotonin, norepinephrine, dopamine—and other chemical messengers that are involved in your emotional reactions. They *think* that one or more of these neurotransmitters fail to dock on a neuron in the correct numbers. As a result, illness *can* develop. Antidepressants are *believed* to work by altering the balance of neurotransmitters zipping around your synapses, thus changing the chemistry to your advantage. [151]

Three of the four words I have emphasised in the above passage demonstrate uncertainty and faith rather than evidence-based science; believe, think, believed. The fourth represents a seamless shift from theory to fact; "as a result, illness *can* develop." This is inconsistent with the tone of uncertainty created by the other three words. The authors should have remained consistent in their writing; "might develop" would have been accurate; "can develop" is misinformation. The authors' statement that the interference effected by antidepressants change "the chemistry to your advantage" is a Wishful Thinking logical fallacy, since we have no way of verifying this scientifically.

Internationally known neuroscientist Dr. Candace Pert was quoted in 1984 as saying:

> People who act crazy are acting that way because they have too much or too little of some chemicals in their brains. [152]

This is an unsubstantiated statement since there is no scientific evidence that confirms this to be true.

Best-selling British medical doctor and author Dr. Miriam Stoppard OBE has acknowledged that depression "is quite difficult to understand". [153] However, she mentioned the existence of brain chemical deficiencies as a distinct probability:

> The cause of depression is complex but is probably related to a reduction in the levels of certain chemicals in the brain, called neurotransmitters . . . the best known . . . is serotonin. [154]

Readers will likely take her statement as credible and be influenced by its contents, particularly her statement that chemical abnormalities are "probably related" to depression, for which no supporting evidence exists.

Living with M.E.: the chronic fatigue/post-viral syndrome is a 1999 book written by medical doctor Charles Shepherd, then Medical Director of the M.E. Association. According to Dr. Shepherd:

> Neurotransmitter deficiencies are known to occur in a number of psychiatric and brain disorders, particularly depression (serotonin and noradrenaline). [155]

There is absolutely no reliable scientific evidence to support this unequivocally-made assertion. According to the 2002 medical textbook *Textbook of Medicine*:

> Psychiatric disease constitutes a large proportion of disability and illness in society . . . Changes in neurotransmitter biochemistry in depression are important; current views emphasize a reduction of catecholamine levels at postsynaptic nerve endings. [156]

Changes in neurotransmitter biochemistry have never been identified in depression. They are important not because they have been scientifically found to be deficient or central to depression, but because drug companies, doctors and others have made them important in their assertions for over thirty years. Speaking about SSRI antidepressants during a 2011 TED presentation, neuroscientist Molly Crockett claimed:

> These drugs basically work by enhancing the actions of serotonin in the brain. [157]

This assertion is both a Begging the Question logical fallacy [158] and a False Cause logical fallacy. [159] It is a Begging the Question logical fallacy because Crockett is mistakenly claiming that antidepressants work by enhancing serotonin function when all that has been established is that these substances interfere with serotonin function. It is a False Cause logical fallacy because something that has not been reliably identified as existing cannot be unequivocally claimed to cause anything. Earlier in her TED talk Molly Crockett described her research in terms far more suggestive of interfering than enhancing (italics mine):

> We wanted to know whether *tinkering* with a specific brain chemical called serotonin would change people's judgements of right and wrong. [160]

NOTES TO CHAPTER FIVE

1. Irving Kirsch, *The Emperor's New Drugs: Exploding the Antidepressant Myth*, London; Random House, 2009, pps. 90-93.
2. Marcia Angell, "Drug Companies and Doctors: A Story of Corruption", *New York Review of Books*, 15 January 2009.
3. The American Psychiatric Association, http://www.psychiatry.org/depression, accessed 09 April 2014.
4. American Psychiatrists Association, "Let's Talk Facts Brochures", "Depression", http:// www. psychiatry.org/mental-health/lets-talk-facts-brochures, accessed 04 October 2014.
5. Royal College of Psychiatrists, 2006, referred to in Joanna Moncrieff, *The Myth of the Chemical Cure: A critique of Psychiatric Drug Treatment*, Basingstoke: Palgrave Macmillan, 2009, pps. 10-11.
6. See note 54 in the notes to chapter two and the associated text for Dorothy Rowe's comments on the removal of references to biochemical imbalances from the Royal College of Psychiatrists' website.
7. Royal College of Psychiatrists website, http://www.rcpsych.ac.uk/healthadvice/problemsdisorders/ copingwithphysicalillness.aspx, accessed 04 June 2014.
8. "Antidepressants", Royal College of Psychiatrists website, http://www.rcpsych.ac.uk/ healthadvice/treatmentswellbeing/antidepressants.aspx, accessed 04 October 2014.
9. Morris Lipton, "Affective Disorders: Progress, But Some Unresolved Questions Remain", *American Journal of Psychiatry*, September 1970, p. 33.
10. E. Anderson, & W. Trethowen, *Psychiatry*, London: Bailliere Tindall, 1973, p. 11.
11. "About Mayo Clinic", Mayo Clinic website, http://www.mayoclinic.org/about-mayo-clinic, accessed 01 October 2014.
12. "Antidepressants—How they help relieve depression", video and transcript, "Diseases and Conditions" webpage, mayo Clinic website, http://www.mayoclinic.org/diseases-conditions/depression/multimedia/antidepressants/vid-20084764, accessed 01 October 2014.
13. Nancy Andreasen, *The Broken Brain: The Biological Revolution in Psychiatry*, New York: Harper & Row, 1985, p. 221.
14. Nancy Andreasen, *The Broken Brain: The Biological Revolution in Psychiatry*, New York: Harper & Row, 1985, p. 133.
15. Nancy Andreasen, *The Broken Brain: The Biological Revolution in Psychiatry*, New York Harper & Row, 1985, p. 205-6.
16. Nancy Andreasen, *The Broken Brain: The Biological Revolution in Psychiatry*, New York Harper & Row, 1985, p. 256.
17. Francis Mark Mondimore, *Depression: The Mood Disease*, Third Edition, Baltimore: The Johns Hopkins University Press, 2006, p. 9.
18. Francis Mark Mondimore, *Depression: The Mood Disease*, Third Edition, Baltimore: The Johns Hopkins University Press, 2006.

19. Daniel Carlat, *Unhinged: The Trouble with Psychiatry—a Doctor's Revelations about a Profession in Crisis,* London: Free Press, 2010, p. 9.
20. Lauren Slater, *Prozac Diary,* New York: Penguin Books, 1999.
21. Michael J. Norden, *Beyond Prozac: Brain Toxic Lifestyles, Natural Antidotes and New Generation Antidepressants,* New York: Regan Books (HarperCollins), 1995.
22. Michael J. Norden, *Beyond Prozac: Brain Toxic Lifestyles, Natural Antidotes and New Generation Antidepressants,* New York: Regan Books (HarperCollins), 1995, p. xiv.
23. Michael J. Norden, *Beyond Prozac: Brain Toxic Lifestyles, Natural Antidotes and New Generation Antidepressants,* New York: Regan Books (HarperCollins), 1995, p. 10.
24. Michael J. Norden, *Beyond Prozac: Brain Toxic Lifestyles, Natural Antidotes and New Generation Antidepressants,* New York: Regan Books (HarperCollins), 1995, p. 16.
25. Michael J. Norden, *Beyond Prozac: Brain Toxic Lifestyles, Natural Antidotes and New Generation Antidepressants,* New York: Regan Books (HarperCollins), 1995, p. 21.
26. Michael J. Norden, *Beyond Prozac: Brain Toxic Lifestyles, Natural Antidotes and New Generation Antidepressants,* New York: Regan Books (HarperCollins), 1995, p. 11.
27. Michael J. Norden, *Beyond Prozac: Brain Toxic Lifestyles, Natural Antidotes and New Generation Antidepressants,* New York: Regan Books (HarperCollins), 1995, p. 18.
28. Michael J. Norden, *Beyond Prozac: Brain Toxic Lifestyles, Natural Antidotes and New Generation Antidepressants,* New York: Regan Books (HarperCollins), 1995, p. 1
29. Michael J. Norden, *Beyond Prozac: Brain Toxic Lifestyles, Natural Antidotes and New Generation Antidepressants,* New York: Regan Books (HarperCollins), 1995.
30. For information on Begging the Question logical fallacies see note 22 in the Notes to the Introduction.
31. Elliot S. Valenstein, *Blaming the Brain: The Truth About Drugs and Mental Health,* New York: The Free Press, 1998, p. 3.
32. C. Thompson, *Medical Dialogue,* December 2007.
33. For information on Begging the Question logical fallacies see note 22 in the Notes to the Introduction.
34. A Proof of Tradition logical fallacy is the common logical error of concluding that something is true because one has become so familiar with it over a long period of time. It is also known as an Argumentum ad antiquitatem logical fallacy. http://infidels.org/library/modern/mathew/ logic.html #antiquitatem, accessed 04 January 14.
35. Daniel Amen, *Change Your Brain, Change Your Life: The Breakthrough Program for Conquering Anxiety, Depression, Obsessiveness, Anger, and Impulsiveness,* Harmony, 1999, p. 47.
36. In Philip Hickey Ph.D., "Psychiatry DID Promote the Chemical Imbalance Theory", 06 June 2014, http://www.madinamerica.com/2014/06/psychiatry-promote-chemical-imbalance-theory/, accessed 14 June 2014.
37. Richard Harding, "Unlocking the Brain's Secrets", in *Family Circle* magazine, 20 November 2001, p. 62.
38. A False Dilemma logical fallacy occurs when a restricted number of possibilities are presented when more options exist. I include several examples in this book where just two and sometimes three possibilities are considered and other valid possibilities are not mentioned. http://www.logicallyfallacious.com/index.php/logical-fallacies/94-false-dilemma, accessed 12 May 2014.
39. Nada L. Stotland, "About Depression in Women", in *Family Circle* magazine, 20 November 2001, p. 65.
40. Jesse Wright & Monica Ramirez Basco, *Getting Your Life Back: The Complete Guide to Recovery from Depression,* Free Press, 2002, p. 198.
41. For information on Begging the Question logical fallacies see note 22 in the Notes to the Introduction.
42. A False Cause logical fallacy occurs when a real or perceived relationship between things is taken to mean that one is the cause of the other. In the event that two things occur together, it should not be presumed that one causes the other without adequate evidence. It is also known as the cause versus correlation logical fallacy. Regarding depression, no evidence exists either that there are such abnormalities, or consequently that that any such abnormalities cause depression. To claim or imply that both are established facts is a remarkable leap of faith, based on no scientific evidence whatsoever. https://yourlogicalfallacyis.com/false-cause, accessed 07 May 2014. Also

http://atheism.about.com/library /FAQs/skepticism/blfaq_fall_correlation.htm, accessed 03 January 2014.

43. Virginia Edwards, *Depression: What You Really Need to Know,* London: Constable & Robinson Ltd., London, 2003, pps. 75-76.

44. Virginia Edwards, *Depression: What You Really Need to Know,* London: Constable & Robinson Ltd., 2003, pps. 75-76.

45. James Whitney Hicks, *50 Signs of Mental Illness: A Guide to Understanding Mental Health*, Yale: Yale University Press, 2005, p. 3.

46. For information on Begging the Question logical fallacies see note 22 in the Notes to the Introduction.

47. James Whitney Hicks, *50 Signs of Mental Illness: A Guide to Understanding Mental Health*, Yale: Yale University Press, 2005, p. 100.

48. Sabina Dosani, *Defeat Depression: Tips and Techniques for Healing a Troubled Mind,* Oxford: The Infinite Ideas Company Ltd: 2005, pps 110 and 55.

49. Sabini Dosani, *Defeat Depression: Tips and Techniques for Healing a Troubled Mind*, Oxford: The Infinite Ideas Company Ltd: 2005, p. 55.

50. Rebecca Fox-Spencer, *A Simple Guide to Depression,* Long Hanborough: CSF Medical Publications Ltd, 2005, p. 14.

51. G.S. Malhi et al, "Structural and Functional Models of Depression: From Sub-types to Substrates", *Acta Psychiatrica Scandinavica* vol. 111, no.2 (2005): 94-105 (p. 97).

52. G.S Malhi et al, "Structural and Functional Models of Depression: From Sub-types to Substrates", *Acta Psychiatrica Scandinavica* vol. 111, no.2 (2005): 94-105 (p. 97).

53. A detailed discussion of the effectiveness of antidepressants is beyond the scope of this book. I will address this fully in a future book. I include here some brief comments. Despite the conviction held by most doctors and many people that the effectiveness of antidepressants has been established beyond all doubt, their effectiveness has been questioned almost since they first became available. See R.P. Greenberg & S. Fisher, 1989, "Examining Antidepressant Effectiveness: Findings, Ambiguities and some Vexing Puzzles", in *The Limits of Biological Treatments for Psychological Distress*, S. Fisher & R.P. Greenberg, eds, Hillsdale N.J.: Lawrence Erlbaum Associates, 1989, pp 1-38; D.O. Antonuccio et al, "Raising Questions About Antidepressants", *Psychother.Psychosom.*, vol. 68, no, 1, 1999, pp. 3-14; and J. Moncrieff & I. Kirsch, "Efficacy of Antidepressants in Adults", *British Medical Journal*, vol. 331, no. 7509, 2005, pp. 155-7.
According to a large scale comprehensive 1969 NIMH review of antidepressant clinical trials, the authors concluded that in "well-designed studies the differences between the effectiveness of antidepressant drugs and placebo are not impressive" (A. Smith, E. Traganza & G. Harrison, G., 'Studies on the Effectivemess of Antidepressant Drugs', *Psychopharmacol.Bull.*, 1969, Suppl-53). It is widely recognized within medicine that the effectiveness of newer antidepressants such as Prozac is no greater than the older antidepressants that were the subject of this 1969 review.
Irving Kirsch, *the Emperor's New Drugs,* found that 80 percent of the effect of antidepressants was due to the placebo effect. The results of his study, are *below* the threshold of effectiveness recommended by some governmental bodies including the National Institutes for Health and Clinical Excellence in Britain. See Irving Kirsch, Thomas J. Moore et al, "The Emperor's New Drugs: An Analysis of Antidepressant Medication Data Submitted to the U.S. Food and Drug Administration, *Prevention & Treatment*, Volume 5, Article 23, posted 15 July 2002.
In 1998, eleven years after the launch of Prozac the FDA's own director of clinical research in the psychiatry drug department questioned whether antidepressants should continue to be approved based on the weakness of the evidence. See Leber, "Approvable Action on Forest Laboratories Inc.", discussed in Gary Greenburg, *Manufacturing Depression: The Secret History of a Modern Disease,* London: Bloomsbury, 2010, p.204.
Research suggests that the use of antidepressants may make people more vulnerable to relapse. People diagnosed with depression and treated with antidepressants demonstrate a degree of vulnerability to relapse that is not shown by recovered patients who have been treated without drugs. See H.G. Ruhe et al, "Mood is Indirectly Related to Serotonin, Norepinephrine and Dopamine Levels in Humans: a Meta-analysis of Monoamine Depletion Studies", *Molecular Psychiatry*, 12 (2007): 331-59, and Fava, Giovanni A., 'Can Long-Term Treatment with Antidepressant Drugs Worsen the Course of Depression?', *Journal of Clinical Psychiatry* 64 (2003): 123-33).

54. See note 53 in the Notes to this chapter and note 22 in the Notes to Chapter Three.
55. Francis Mondimore, *Depression: The Mood Disease*, 3rd edition, Baltimore: The Johns Hopkins University Press, 2006, p. 9.
56. Siobhan Barry, *Understanding Mental Health*, Dublin: Blackhall Publishing, 2006, p. 58.
57. For information on False Cause logical fallacies see note 42 in the Notes to this chapter.
58. For information on Begging the Question logical fallacies see note 22 in the Notes to the Introduction.
59. Richard A. Friedman, "On the Horizon; Personalized Depression Drugs", *New York Times*, 19 June 2007.
60. For information on False Cause logical fallacies see note 42 in the Notes to this chapter.
61. For information on Begging the Question logical fallacies see note 22 in the Notes to the Introduction.
62. Jonathan Leo & Jeffrey Lacasse, "The Media and the Chemical Imbalance Theory of Depression", *Society*, 2008, 45:35-45, 2008. http://link.springer.com/article/10.1007/s12115-007-9047-3/full-text.html, accessed on 29 December 2013.
63. A transcript of this interview with Daniel Carlat is available at http://www.npr.org/templates/transcript/transcript.php?storyId=128107547.
64. Daniel Carlat, *Unhinged: The Trouble with Psychiatry—a Doctor's Revelations about a Profession in Crisis*, London: Free Press, 2010.
65. Jeffrey Lieberman, "Causes of Depression" video, The University Hospital of Columbia and Cornell, 19 June 2012, https://www.youtube.com/watch?v=Il7VFP_ugjM, accessed 12 August 2014.
66. For information on Begging the Question logical fallacies see note 22 in the Notes to the Introduction.
67. For information on False Cause logical fallacies see note 42 in the Notes to this chapter.
68. Jeffrey Lieberman, "Causes of Depression" video, The University Hospital of Columbia and Cornell 19 June 2012, https://www.youtube.com/watch?v=Il7VFP_ugjM, accessed 12 August 2014.
69. A Weak Analogy logical fallacy occurs when an analogy is used to prove or disprove an argument, but the analogy is too dissimilar to be a proper analogy. It is also known as a false, bad, questionable or faulty analogy. See http://www.logicallyfallacious.com/index.php/logical-fallacies/182-weak-analogy, accessed 13 August 2014. A weak analogy logical fallacy occurs when two things are said to be like each other in a way that they are not like each other, or an analogy is made between two things that are not similar enough to correctly qualify as an analogy. See http://www. seekfind. net/Logical_Fallacy_of_False_or_Faulty_Analogy__Weak_Analogy__ Bad_Analogy__Appeal_ to _the_Moon.html#.U-r_5fldXco, accessed 13 August 2014.
70. Tim Cantopher, in *The Guardian* special report on antidepressants, *The Guardian*, 21 November 2013.
71. Irish Health.com website, "about irishhealth.com", http://www.irishhealth.com/about. html, accessed 31 August 2014.
72. Psychiatrists Professor Brian Lawlor and Professor Patrick McKeon, irishhealth.com Expert Video Panel, "about irishhealth.com", http://www.irishhealth.com/about.html, accessed 01 September 2014.
73. Irish Health.com website, "about irishhealth.com: editorial policy", http://www.irishhealth.com /about.html, accessed 01 September 2014.
74. Irishhealth.com website, "Depression: What causes depression?", http://www.irishhealth.com /article.html?con=304, accessed 01 September 2014.
75. Irishhealth.com website, "Depression: How is depression treated?", http://www.irishhealth. com/article.html?con=304, accessed 01 September 2014.
76. For information of Begging the Question logical fallacies see note 22 in the notes to the Introduction.
77. Irishhealth.com website, "Depression: How is depression treated?", http://www.irishhealth. com/article.html?con=304, accessed 01 September 2014.
78. Irishhealth.com website, "Depression Clinic: How antidepressants work" webpage, http://www. irishhealth.com/clin/depression/antidepressants.html, accessed 01 September 2014.
79. Irish Health.com website, "About irishhealth.com", http://www.irishhealth.com/about.html, accessed 31 August 2014.

80. Kwame McKenzie, *Understanding Depression*, 2006, Family Doctor Publications in association with the British Medical Association, 2006, p. 72.
81. Kwame McKenzie, *Understanding Depression*, 2006, Family Doctor Publications in association with the British Medical Association, 2006, p. 17.
82. Kwame McKenzie, *Understanding Depression*, 2006, Family Doctor Publications in association with the British Medical Association, 2006, p. 17.
83. Kwame McKenzie, *Understanding Depression*, Poole: Family Doctor Publications in association with the British Medical Association, 2006, p. 74.
84. Kevin M. O'Shaughnessy, ed., *New Guide to Medicines and Drugs: The Complete Home Reference to Over 2,500 Medicines*, British Medical Association, London: Dorling Kindersley, 2011, p. 40.
85. Kevin M. O'Shaughnessy, ed., *New Guide to Medicines and Drugs: The Complete Home Reference to Over 2,500 Medicines*, British Medical Association, London: Dorling Kindersley, 2011, p. 40.
86. Kevin M. O'Shaughnessy, ed., *New Guide to Medicines and Drugs: The Complete Home Reference to Over 2,500 Medicines*, British Medical Association, London: Dorling Kindersley, 2011, p. 40.
87. http://www.mirror.co.uk/3am/celebrity-news/itv-tops-daytime-viewing-figures-204810, accessed 28 April 2014.
88. http://www.itv.com/thismorning/health/dr-chris-answers-your-depression-questions.
89. http://www.itv.com/thismorning/health/dr-chris-answers-your-depression-questions.
90. http://www.itv.com/thismorning/health/dr-chris-answers-your-depression-questions.
91. For information on Begging the Question logical fallacies see note 22 in the Notes to the Introduction.
92. For information on False Cause logical fallacies see note 42 in the Notes to this chapter.
93. "Dr. Chris talks about Depression", 14 June 2011, YouTube video, http://www.youtube. com/watch?v=GVL1WHqISJk, accessed 21 April 2014.
94. For information on Begging the Question logical fallacies see note 22 in the Notes to the Introduction.
95. For information on False Cause logical fallacies see note 42 in the Notes to this chapter.
96. Julie Leonovs, "Open Letter Re: *This Morning's* Feature on Depression", 15 April 2014, http://www.madinamerica.com/2014/04/open-letter-re-morning-feature-depression/, accessed 20 April 2014.
97. Julie Leonovs, "Open Letter Re: *This Morning's* Feature on Depression", 15 April 2014, http://www.madinamerica.com/2014/04/open-letter-re-morning-feature-depression/, accessed 20 April 2014.
98. Joanna Moncrieff, http://www.madinamerica.com/2014/04/open-letter-re-morning-feature-depression/, accessed 20 April 2014.
99. See note 14 in the Notes to Chapter Fourteen and the corresponding text.
100. "Dr. Chris talks about Depression", 14 June 2011, YouTube video, https://www.youtube.com/watch?v=GVL1WHqISJk, accessed 21 April 2014.
101. Dawn Harper, medical expert on ITV's *This Morning*, during a discussion on depression on 12 August 2014.
102. For information on Begging the Question logical fallacies see note 22 in the Notes to the Introduction.
103. For information on Begging the Question logical fallacies see note 22 in the Notes to the Introduction.
104. For information on False Cause logical fallacies see note 42 in the Notes to Chapter Five.
105. For information on False Cause logical fallacies see note 42 in the Notes to Chapter Five.
106. See note 38 in the notes to Chapter Eleven.
107. From the presentation at the launch of the Council for Evidence-based Psychiatry (CEP) at the House of Lords, 30 April 2014. Pending publication; information regarding this survey is available from CEP on request, http://vimeo.com/93520896, accessed 22 September 2014.
108. Greg Castello, "Depression, Anxiety, OCD and More: Serotonin the Master chemical", YouTube video, 12 May 2013, https://www.youtube.com/watch?v=6YO6SMGHn_M, accessed 08 June 2014.
109. Greg Castello, "Depression, Anxiety, OCD and More: Serotonin the Master chemical", YouTube video, 12 May 2013, https://www.youtube.com/watch?v=6YO6SMGHn_M, accessed 08 June 2014.

110. Greg Castello, "Depression, Anxiety, OCD and More: Serotonin the Master chemical", YouTube video, 12 May 2013, https://www.youtube.com/watch?v=6YO6SMGHn_M, accessed 08 June 2014.

111. Greg Castello, "Depression, Anxiety, OCD and More: Serotonin the Master chemical", YouTube video, 12 May 2013, https://www.youtube.com/watch?v=6YO6SMGHn_M, accessed 08 June 2014.

112. Greg Castello, "Depression, Anxiety, OCD and More: Serotonin the Master chemical", YouTube video, 12 May 2013, https://www.youtube.com/watch?v=6YO6SMGHn_M, accessed 08 June 2014.

113. Greg Castello, "Depression, Anxiety, OCD and More: Serotonin the Master chemical", YouTube video, 12 May 2013, https://www.youtube.com/watch?v=6YO6SMGHn_M, accessed 08 June 2014.

114. Greg Castello, "Depression, Anxiety, OCD and More: Serotonin the Master chemical", YouTube video, 12 May 2013, https://www.youtube.com/watch?v=6YO6SMGHn_M, accessed 08 June 2014.

115. Greg Castello, "Depression, Anxiety, OCD and More: Serotonin the Master chemical", YouTube video, 12 May 2013, https://www.youtube.com/watch?v=6YO6SMGHn_M, accessed 08 June 2014.

116. Greg Castello, "Depression, Anxiety, OCD and More: Serotonin the Master chemical", YouTube video, 12 May 2013, https://www.youtube.com/watch?v=6YO6SMGHn_M, accessed 08 June 2014.

117. Greg Castello, "Depression, Anxiety, OCD and More: Serotonin the Master chemical", YouTube video, 12 May 2013, https://www.youtube.com/watch?v=6YO6SMGHn_M, accessed 08 June 2014.

118. Greg Castello, "Depression, Anxiety, OCD and More: Serotonin the Master chemical", YouTube video, 12 May 2013, https://www.youtube.com/watch?v=6YO6SMGHn_M, accessed 08 June 2014.

119. Greg Castello, "Depression, Anxiety, OCD and More: Serotonin the Master chemical", YouTube video, 12 May 2013, https://www.youtube.com/watch?v=6YO6SMGHn_M, accessed 08 June 2014.youtube video, 12 May 2013, https://www.youtube.com/watch?v=6YO6SMGHn_M, accessed 08 June 2014.

120. "From *Beyond Prozac* to *Selfhood* and beyond: A Conversation with Terry Lynch", Athlone Literary Festival, 2013. https://www.youtube.com/watch?v=85Ync0GeIhQ, accessed 13 August 2013.

121. Greg Castello, "Depression, Anxiety, OCD and More: Serotonin the Master chemical", YouTube video, 12 May 2013, https://www.youtube.com/watch?v=6YO6SMGHn_M, accessed 08 June 2014.

122. Daniel Carlat, *Unhinged: The Trouble with Psychiatry—a Doctor's Revelations about a Profession in Crisis*, London: Free Press, 2010, pps. 75 and 81.

123. Caroline Shreeve, *Dealing with Depression: Understanding and Overcoming the Symptoms of Depression*, London: Piatkus, 2010, p. 5.

124. Caroline Shreeve, *Dealing with Depression: Understanding and Overcoming the Symptoms of Depression*, London: Piatkus, 2010, p. 39.

125. Caroline Shreeve, *Dealing with Depression: Understanding and Overcoming the Symptoms of Depression*, Lon don: Piatkus, 2010, p. 31.

126. For information on Begging the Question logical fallacies see note 22 in the Notes to the Introduction.

127. For information on False Dilemma logical fallacies see note 38 in the Notes to this chapter.

128. Harry Barry, *Flagging the Problem: A New Approach to Mental Health*, Dublin: Liberties Press, 2007, pps. 135, 33-34, 83, 145.

129. For information on Begging the Question logical fallacies see note 22 in the Notes to the Introduction.

130. Harry Barry, *Flagging the Problem: A New Approach to Mental Health*, Dublin: Liberties Press, 2007, p. 144-5.

131. For information on False Cause logical fallacies see note 42 in the Notes to this chapter.

132. For information on Begging the Question logical fallacies see note 22 in the Notes to the Introduction.

133. Harry Barry, *Flagging the Problem: A New Approach to Mental Health*, Dublin:Liberties Press, 2007, p. 77.

134. Harry Barry, *Flagging the Problem: A New Approach to Mental Health*, Dublin:Liberties Press, 2007, p. 77.

135. Harry Barry, *Flagging the Problem: A New Approach to Mental Health*, Dublin: Liberties Press,2007, p. 77.

136. Harry Barry, *Flagging Depression: A Practical Guide*, Dublin: Liberties Press, 2012, pps 232-3.

137. Muiris Houston, *Irish Times*, 17 December 2001.

138. Muiris Houston, *Irish Times*, 17 December 2001.

139. Rolf Dobelli, *The Art of Thinking Clearly*, London: Hodder & Stoughton Ltd., 2013, p. 23.

140. Rolf Dobelli, *The Art of Thinking Clearly*, London: Hodder & Stoughton Ltd., 2013, p. 23.

141. Colm Toibin, April 2008, http://corkuniversitypress.typepad.com/cork_university_press/2008/04/psychiatrist-he.html, accessed 02 January 2014.

142. A straw man argument is one that misrepresents a position in order to make it appear weaker than it actually is, refutes the misrepresentation of the position, and then concludes that the real position has been refuted. Whether the intention is deliberate or not, this is a fallacy, because the position that has been claimed to be refuted is different to that which has actually been refuted. In this case, by implying that Ivor Browne and I were evangelists, it could be argued that Muiris Houston sought to discredit us and in turn discredit our position.

    The "yourlogicalfallacyis" website describes the purpose of using a straw man fallacy argument: "By exaggerating, misrepresenting, or just completely fabricating someone's argument, it is much easier to present your position as being reasonable".

    http://www.logicalfallacies.info/ambiguity/straw-man/, accessed 02 January 2014.

    https://yourlogicalfallacyis.com/strawman, accessed 02 January 2014.

143. American Medical Association, *Essential Guide to Depression,* 1998, Simon & Schuster: New York, p. 65.

144. For information on Begging the Question logical fallacies see note 22 in the Notes to the introduction.

145. *Essential Guide to Depression,* American Medical Association, 1998, Simon & Schuster: New York, p. 64.

146. *Essential Guide to Depression,* American Medical Association, 1998, Simon & Schuster: New York, p. 153.

147. For information on Red Herring logical fallacies see note 23 in the Notes to the Introduction.

148. *Essential Guide to Depression, American* Medical Association, Simon & Schuster: New York, 1998, p. 153.

149. *Essential Guide to Depression, American* Medical Association, Simon & Schuster: New York, 1998, p. 153.

150. For information on Wishful Thinking logical fallacies see note 115 in the Notes to Chapter Two.

151. American Medical Association, *Essential Guide to Depression*, New York: Simon & Schuster, 1998, p. 153.

152. Candace Pert, quoted in the *Baltimore Evening Sun* (special reprint) 23-24 July 1984, p.3, quoted by Elliot S. Valenstein, *Blaming the Brain: The Truth About Drugs and Mental Health,* New York: The Free Press, 1998, p. 152.

153. Miriam Stoppard, *Family Health Guide*, Dorling Kindersley, London, 2005, p. 285.

154. Miriam Stoppard, *Family Health Guide,* Dorling Kindersley, London, 2005, p. 198.

155. Charles Shepherd, *Living with M.E.: the chronic fatigue/post-viral syndrome,* London: Vermilion, 1999.

156. R.L. Soulami & J. Moxham, eds., *Textbook of Medicine,* 4th edition, Churchill Livingstone, 2002, pps. 205 and 221.

157. Molly Crockett, TED talk, uploaded 04 October 2011, https://www.youtube.com/watch?v=X2oZwveMpSM, accessed 08 June 2014.

158. For information on Begging the Question logical fallacies see note 22 in the Notes to the Introduction.

159. For information on False Cause logical fallacies see note 42 in the Notes to Chapter Five.

160. Molly Crockett, TED talk, uploaded 04 October 2011, https://www.youtube.com/watch?v=X2oZwveMpSM, accessed 08 June 2014.

6. DRUG COMPANIES, DRUG REGULATORY AUTHORITIES AND PHARMACISTS

For more than half a century, the drug companies who manufacture antidepressants have enthusiastically promoted the notion that depression is caused by biochemical brain abnormalities as either a fact or so-close-to-a-fact-as-makes-no-difference. None of this is factually accurate, but it has greatly helped drug companies to make billions every year for the past twenty-seven years since the launch of Prozac. By the late 2000s, antidepressant production had become a thriving industry generating 19 billion dollars annually. The widely accepted notion that depression is caused by a chemical imbalance that is corrected by antidepressants has been vitally important for the manufacturers of antidepressants. The public acceptance of the veracity of this notion has led to the widespread public acceptance of antidepressants, as a supposedly logical and scientific rationale for taking them. Here are some examples of misinformation originating from drug companies.

ELI LILLY

Eli Lilly manufacture Prozac, the first of a long list of blockbuster antidepressant drugs. The following appeared in a Prozac advertisement in *People* magazine in 1998, ten years after Prozac was first launched:

> When you are clinically depressed, one thing that can happen is the level of serotonin—a chemical in your body—may drop. So you may have trouble sleeping. Feel unusually sad and irritable. Find it hard to concentrate. Lose your appetite. Lack energy. Or have trouble feeling pleasure . . . to bring serotonin levels closer to normal, the medicine doctors now prescribe most often is Prozac. [1]

This advertisement is misleading on several counts. There is no reliable evidence to confirm that serotonin brain levels drop when one is clinically depressed or more accurately, when a doctor has decided that you are clinically depressed. This advertisement is constructed to convey the impression that the listed experiences are the result of a drop in serotonin levels. This is without foundation, and attributes qualities to the drug that it is not known to possess. Neither Prozac nor any other antidepressants are known to bring serotonin "closer to normal". Since no one knows what "normal" serotonin levels are to begin with and abnormalities in serotonin levels have never been established and the drug manufacturers were well aware of these realities, this is a highly misleading statement.

In his 1998 book *Blaming the Brain: The Truth About Drugs and Mental Health*, neuroscientist Elliot Valenstein described one of Eli Lilly's marketing strategies for Prozac. Valenstein wrote that Eli Lilly produced tearaway sheets which were widely distributed to psychiatrists to give to the patients for whom they prescribed the drug.

The sheets contained blatant misinformation. The statement "when your serotonin is in short supply, you may suffer from depression" appeared alongside an image of a sad face that included the words "serotonin in short supply", the image also included the brain with few serotonin "spots". Beneath this was the statement "when you have enough serotonin, symptoms of depression may lift". Next to this was an image of a happy smiling face with the caption "serotonin in good supply" and an image of the brain with many dots portraying serotonin. The main heading on the sheet read "Like diabetes or arthritis, depression is a physical illness". [2]

According to the 2006 "How Prozac works" website:

> A growing amount of evidence supports the view that people with depression have an imbalance of the brain's neurotransmitters, the chemicals that allow nerve cells in the brain to communicate with each other. [3]

These claims are simply not true. The truthful position is that "no" rather than "a growing amount of" evidence supports this view. There is no shortage of theory supporting this notion, but there is a total absence of reliable factual scientific evidence for these claims. No such evidence exists. The next line read:

> Many scientists believe that an imbalance of serotonin, one of these neurotransmitters, may be an important factor in the development and severity of depression. Prozac may help to correct this imbalance by increasing the brain's own supply of serotonin. [4]

Here is another example of the flawed logic of seamlessly moving from a *belief* regarding serotonin to "this imbalance" being presented as a *fact* in the very next sentence. I was unable to locate these passages despite an extensive search in May 2014, which suggests that this wording may have been quietly removed since psychiatrist Joanna Moncrieff accessed it in 2006.

In 2014 the Irish Lilly website contained the following:

> Depression is believed to be associated with an imbalance of chemicals, called neurotransmitters, which help to send messages to the brain . . . The goal of treatment is to relieve the symptoms of depression, restore normal mood and return the individual to their normal activities and interests. [5]

In October 2014 the British Lilly website contains similar statements:

> Depression is believed to be caused by an imbalance of chemicals, called neurotransmitters, which help send messages in the brain . . . The goal of treatment is to restore a balance of emotions, relieve symptoms and return the individual to their pre-depression self in thoughts, function, and general outlook on life. [6]

On the Irish Lilly website, depression is believed to be *associated* with an imbalance of chemicals, whereas on the UK site, depression is believed to be *caused* by an imbalance of chemicals. If depression was known to be caused by an "imbalance of chemicals" as stated, the key stated goal of treatment would be to rebalance these chemicals, as it is a core goal of any illness characterized by chemical imbalances.

LUNDBECK

The drug company Lundbeck manufactures citalopram, which is sold under several trade names including Cipramil. Under the heading "What causes depression?" on the Lundbeck website, it is claimed:

> It is known that chemical changes in the brain contribute to producing the symptoms of depression . . . Depression is thought to be associated with changes to the levels of three principal chemicals in the brain that control a variety of body processes . . . If the levels of these chemicals are upset, this can lead to medical problems, such as depression . . . Many of the medications used to treat depression work by helping to return the levels of chemicals in the brain back to normal. [7]

In my opinion, this passage is quite mischievous, contradictory and misleading. The drug company followed their claim that chemical changes in the brain are "known" to occur with a statement that depression is "thought" to be associated with certain chemical changes. Something cannot be simultaneously both "known" and "thought" to exist. Claims that serotonin, noradrenaline and dopamine are "three principal chemicals in the brain" when so little is known about the brain and brain function are highly questionable. There is no scientific evidence whatsoever that "if the levels of these chemicals are upset, this can lead to medical problems, such as depression". The idea that depression is a "medical problem" is subtly planted in this sentence. Informing people that antidepressants "work by helping to return the levels of chemicals in the brain back to normal" is a blatant falsehood.

The Lundbeck website also contains a downloadable patient brochure called "Feeling Better", in which the following claims appear:

> Anxiety disorders and depression are illnesses. Depression takes root when the brain doesn't function properly and its levels of serotonin—a chemical "messenger"—are thrown out of balance. [8]

There is no reliable scientific evidence that anxiety or depression are "illnesses", or that "depression takes root" when the brain does not function properly. Brain chemicals have never been shown to have been "thrown out of balance". Lundbeck also produce the "educational" leaflet titled "Mind yourself at work: Depression in the workplace— a guide for employees". Readers of this leaflet are informed that:

> Low levels of the neurotransmitters such as serotonin, noradrenaline and dopamine have been implicated in depression. Antidepressant drugs re-balance the levels of neurotransmitters and relieve the symptoms of depression. [9]

The clever use of the word "implicated" plants the idea in the reader's mind that there is reliable evidence linking depression to low neurotransmitter levels. Actually, the link is far more tenuous, existing only in the minds of researchers, doctors and others who would very much like this notion to be true. Lundbeck's assertion that "antidepressant drugs re-balance the levels of neurotransmitters" is a falsehood. It cannot rightly be claimed that any substance re-balances something that has never been identified to be out of balance.

A 2006 booklet on depression produced by Lundbeck Australia titled "Depression: What You Should Know" informed its readers that:

> Depression is ultimately thought to be caused by an imbalance of special chemical substances in the brain, called neurotransmitters . . . Depression is an illness that is thought to result from a chemical imbalance in the brain. [10]

A booklet titled "Feeling Better: Dealing With Anxiety In The Workplace" is sponsored by Lundbeck in association with Standard Life, RBC Insurance and DesJardins Financial Security. I have a hunch that apart from Lundbeck, the other major sponsors were not aware that the following contents of their sponsored booklet are fallacious:

> Anxiety disorders and depression are illnesses. Depression takes root when the brain doesn't function properly and its levels of serotonin—a chemical "messenger"—are thrown out of balance. [11]

No scientific evidence has ever confirmed that either anxiety or depression are "illnesses", or that "depression takes root" when the brain does not function properly. Brain chemicals have never been shown to have been "thrown out of balance".

"Lean on me" is a major depression campaign sponsored by Lundbeck. According to the campaign website, Lundbeck is partnered in this initiative by the European Depression Association, The World Organization of Family Doctors (WONCA), The World Federation for Mental Health and Aware, an Irish mental health organization. That these respected sponsors did not object to misinformation appearing on the campaign website is testament to the pervasive nature of the depression delusion. Under the heading "What causes depression?" on the "Lean on me" website it is claimed:

> It is known that chemical changes in the brain contribute to producing the symptoms of depression . . . Depression is thought to be associated with changes to the levels of three principal chemicals in the brain that control a variety of body processes, including serotonin, noradrenaline and dopamine . . . If the levels of these chemicals are upset, this can lead to medical problems, such as depression

. . . Many of the medications used to treat depression work by helping to return the levels of chemicals in the brain back to normal". [12]

This passage is contradictory and seriously misleading. The baseless claim that chemical changes in the brain are "known" to occur in depression is directly followed by a statement that depression is "thought" to be associated with certain chemical changes. As I mentioned earlier, something cannot simultaneously be both "known" and "thought" to exist. Claims that serotonin, noradrenaline and dopamine are "three principal chemicals in the brain", when so little is known about the brain and brain function, are somewhat premature. There is no evidence whatsoever that "if the levels of these chemicals are upset, this can lead to medical problems, such as depression". The idea that depression is a "medical problem" is subtly planted in this sentence. Informing the public that antidepressants "work by helping to return the levels of chemicals in the brain back to normal" is a blatant falsehood. An image of the human brain is strategically placed right beside these passages of false information, the intention presumably being to reinforce the notion that depression is known to be a brain disease. The official "Lean on me" booklet contains the following false information:

Antidepressants re-balance the levels of brain neurotransmitters. [13]

GLAXOSMITHKLINE

In their drive to push their products, drug companies who manufacture antidepressant substances have regularly resorted to misinformation. Here are some examples of the blatant misinformation propagated by GlaxoSmithKline, the manufacturers of Seroxat, known as Paxil in some countries including the United States. As I discussed in chapter one, GlaxoSmithKline is one of the major pharmaceutical companies that in recent years has withdrawn from psychiatry research.

While working as a GP up to 1989, I received sample packs from SmithKline Beecham as the company was then known, manufacturers of Seroxat. Titled "Understanding Depression", these were promoted as information packs for patients. Each pack consisted of a booklet titled *A Patient's Guide to Depression: What it is and How it Can be Treated*, a cassette tape about depression and a letter from Irish psychiatrist Dr. Pat McKeon, then director of Irish mental health organization Aware. The pack contained a letter on Aware's headed paper with the heading in big bold underlined print:

Depression: A Treatable but Hidden Illness.

According to the pack booklet, *A Patient's Guide to Depression: What it is and How it Can be Treated*:

Nowadays, it is felt that scientific evidence points to an imbalance of certain brain chemicals called "neurotransmitters" which is the actual cause of depression. These are biological substances that are naturally found in the brain which carry signals between the nerve cells of the brain. When these are out of balance, they do not regulate the signals as they would normally do, and this can affect a person's mood. One such chemical or neurotransmitter is serotonin. Fortunately, there are several medicines that can correct the chemical imbalance that is thought to lead to depression.

The author of this booklet is not identified. It was produced by SmithKline Beecham as part of "Inform", a "SmithKline Beecham information programme". This and other parts of the booklet might have been more accurately titled a misinformation programme. The passage above contains several inaccurate statements and claims. The line, "it is felt that scientific evidence points to an imbalance of certain brain chemicals called 'neurotransmitters' which is the actual cause of depression" is ambiguous. "Felt" is generally not a word used in a scientific context; research either does or does not point to an imbalance of certain brain chemicals. The sentence beginning with "When they are out of balance" is fallacious, because the premise upon which it is built—brain chemicals being out of balance—has never been established to exist. It is therefore a Begging the Question logical fallacy. [14] The authors repeat this untruth two sentences later, referring to medicines "that can correct the chemical imbalance". The accompanying letter on Aware headed paper and signed by a leading Irish psychiatrist gave the pack an aura of authority and credibility. Aware is one of Ireland's best known mental health organizations. Since he was prepared to sign a letter on Aware headed paper that accompanied each information pack and endorsed it, I presume that psychiatrist Pat McKeon read the information pack and was satisfied with its contents.

The following appeared in a drug advertisement in *Newsweek* magazine in 2001 (italics theirs):

Chronic anxiety can be overwhelming. But it can also be overcome . . . *Paxil,* the most prescribed medication of its kind for generalized anxiety, works to correct the chemical imbalance believed to cause the disorder. [15]

This wording misleadingly conveys the message that a chemical imbalance has been identified that is believed to cause "the disorder". The truth is that no such chemical imbalance has been identified. Like the other advertisements mentioned above, the Paxil advertisement appears credible at first glance. Brief as this advertisement is, it too contains misinformation. The second sentence above doesn't make sense logically, but the incongruence is so subtle that many people may not notice it, which may have been the advertiser's intention. How can a substance be stated to correct a chemical imbalance whose existence has not been established but is merely "believed" to be present and therefore is totally a matter of faith? If truth was the advertiser's priority, the second half of that sentence would have been read something like "may be working to correct the assumed chemical imbalance, in the event that such an imbalance is ever found to exist".

The manufacturer's prescribing information for Paxil in 2003 stated the following. Paroxetine is the generic name for the active ingredient in Seroxat and Paxil (italics mine):

> The efficacy of paroxetine in the treatment of major depressive disorder, social anxiety disorder, obsessive-compulsive disorder (OCD), panic disorder (PD), generalized anxiety disorder (GAD), and post-traumatic stress disorder (PTSD), is *presumed* to be linked to potentiation of serotonergic activity in the central nervous system resulting from inhibition of neuronal uptake of serotonin. [16]

Translating this passage into plain English, this drug company stated that their drug works by enhancing serotonin function by inhibiting the reuptake of serotonin, resulting in more serotonin in brain synapses, the space between brain cells. As discussed earlier, no scientific evidence has confirmed a problem with serotonin function to begin with that needs enhancing.

The GlaxoSmithKline website in 2008 contained the following misinformation:

> Paxil helps balance your brain's chemistry. Just as a cake recipe requires you to use flour, sugar, and baking powder in the right amounts, your brain needs a fine chemical balance in order to perform at its best. Normally, a chemical messenger in your brain, called serotonin, helps send messages from one brain cell to another. This is how the cells in your brain communicate. Serotonin works to keep these messages moving smoothly. However, if serotonin levels become unbalanced, communication may become disrupted and lead to depression, anxiety, and PMDD (Pre-Menstrual Dysphoric Disorder). Paxil CR helps maintain a balance of serotonin levels, which may help cell-to-cell communication return to normal.[17]

This passage is highly misleading. Paxil does not help balance brain chemistry. Serotonin levels have never been identified as "unbalanced". Since communication between nerve cells has never been demonstrated to be "disrupted" in depression, claims that such disruption can "lead to depression" and other psychiatric diagnoses may appear persuasive but it is patent nonsense. Paxil CR has never been demonstrated to "maintain a balance of serotonin levels". "Cell-to-cell communication" has never been demonstrated to be abnormal and therefore in need of a "return to normal". This amounts to *six* instances of misinformation in just one passage. Also, with all due respect to all you bakers out there, comparing brain function to baking a cake is bizarre and inappropriate.

The following appeared on the paxilcr.com website up to May 2009:

> Scientific evidence suggests that depression and certain anxiety disorders may be caused by a chemical imbalance in the brain. Paxil CR helps balance your brain's chemistry. Normally, a chemical messenger in your brain, called serotonin, helps send messages from one brain cell to another. This is how the cells in your brain communicate. Serotonin works to keep the messages moving smoothly. However, if serotonin levels become unbalanced, communication may become disrupted

and lead to depression, anxiety and PMDD (Pre-Menstrual Dysphoric Disorder). Paxil CR helps maintain a balance of serotonin levels, which may help cell-to-cell communication return to normal. Paxil CR is with you throughout the day to help you manage and treat your condition. [18]

Again, there are several examples of misinformation and fabrication in this passage. It is medical and drug company theory that suggests a chemical imbalance cause for anxiety and depression, not scientific evidence. It is grossly misleading to claim that "Paxil CR helps balance your brain's chemistry" since no such imbalances have been identified. Paxil CR does not "help maintain a balance of serotonin levels". These drugs raise serotonin levels in the spaces between nerve cells, but it has never been established whether doing so is necessary or therapeutic. We have no idea what constitutes normal levels of these chemicals, let alone abnormal levels.

The four sentences in this passage about how brain cells communicate messages are grossly misleading. The first sentence begins with the word "normally", sowing seeds of normality and abnormality in the reader's mind. The use of this word implies that medical science has a deep and comprehensive understanding of how brain cells communicate and serotonin's precise role in this complex process, which it most certainly does not, but the general reader would not know this. Claiming that "this is how the cells in your brain communicate" is therefore an astonishingly presumptuous statement, given the current primitive level of understanding of the human brain.

FOREST PHARMACEUTICALS

Forest Pharmaceuticals manufacture two commonly prescribed antidepressants, Lexapro (generic name escitalopram) and Celexa (generic name citalopram). According to the "How Lexapro works" section of the Forest Pharmaceuticals website in 2005 (emphasis theirs):

The nerve cell picks up the serotonin and sends some of it back to the first nerve cell, similar to a conversation between two people. In people with depression and anxiety, there is an imbalance of serotonin—too much serotonin is absorbed by the first nerve cell, so the next nerve cell does not have enough; as in a conversation, one person might do all the talking and the other does not get to comment, leading to a communication imbalance. LEXAPRO blocks the serotonin from going back into the first nerve cell. This increases the amount of serotonin available for the next nerve cell, like a conversation moderator. LEXAPRO appears to work by increasing the available supply of serotonin. Here's how: The naturally occurring chemical serotonin is sent from one nerve cell to the next. The blocking action helps balance the supply of serotonin, and communication returns to normal. In this way, LEXAPRO improves symptoms of depression. [19]

What a colourful piece of creative writing this is. None of it is true. No imbalance of serotonin has ever been identified in people diagnosed with depression or experiencing anxiety. It has not been established that too much serotonin is absorbed by one cell and not enough by the next. This fanciful notion may appear impressive but it is without foundation. Analogies are intended to compare and contrast things that have many shared characteristics and some differences. Using a conversation as an analogy for brain transmitter function in depression is about as appropriate as using and analogy to compare rain to sausages; they have little in common. But with the limited information the lay reader has at their disposal, the majority of those who read the advertisement are not likely to realize this. It is not true to say that the blocking action of Lexapro helps balance the supply of serotonin. This is an outrageous claim, one that sells a lot of antidepressants but for which there is no scientific basis. SSRIs do interfere with the reuptake of serotonin in the spaces between brain nerve cells, that much is true. But doctors have no idea whether this interference in brain function is beneficial or harmful. On the balance of probability it is more likely to be harmful, as it is a clumsy man-made interference in a sensitive and highly complex brain dynamic that remains largely a mystery. To present such conjecture as fact is grossly misleading. According to a Lexapro press release:

> While the brain chemistry of depression is not fully understood, research suggests that depression is caused by an imbalance of certain chemicals in the brain, most notably serotonin. [20]

It is misleading to state that the brain chemistry of depression is not *fully* understood, when in truth it is really not understood at all. It is also misleading to state that "research suggests" that "depression is caused by an imbalance" of brain chemicals. It is drug companies, doctors and researchers who suggest this, not the research itself. As outlined in detail earlier, the research itself does not suggest this at all and indeed contradicts this notion. No reliable scientific evidence for this theory has ever been identified. The following was on the Lexapro website up to May 2009:

> Whatever the circumstances, depression is caused by an imbalance of certain chemicals in the brain. Normally, these "chemical messengers" help nerve cells communicate with one another by sending and receiving messages. They may also influence a person's mood. In the case of depression, the available supply of the chemical messengers is low, so nerves can't communicate effectively. This often results in symptoms of depression. [21]

This passage contains false claims. The hypothesis that depression may be caused by a chemical imbalance is misrepresented as an established fact: "depression is caused by an imbalance of certain chemicals in the brain". Claiming this to be the case "whatever the circumstances" is in my opinion a display of breathtaking arrogance, given that such imbalances have not been found in *any* circumstances. It is therefore a Begging the Question logical fallacy. [22] Stating as a fact that "the available supply of chemical messengers is low" is a falsehood, since this has never been established. Stating as a fact that low levels of chemical messengers "results in symptoms of depression" is a striking example of a False Cause logical fallacy. [23]

Forest Pharmaceuticals also manufacture the antidepressant Celexa, a commonly prescribed antidepressant in some countries including the United States. From the "Frequently Asked Questions" of manufacturer Forest Pharmaceuticals website in 2005:

> Celexa helps to restore the brain's chemical imbalance by increasing the supply of a chemical messenger called serotonin. Although the brain chemistry of depression is not fully understood, there does exist a growing body of evidence to support the view that people with depression have an imbalance of the brain's neurotransmitters. [24]

It cannot be rightly stated as a known fact that Celexa "helps to restore the brain's chemical imbalance" when no such chemical imbalance has ever been identified to exist. No "growing body of evidence" exists that supports "the view that people with depression have an imbalance of the brain's neurotransmitters". This is a series of misleading fabrications, designed to persuade doctors and the public. It is outrageous that this company and others have been allowed to get away with such practices for over a quarter of a century.

PFIZER

The drug company Pfizer was the original manufacturer of sertraline, which was marketed in some countries as Zoloft and in others as Lustral. According to a 2011 statement by Pfizer:

> Zoloft works to correct a chemical imbalance in the brain which may be related to symptoms of depression or certain anxiety conditions. [25]

Translating this quote into plain English and adding a sprinkling of truth, according to Pfizer, Zoloft works to correct a chemical imbalance in the brain that has never been established to exist, yet the drug makers know for sure it is there. Not only do they know that, they also apparently know that depression is likely to be related to this chemical imbalance that they know exists though it has never been identified to exist. The following was present on the Zoloft.com website in 2009:

> Because it is linked with so many functions in our body, serotonin has an effect on a wide range of conditions such as depression. This tie between serotonin and depression has led scientists to an interesting find. Scientists believe people with depression could have an imbalance of serotonin in the brain. That means the level of serotonin is "off". So the nerve cells can't communicate, or send messages to each other the right way. This lack of contact between cells might cause depression. Zoloft helps fix this. Zoloft helps the nerve cells send messages to each other the way they normally should. [26]

Many inaccuracies and falsehoods occur in this passage. As outlined earlier, it has not been established scientifically that serotonin has an effect on depression. There is no such "tie between serotonin and depression", other than the hypothetical tie that has been invented by the pharmaceutical industry and many enthusiastic medical researchers and practitioners. The "interesting find" referred to in the second sentence turns out in the next sentence not to be a find at all but merely an unsubstantiated belief; "Scientists believe people with depression could have an imbalance of serotonin in the brain". A belief is not a find.

The next four sentences are logically flawed for several reasons. Being grounded upon and consequent to a premise which is itself wholly speculative, these four sentences cannot be taken as facts, yet they are misleadingly presented as such. Describing levels of serotonin as "off" is an unverified claim, but the vagueness and unscientific nature of the word "off" does reveal the dearth of true scientific facts these people have at their disposal to support their claims. The four sentences in which the supposed problems within the brain communication systems are set out are utterly fictional, though misleadingly presented as known scientific facts. The claim that "Zoloft helps fixes this" and the preceding sentences are striking examples of logical gymnastics. The manufacturers are claiming as a fact that Zoloft helps to fix something that has not been identified to be broken. There is not a shred of reliable scientific evidence that confirms or even suggests that "the nerve cells can't communicate, or send messages to each other the right way." Therefore, claiming that "this lack of contact between cells might cause depression" when no such lack of contact has been established in the first place is logical nonsense. But the reader is unlikely to know this, and is likely to believe this information as accurate and trustworthy. According to a 2004 Zoloft advertisement:

> While the cause is unknown, depression may be related to an imbalance of natural chemicals between nerve cells in the brain. Prescription Zoloft works to correct this imbalance. You shouldn't have to feel this way anymore. [27]

The advertisers begin with a truth. The assumed biological cause of depression is unknown; the assumed biological cause that the medical profession and the pharmaceutical industry keep emphasizing has not been verified scientifically. Having acknowledged this, the company focuses solely on just one possible cause, one which they claim their drug acts upon, for which there is no objective evidence. It seems quite a coincidence that the only mentioned possible cause happens to be beneficial in regard to the drug companies own interests; producing substances that are called antidepressant drugs. As with the previous advertisement, this one also contains a similarly subtle and apparently innocuous comment that is utterly incongruous. The advert states unequivocally that Zoloft corrects an imbalance of natural chemicals, even though this imbalance has not been demonstrated to exist. The last sentence conveys an impression of empathy. The caring drug company doesn't want you to suffer any more. Take their tablet, and your suffering will be over.

Wyeth is the manufacturer of the antidepressant Effexor, in which the active ingredient is venlafaxine. From the Wyeth website in 2009:

> Effexor SR is believed to treat depression and anxiety symptoms by affecting the levels of naturally occurring chemicals in the brain—serotonin and norepinephrine. It is believed that correcting an imbalance of these two chemicals may relieve symptoms of depression. [28]

Again, the subtle deceptive persuasion. It is correct that Effexor is "believed" to affect brain chemical levels, beneficially of course. Referring to these chemicals as "naturally occurring" was a clever strategy. Of course they are naturally occurring. The use of this term suggests to the reader that Effexor's action too is natural—which is not the case— and therefore appropriate and safe. The authors of the sentence, "It is believed that correcting an imbalance of these two chemicals", failed to mention the fact that no such imbalance had been demonstrated to exist.

Direct-to-consumer advertising is permitted in the United States and New Zealand. This practice provides drug companies with the opportunity to address the consumer directly and put misleading ideas into their heads about brain chemical imbalances in depression. In a 2008 internet article, integrative therapist Chris Kresser expressed concern regarding misleading drug company direct-to-consumer advertising in America:

> For example, Pfizer's television advertisement for Zoloft states that "depression is a serious medical condition that may be due to a chemical imbalance" and that "Zoloft works to correct this imbalance". Other SSRI advertising campaigns make similar claims. The Effexor website even has a slick video explaining that "research suggests an important link between depression and an imbalance in some of the brain's chemical messengers", and that "Two neurotransmitters believed to be involved in depression are serotonin and norepinephrine". The video goes on to explain that Effexor works by increasing serotonin levels in the synapse, which is "believed to relieve symptoms of depression over time". [29]

DRUG REGULATORY AUTHORITIES

Effective regulation of the pharmaceutical industry is vitally important. The pharmaceutical industry is a powerful global entity. The U.S. Food and Drug Administration (FDA) requires that advertisements "cannot be false or misleading" and "must present information that is not inconsistent with the product label". [30] FDA regulations have not prevented drug companies putting many falsehoods regarding depression and neurotransmitters into the public arena, a sample of which I presented earlier. Having reviewed this area in detail, researchers Jeffrey Lacasse and Jonathan Leo concluded in 2005:

The incongruence between the scientific literature and the claims made in FDA-regulated SSRI advertisements is remarkable, and possibly unparalleled. [31]

I mentioned earlier the Irish Medicines Board's 2003 decision to advise the makers of Seroxat to correct false information that had been on their patient information leaflet since the drug was launched twelve years previously. In October 2002 I became aware that the patient information leaflet that accompanied every pack of Seroxat sold in Ireland had for the previous eleven years contained wording which seriously misinformed anyone who read it. The wording in question was:

> This medicine works by bringing the levels of serotonin back to normal. Seroxat is one of the antidepressants that works by returning your serotonin levels to normal. [32]

I immediately knew that these statements were untrue. I wrote to the Irish Medicines Board, expressing alarm that international regulatory bodies would permit such a situation to occur. The following extract from my first letter to the Irish Medicines Board outlined the true situation:

> Patients on Seroxat *never* have their serotonin levels measured prior to treatment to assess whether their serotonin levels are normal or abnormal to begin with. Patients *never* have their serotonin levels checked while on treatment to see whether their so-called "abnormal" serotonin levels have returned to normal. It has not been scientifically established what the normal range of serotonin actually is; and obviously if we don't know what constitutes "normal" serotonin levels, our knowledge of what constitutes "abnormal" serotonin levels is inevitably seriously deficient.
>
> When treatment with Seroxat (and the other SSRIs) is stopped, no attempt is made by the doctor to assess serotonin levels. If Seroxat was working all along by "returning your serotonin levels to normal" as the leaflet so emphatically states, what happened to one's serotonin level when Seroxat is stopped? Does it somehow miraculously remain "normal" in the absence of treatment? Or does it become "abnormal" again?
>
> The bottom line here is that we doctors haven't a clue what happens to our patients' serotonin levels when the drug is stopped because we have no way of measuring our patients' serotonin levels, and we do not know what constitutes "normal" or "abnormal" levels. The bottom line is that we doctors have no idea whether the patients we treat with Seroxat (and other SSRIs) have a normal, low or raised serotonin level at any stage of the entire process of diagnosis and treatment. And we have absolutely no idea how our patients' serotonin levels are responding to the treatment on an ongoing basis. In twenty years as a medical doctor, I have never, ever heard of a patient anywhere having their serotonin levels checked. [33]

The Irish Medicines Board did not take issue with any point I raised. In their November 2002 reply, the Irish Medicines Board informed me that:

> The Irish Medicines Board has been reviewing this matter with its experts for some time and is in agreement that the statement that SSRIs "work by bringing the levels of serotonin back to normal" is not consistent with the literature. The company has been asked to review the patient information leaflet accordingly. Thank you for your interest in this matter. [34]

In November and December of 2002, I wrote two further letters to the Irish Medicines Board. Among other issues, I asked the Board how it could have transpired that such information, acknowledged by the Irish Medicines Board as "not consistent with the scientific literature", was ever allowed to appear on the patient information leaflet, and how it could have remained there for the previous eleven years. I felt that the replies from the Irish Medicines Board to these and other questions were neither comprehensive nor satisfactory. Then in May 2003 I received a letter from the Irish Medicines Board (italics theirs):

> Dear Dr. Lynch, Further to my letter of 10 February 2003, I now wish to confirm that the package leaflet for the Seroxat range has been revised. Regarding mechanism of action, the original phrase "*Seroxat . . . works by bringing serotonin levels back to normal*" has been replaced by "Seroxat works . . . by altering serotonin function. There is evidence that such function is disturbed in depression". [35]

I was far from satisfied with this new wording, and I was struck by the fact that the Irish Medicines Board appeared satisfied with it. GlaxoSmithKline had merely substituted one falsehood for another, under the direct view of the Irish Medicines Board. To state that "there is evidence" that serotonin "function" is "disturbed in depression" is as untrue as their previous claims that Seroxat brought serotonin levels back to normal. The drug company had in effect run rings around the Irish drug regulatory authority. This whole episode demonstrated to me how powerful drug companies are and how important it is for their interests to maintain the biochemical imbalance delusion as a real entity in people's minds. The drug company received no sanction or penalty for misleading the public so blatantly for eleven years, and were in effect given the green light by the Irish drug regulatory authorities to continue misleading the Irish public into the future.

When the Irish Medicines Board wrote to inform me of the changed wording, I presumed that this change was being applied in many countries and was the result of a broader review. The fact that the Irish wording change has been referred to widely by many international authors since then suggests that it may not have been a widely international move.

Drug regulatory authorities internationally have failed to prevent drug companies from promoting falsehoods—that brain chemical imbalances occur in depression, and that antidepressants correct these imbalances—as facts since Prozac became available in 1988. These regulatory bodies might have stemmed the explosion of depression diagnoses and antidepressant prescribing if they had insisted that drug companies stick to the truth in their pronouncements about depression and medication.

PHARMACISTS

Pharmacists play an important role in health care, regularly providing expert information regarding medications to patients. In practice, pharmacists tend to work with and support the prescriptions written by doctors. It is therefore not surprising that some pharmacy journals and websites promote the brain chemical imbalance misinformation to their clients. Compared to some groups and professions involved in depression, in my experience pharmacists are certainly not the worst offenders.

U.S. *Pharmacist* is a prominent monthly pharmacy journal. According to its website, *U.S. Pharmacist*:

> Is a monthly journal dedicated to providing the nation's pharmacists with up-to-date, authoritative, peer-reviewed clinical studies relevant to contemporary pharmacy practice in a variety of settings, including community pharmacy, hospitals, managed care systems, ambulatory care clinics, home care organizations, long-term care facilities, industry and academia. The publication is also useful to pharmacy technicians, students, other health professionals and individuals interested in health management. [36]

The message is that *U.S. Pharmacist* is a high quality journal trusted by the wide range of pharmacy activities within America. No doubt the journal does generally live up to these expectations. However, *U.S. Pharmacist* is promoting misinformation on its website regarding claimed brain chemical abnormalities in depression:

> In depression . . . critical neurotransmitters are out of balance. [37]

No reliable scientific evidence has ever established that "critical neurotransmitters are out of balance".

Short Hills Pharmacy in New Jersey USA has been serving the local community for over 80 years. According to their website, this pharmacy is:

> Staffed with highly experienced pharmacists, committed to providing you with knowledgeable advice and counselling about your prescription and over-the-counter medication needs. [38]

Yet, regarding depression, this pharmacy's website contains the following misinformation about brain chemicals and depression:

> Researchers aren't sure whether malfunctioning neurotransmitters (brain chemicals that regulate mood) cause depression or whether it's changes in mood that affect brain chemistry. [39]

This sentence wrongly conveys the message that "malfunctioning neurotransmitters" are an established fact in depression; all that remains is to ascertain whether these brain chemical abnormalities are the cause or the effect of depression. This is clearly misinformation, since no such abnormalities have been established to occur. This assertion from a reputable and respected U.S. pharmacy is both a Begging the Question logical fallacy [40] and a False Cause logical fallacy. [41]

NOTES TO CHAPTER SIX

1.   Eli Lilly, Prozac advertisement, *People* magazine, January 1998, p. 40.
2.   As quoted in Elliot S. Valenstein, *Blaming the Brain: The Truth About Drugs and Mental Health*, New York: The Free Press, 1998, p. 180.
3.   "How Prozac works", http://www.prozac.com/how_prozac_works.jsp?reqNavId=2.2, accessed 06 February 2006 by Joanna Moncrieff, quoted in her 2006 *British Journal of Psychiatry* editorial article "Psychiatric drug promotion and the politics of neoliberalism", 188, 301-302, Editorial.
4.   Accessed by Joanna Moncrieff in 2006, in Joanna Moncrieff, *The Myth of the Chemical Cure: A critique of Psychiatric Drug Treatment,* 2009, Basingstoke: Palgrave Macmillan, p. 59; and Eli Lilly's website, http://www.prozac.com/how_prozac_works.jsp?reqNavId=2.2, accessed 6th February 2006 by Joanna Moncrieff, in her 2006 *British Journal of Psychiatry* editorial article "Psychiatric drug promotion and the politics of neoliberalism", 188, 301-302, Editorial.
5.   Eli Lilly website, https://www.lilly.ie/your-health/major-depressive-disorder, accessed 19 March 2014.
6.   "Depression", Lilly UK website, https://www.lilly.co.uk/en/about/what-we-do/biomedicines/depression.aspx, accessed 05 October 2014.
7.   "What Causes Depression", Lundbeck website, http://www.leanonme.net/ie/about-depression/what-causes-depression, accessed 09 April 14.
8.   "Feeling Better" brochure, Lundbeck website, https://www.lundbeck.com/upload/ca/en/files/pdf/MentalHealth-%2520eng.pdf, accessed 29 March 2014, p. 7.
9.   Lundbeck website, "Mind yourself at work: Depression in the workplace—a guide for employees", https://www.lundbeck.com/upload/ie/files/pdf/leaflets/Mind_yourself_at_work_leaflet.pdf, p. 5, accessed 05 October 2014.
10.   Lundbeck Australia Pty Ltd., "Depression: What You Should Know", pps 3 & 14, June 2006, https://www.lundbeck.com/upload/au/files/pdf/MDD_Booklet.pdf, accessed 05 October 2014.
11.   "Feeling Better: Dealing With Anxiety In The Workplace", published in association with Rogers Publishing Ltd., p. 7, https://www.desjardinslifeinsurance.com/en/life-events/Documents/Feeling%20better.pdf, accessed 06 October 2014.
12.   "What causes depression?" webpage, Leanonme website, http://www.leanonme.net/ie/about-depression/what-causes-depression, accessed 06 October 2014.
13.   "Lean on Me – to Win: A Winning Mentality for a Positive Mind", p. 13, http://www.leanonme.net/upload/ie/pdf/LOMTW.pdf, accessed 06 October 2014.
14.   For information on Begging the Question logical fallacies see note 22 in the Notes to the Introduction.
15.   Glaxosmithkline, Paxil Advertisement. *Newsweek* 61, October 2001.
16.   Glaxosmithkline, Paxil Prescribing Information. Research Triangle Park, North Carolina: Glaxosmithkline, 2003.
17.   GlaxoSmithKline, SSRIs like Paxil CR help to balance serotonin, http://www.paxilcr.com/how_paxilcr_works/how_paxilcr_works.html, viewed on September 6, 2008 by Christian Perring Ph. D., "'Madness' and 'Brain Disorders': Stigma and Language" http://www.inter-disciplinary.net/wp-content/uploads/2008/12/perring-paper.pdf.

18. paxilcr.com website, 01 May 2009, http://www.anxietycentre.com/downloads/Chemical-Imbalance-Theory-is-False.pdf, accessed 24 February 2014.

19. Forest Pharmaceuticals, "How Lexapro (escitalopram) works", New York: Forest Pharmaceuticals, 2005. Available: http://www. lexapro.com/english/about_lexapro. Cited by Jeffrey R. La-casse & Jonathan Leo, "Serotonin and Depression: A Disconnect between the Advertisements and the Scientific Literature", *PLoS Med* 2(12): e392. doi:10.1371/journal.pmed.0020392, access-ed 12 may 2014.

20. Lexapro press release, http://psychroaches.blogspot.ie/2011/04/chemical-imbalance-mythfraud. html, accessed 24.02.14.

21. Taken from the Lexapro website on May 1st 2009, http://www.anxietycentre.com/downloads /Chemical-Imbalance-Theory-is-False.pdf, accessed 24.02.14.

22. For information on Begging the Question logical fallacies see Note 22 in the Notes to the Introduction.

23. For information on False Cause logical fallacies see note 42 in Chapter Five.

24. Forest Pharmaceuticals website, Frequently Asked Questions, New York: Forest Pharmaceuticals, 2005, http://www.celexa.com/Celexa/faq.aspx, accessed on 17 October 2005 by Jeffrey R. Lacasse and Jonathan Leo, "Serotonin and Depression: A Disconnect between the Advertisements and the Scientific Literature", *PLoS Med* 2(12): e392. doi:10.1371/journal.pmed.0020392, accessed 24 February 2014.

25. "What is Zoloft?", cited in http://psychroaches.blogspot.ie/2011/04/chemical-imbalance-mythfraud.html, accessed 12 May 2014.

26. zoloft.com website, 01 May 2009, http://www.anxietycentre.com/downloads/Chemical-Imbalance-Theory-is-False.pdf, accessed 24.02.14.

27. Zoloft advertisement, March 2004, Pfizer, Burbank (California), NBC, cited by Jeffrey R. Lacasse & Jonathan Leo, "Serotonin and Depression: A Disconnect between the Advertisements and the Scientific Literature". *PLoS Med* 2(12): e392. doi:10.1371/journal.pmed.0020392, accessed 2 February 2014.

28. Wyeth 2006, effexorxr.com/condition.asp website as of 01 May 2009, http://www.anxietycentre.com/downloads/Chemical-Imbalance-Theory-is-False.pdf, accessed 24 February 2014.

29. Chris Kresser, "The 'Chemical Imbalance' Myth", 2008, http://chriskresser.com/the-chemical-imbalance-myth, accessed 26.02.14.

30. United States General Accounting Office (2002) "Prescription drugs: FDA oversight of direct-to-consumer advertising has limitations." Washington (D.C.): United States General Accounting Office.

31. J.R. Lacasse & J. Leo, "Serotonin and depression: A Disconnect between the Advertisements and the Scientific Literature", 08 November 2005, *PLoS Med*, 2(12) e392.

32. Seroxat Patient Information Leaflet, 2002.

33. Letter from me to Irish Medicines Board, 19 October 2002.

34. Letter from Irish Medicines Board to me, November 2002.

35. Letter from Irish Medicines Board to me, May 2003.

36. U.S. Pharmacist website, http://www.uspharmacist.com/content/d/feature/ c/31081/, accessed 15 September 2014.

37. Charles Brown, Professor Emeritus of Clinical Pharmacy, "Pharmacotherapy of Major Depressive Disorder", *U.S. Pharmacist,* http://www.uspharmacist.com/content/d/feature/c/31081/, access-ed 15 September 2014.

38. Short Hills Pharmacy, New Jersey, website, https://www.shorthillspharmacy.com/index.php, accessed 15 September 2014.

39. Short Hills Pharmacy website, New Jersey, "Depression", https://www.shorthillspharmacy. com /library.php?id=644934, accessed 15 September 2014.

40. For information on Begging the Question logical fallacies see note 22 in the Notes to the Introduction.

41. For information on False Cause logical fallacies see note 42 in the Notes to Chapter Five.

7. PSYCHOLOGY, PSYCHOTHERAPY AND BRAIN CHEMICAL IMBALANCES

The magnitude of the depression delusion is demonstrated by the fact that many mental health professionals outside the medical profession such as psychology have embraced the delusion as truth. Many members of the professions of psychology, psychotherapy and counselling have raised serious questions about the assumed brain chemical deficiency in depression, the validity of the *Diagnostic and Statistical Manual of Mental Disorders* and the dominance of biological approach to mental health. However, given the long-term and widespread promotion of depression as a brain chemical imbalance, it is not surprising that misinformation regarding depression and brain chemicals has to some extent also permeated the world of psychology, counselling and psychotherapy. It is significant that some psychologists and therapists mistakenly accept the brain chemical abnormality idea as either an established fact or as a likely occurrence in depression. Perhaps because psychology is more aligned to psychiatry than psychotherapy, in my research for this book I found more examples of the depression brain chemical imbalance delusion in psychology than in psychotherapy.

It is easy to understand why many psychologists and psychotherapists might believe that brain chemical imbalances are known to occur in depression. These professionals are not immune to the effects of repetition of the widely assumed link between depression and serotonin they regularly encounter in conversation, magazines, books and the media. Aware of their place on the mental health pyramid—at the top of which are doctors, psychiatrists particularly—many psychologists, psychotherapists and counsellors defer to the supposedly superior knowledge of these doctors. Many do so even when intuitively they feel that the brain chemical abnormality explanation does not tally with their daily work experience with clients or their own understanding of depression.

While many psychologists and psychotherapists do very good work with people diagnosed with depression without reference to the brain chemical imbalance notion in depression, the pervasive nature of the depression brain chemical imbalance belief can at times affect their work. For example, many people who attend them will already have received a diagnosis of depression from their doctor and a prescription for antidepressant medication. Many will have been told by their doctors that they have a brain chemical deficiency and the drug will correct this imbalance. Given that doctors are generally seen as higher in the chain of expertise, few psychologists and therapists feel in a position to challenge these assertions, either with the person with whom they are working or with the doctor who put this idea into the person's mind. A young woman currently attending me had been diagnosed with depression for two years. The list of professionals she had previously attended included her GP, a psychiatrist and two counsellors. She recently told me that I was the first professional she attended who did not tell her that she had a brain chemical imbalance. Off all medication for the past six months and thriving, she never did have a chemical imbalance.

PSYCHOLOGY

While the predominant view that brain chemical imbalances exist in depression is not universally accepted within the field of psychology, belief in this notion is not uncommon within this profession. For example, according to the *Psychology Today* website (italics mine), "Important neurotransmitters *appear* to be out of balance" in depression. [1]

HOOK, LINE AND SINKER

In 2002, two psychologists—Professor Brent D. Slife and Dr. Colin M. Burchfield Ph.D.—and a psychiatrist, Associate Professor Dawson W. Hedges, were invited to address the Rocky Mountain Psychological Association in Park City, Utah. All three were at that time affiliated to the Department of Psychology at Brigham Young University, Utah, USA. Their address was titled "Hook, Line and Sinker: Psychology's Uncritical Acceptance of Biological Explanation". [2] According to these three professionals (brackets mine):

> Both the experimental and the applied aspects of our discipline are moving headlong toward exclusively materialist (biological) explanations, with almost no critical examination . . . debates rarely, if ever, broach the fundamental issues, such as "should we explain people in solely biological terms?" . . . Even in my relatively short professional career, many psychologists seem to have changed the diagnosis of depression from a mostly psychological disorder, with psychological causes and treatments, to a biological disorder . . . Psychology is taking a "headlong plunge" into this tidal wave.

Regarding the biochemical abnormality theory of depression, the authors stated that:

> Psychology has accepted such explanation without evidence. In fact, psychology has accepted such explanations despite considerable evidence to the contrary.

The authors continued (italics theirs):

> Because we assume philosophically the sufficiency of the biological *before* investigation, we do not need to critically examine biological research *after* investigation. The sufficiency of biological explanation is a truism, already accepted "hook, line and sinker" in our background assumptions about the world, before any data has been gathered. Data gathering, in this sense, is basically window dressing, validating what we already know to be true. The problem is that we do not know it to be true. As scientists, we cannot accept it as true until it has been thoroughly tested. However, there is an even more compelling reason to make us certain that it is thoroughly tested—this form of materialism can rob us of our humanity.

Within the profession of psychology, these authors are not alone in their conclusion that biological perspectives have become the dominant view in psychology. In a 1989 article, psychologist Robert Plomin described how some biological explanations were enjoying "a wave of acceptance" in psychology that was "growing into a tidal wave". [3]

According to some psychologists, psychology has rapidly become "biologized", meaning that biological explanations have largely replaced psychological explanations within psychology. [4] One psychologist wrote in 1994 that the biological emphasis within psychology and psychotherapy had increased to such a degree that diagnoses were rarely considered other than fundamentally biological problems. [5]

Professor of Psychology at Brooklyn College Matthew H. Erdelyi has created a YouTube video titled "What is depression?". In the seven years since this video was uploaded on 23 August 2007, by September 2014 just short of 1,060,000 people have been exposed to the following blatant misinformation:

> It is important to understand that when someone has depression, there are . . . reduced levels of important chemicals called neurotransmitters . . . People suffering from depression typically have reduced levels of neurotransmitters, especially serotonin. Lower levels of serotonin lead to mood destabilization and depression. [6]

In my opinion, it is extremely worrying that a respected psychology professor would consider it appropriate to include such misinformation on a video that is apparently intended to "educate" the public. Presumably he believed what he said to be true. This professor either knows or should know that reduced levels of serotonin have never been identified as occurring in depression. At the very least, he should have familiarised himself with the facts. It appears that like so many others, this professor has been seduced by the depression brain chemical imbalance delusion. Like so many others, having become a believer he has turned preacher, making claims that belong solely within the realm of fiction and faith rather than fact and evidence-based science.

The eighth edition of *Introduction to Psychology* is a comprehensive 1983 psychology textbook of 701 pages. Two of the three authors were then attached to the University of California, San Diego and the third to Stanford University. According to these authors:

> Mounting evidence indicates that our moods are regulated by a group of chemicals called neurotransmitters . . . A widely accepted hypothesis is that depression is associated with a deficiency . . . of these neurotransmitters. [7]

The authors add that "the evidence is indirect". [8] They continue (brackets mine):

> There is no doubt that affective disorders (of which depression is considered one) involve biochemical changes in the nervous system. The unresolved question is whether the physiological changes are the cause or the result of the psychological changes. [9]

Regarding antidepressant drugs, according to this psychology textbook:

> These drugs energize rather than tranquillize, apparently by increasing the availability of two neurotransmitters (norepinephrine and serotonin) that are deficient in some cases of depression. [10]

Written five years before the launch of Prozac, this book illustrates that the biochemical imbalance notion preceded the arrival of the SSRI drugs. While some of this text is accurate, much of it is not, indicating that these respected psychology academics have unwittingly succumbed to the depression brain chemical imbalance delusion.

Depression being associated with a deficiency of brain neurotransmitter has indeed been a widely accepted hypothesis for almost five decades, but there is no direct evidence to confirm this. Many antidepressants do energize rather than tranquillize. However, it is incorrect to claim that mounting evidence indicates that our moods are regulated by our brain chemicals. This assumption is widespread, but it is without any confirming scientific evidence.

The authors' assertion that "There is no doubt that affective disorders (such as depression) involve biochemical changes in the brain. The unresolved question is whether the physiological changes are the cause or the result of the psychological changes" is problematic. A doubting and questioning attitude is a key characteristic of any true science. To assert that there can be no doubt about something that has no direct evidence to support it is therefore a rather dubious practice scientifically. The primary question here is not whether physiological changes are cause or effect; it is whether they are present at all. In stating as a fact that "the availability of two neurotransmitters . . ." is "deficient in some cases of depression", the authors are misleading their readers and appear to have forgotten their earlier description of the biochemical brain deficiency notion as a "widely accepted hypothesis".

Understanding and Treating Depressed Adolescents and their Families is a 1990 book written by American psychologists Gerald D. Oster and Janice E. Caro. According to these authors:

> Much of the research data has demonstrated that depressed persons have imbalances of neurotransmitters, which are the natural chemicals that allow communication between brain cells. In general, individuals suffering from mood disorders display (a) a deficit of neurotransmitters, which may lead to depression; (b) an excess of them, which may lead to mania; or (c) an imbalance of them. [11]

This passage contains many falsehoods. "Imbalances of neurotransmitters" in "depressed persons" have never been "demonstrated" to exist. It is wholly inaccurate to state with certainty that "individuals suffering from mood disorders display" either "a deficit of neurotransmitters", "an excess of them" or "an imbalance of them". Not one of these assertions is scientifically established as a fact. It is unfortunate that these and other authors and so-called experts did not ascertain the facts before publishing such misinformation. Such is the level of penetration of the depression delusion within the collective consciousness that separating facts from delusion is not an easy task.

In their 1993 book on depression titled *Understanding Depression: A Complete Guide To Its Diagnosis And Treatment*, psychologists Klein and Wender concluded:

> Depression has a biological rather than a psychological cause. [12]

Psychologist Tony Bates is one of Ireland's best known and most respected psychologists. He wrote a chapter titled "Depression" in the 1994 book *Nervous Breakdown*, in which he stated:

> In severe episodes of depression there is a malfunction in the amount of serotonin available. [13]

This assertion is presented as an established fact, without any indication from the author that it is merely an unsubstantiated theory. It appears that Tony Bates believed the supposed link between depression and theorised biochemical brain abnormalities to be an established fact when he wrote this. Presenting a theory as a fact constitutes misinformation, whether intentional or not.

In Tony Bates' later books, the stated certainty regarding serotonin had been relegated to a possibility, which may reflect a shift in the author's understanding. Nevertheless, in his 1999 book *Depression: The Common Sense Approach*, Bates included a sentence which is strictly speaking correct but which overstates the value of its content and may inadvertently misinform the reader:

> Depletion in the availability of certain neurotransmitters has been linked to depression. [14]

The reader might erroneously interpret this to mean that a scientific link has been found between depression and depletion of neurotransmitters. This is not correct. The link is merely conjecture, which remains totally unproven after 50 years of trying and is in fact discredited, as I discussed in chapter three. Neurotransmitter depletion has never even been demonstrated in the human brain, let alone linked scientifically to depression. In his 2011 book *Coming Through Depression*, Tony Bates wrote:

> In severe episodes of depression, there is believed to be a reduction in the amount of serotonin available in the brain which, in turn, causes fatigue, listlessness and sleep disturbance, so characteristic of depression. [15]

While this wording is strictly speaking correct, because it is not balanced by a statement to the effect that there is no direct scientific evidence to confirm this belief, the reader may erroneously conclude that low serotonin is known to cause the experiences listed. This is clearly not the case, since low brain serotonin levels have never been identified in relation to any human experience. One might also conclude that the author accepts the notion of "biological symptoms" arising secondary to serotonin deficiency, a questionable though commonly made assumption that has no established scientific basis. Bates added:

> Depression is often treated with medication to regulate specific biochemical changes in the brain that are believed to play a part in keeping our mood in a depressed state. Research is not clear what exactly these changes are. [16]

The first sentence of this passage conveys the impression that there are known specific biochemical changes in the brain, and that these identified changes are believed to be linked to depression. Yet the next sentence appears to contradict this, intimating that these changes are not yet "exactly" identified. How can something that has not been found to exist be accurately described as "specific biochemical changes"? The sentence, "Research is not clear what *exactly* these changes are (italics mine)" may be erroneously interpreted to mean that these changes do definitely exist, research just hasn't yet *fully* clarified the detail of the changes. At best they are hypothesised biological changes; medical science is nowhere near "exactly" identifying any such biochemical changes.

Joseph Carver Ph.D. is an American psychologist. He is the author of "The 'Chemical Imbalance' in Mental Health Problems", a 2002 article. [17] This article opens with a statement that it "has been developed and written for use as a patient handout. It may be reproduced/copied to provide patient information". [18] This has become an influential paper, often cited by people writing about depression. I have rarely encountered an article containing more fiction and misinformation relating to depression and neurotransmitters. According to Carver:

> As research in neurotransmitters continued, studies between neurotransmitters and mental conditions revealed a strong connection between amounts of certain neurotransmitters in the brain and the presence of specific psychiatric conditions. [19]

In fact, studies between neurotransmitters and mental conditions did not reveal *any* connection between the amount of brain neurotransmitters and the presence of psychiatric conditions. The author continued:

> Research tells us that several neurotransmitters are related to mental health problems . . . Too much or too little of these neurotransmitters are now felt to produce psychiatric conditions such as schizophrenia, depression, bipolar disorder, obsessive-compulsive disorder, and ADHD. [20]

Research does not tell us that lower or higher neurotransmitter levels produce any psychiatric disorders, depression included. The author compared depression to medical conditions, as if the medical approach to these conditions is a precedent that also applies to depression:

> Medical patients with high blood pressure, high blood sugar, or high cholesterol are informed that their body chemistry is too high, or in some cases, too low and must be corrected with medication. [21]

Carver does not point out a core difference between depression and the conditions he mentioned. In all of these conditions with the exception of depression, doctors have something to measure. Doctors also have knowledge of the normal and abnormal levels of what they are measuring. In depression there is no biological marker to measure, no test to measure it with, and no scientific clarity regarding what normal or abnormal levels might be, or even if this approach applies to brain neurotransmitters in depression at all. Carver wrote:

> For many years, mental health professionals have used the term "chemical imbalance" to explain the need for medications that are used to treat mental health conditions. This simple and commonly used explanation recognizes that the condition is a medical problem and that it can be treated with medication. [22]

Using the term "chemical imbalance" to "explain the need for medications" is a classic Begging the Question logical fallacy, since the foundation of the argument is itself conjecture; no such chemical imbalances are known to exist. [23] Carver continued:

> Four neurotransmitters, out of fifty, are well researched and known to be related to psychiatric conditions . . . Serotonin, first isolated in 1933, is the neurotransmitter that has been identified in multiple psychiatric disorders including depression . . . The less serotonin available to the brain, the more severe our depression and related symptoms. [24]

Carver failed to inform the reader that all of this research has yielded no tangible scientific information regarding postulated neurotransmitter abnormalities or evidence of the role of neurotransmitters in depression of other psychiatric diagnoses. It is grossly incorrect to claim that "serotonin . . . has been identified in multiple psychiatric disorders including depression". No scientific evidence exists that confirms his claim that "The less serotonin available to the brain, the more severe our depression and related symptoms". Carver made many further claims:

> When serotonin is low, we experience problems with concentration and attention. We become scatterbrained and poorly organized. Routine responsibilities now seem overwhelming. It takes longer to do things because of poor planning. We lose our car keys and put odd things in the refrigerator. We call people and forget why we called or go to the grocery and forget what we needed. We tell people the same thing two or three times. [25]

This too is nonsense. There is no scientific evidence to back up the author's claim that all of the above happens "when serotonin is low". Low serotonin cannot ever be identified since brain serotonin cannot be measured and we do not know what serotonin levels should or should not be. There are no reliable tests for brain serotonin levels. We do not even know if such concepts are applicable to serotonin and depression. I regularly forget where I put my keys. From time to time in a store I purchase some items, receive the change from the store attendant, and then exit the shop with my purchases still on the counter. I did it again last Sunday, leaving mushrooms and milk needed for breakfast on the counter behind me. I do these things not because my serotonin is low, but simply because my mind and my attention is elsewhere at that moment in time. Carver continued:

> When serotonin is low, we have the following symptoms and behaviours; chronic fatigue . . . sleep disturbance . . . appetite disturbance . . . total loss of sexual interest . . . social withdrawal . . . emotional sadness and frequent crying spells . . . self-esteem and self-confidence is low . . . loss of personality . . . we begin to take everything very personally . . . you talk less, smile less, and sit for hours without noticing anyone . . . your behaviour becomes odd. [26]

Again, no scientific evidence exists that identifies the cause of these experiences and behaviours to be low serotonin, but that certainly isn't the message one picks up from reading this passage. Carver continued:

> Very low levels of serotonin typically bring people to the attention of their family physician, their employer, or other sources of help. Severe serotonin loss produces symptoms that are difficult to ignore . . . When serotonin is severely low, you will experience some if not all of the following; . . . thinking speed will increase . . . the brain will focus on torturing memories . . . you'll become emotionally numb . . . outbursts will begin . . . temper tantrums may surface . . . escape fantasies will begin . . . you'll have evil thoughts . . . you'll develop a Need-for-Change Panic. You'll begin thinking a change in lifestyle (Midlife Crisis!), a divorce, an extramarital affair, or a Corvette will change your mood. [27]

While people may experience or do some or all of the above, asserting that the cause is "very low" or "severely low" serotonin levels is fantasyland stuff in the extreme. The author continued:

> As stress continues and our serotonin level continues to drop, we become more depressed. [28]

To present this utterly unevidenced assertion to a public likely to believe it as a known scientific fact is in my opinion an act of major public misinformation, whether done intentionally or not. According to Carver:

> Mental health professionals use psychological testing, interviews, questionnaires, and patient history to determine first, if a change in the neurotransmitter system is present, then second, what neurotransmitters are involved. [29]

Mental health professionals do use psychological testing, interviews, questionnaires and take histories for their patients. But they do not do so as a means of determining either "a change in the neurotransmitter system" or "what neurotransmitters are involved".

Any such deductions would be logically and scientifically inappropriate. This is an extraordinarily misleading claim. Carver still had more to say:

> Medications are prescribed in an effort to return the brain's neurotransmitter status to normal. Much like a physician may prescribe a medication to lower your cholesterol or increase another body chemical, mental health professionals are concerned with returning your neurotransmitter levels to normal. [30]

No doctor who prescribes any psychiatric medication including antidepressants has any idea what anyone's "brain neurotransmitter status" is. Any doctor who is "concerned with returning your neurotransmitter levels back to normal" when no human being has even been demonstrated to have an abnormal brain neurotransmitter level to begin with cannot be operating according to true scientific principles. No competent doctor would dream of "lowering your cholesterol" or your blood sugar without first identifying through a blood test that your cholesterol or blood sugar was raised and therefore in need of lowering. Carver continued:

> The "chemical imbalance" explanation also reflects the overall theme of treatment—identifying what neurotransmitters are involved in the clinical symptom picture and with medication, attempting to return that neurotransmitter level back to the "normal range" . . . there are times when coping with our experiences and life events changes our neurotransmitter status. [31]

Treatment cannot identify what neurotransmitters are involved. To claim that medication helps "return that neurotransmitter to the 'normal range'" is highly inaccurate and misleading, given that neurotransmitter levels cannot be measured in people on medication and there is no realistic sense of what a postulated "normal" range might be. The author added:

> We are all at-risk for changes in our brain's chemistry. Most commonly, we will experience depression, anxiety, or stress reactions. As our neurotransmitters change, they bring with them additional symptoms, behaviours and sensations . . . Recognizing these changes is an important part of treatment. [32]

Since brain chemistry changes have not been scientifically identified, claiming that "we are all at risk for changes in our brain's chemistry" is an extraordinarily erroneous and scaremongering assertion. There is no reliable scientific evidence based upon which it can be correctly stated that recognizing neurotransmitter changes based on "additional symptoms, behaviours and sensations" is an important part of treatment. This plays no part in assessment and treatment. No such clinical tests or evaluations can be carried out because none have been reliably identified. The author concluded:

> This discussion is offered to explain how the neurotransmitter system in the brain can create psychiatric conditions and mental health problems. [33]

Presented by a psychologist as "a public service", [34] many readers may indeed conclude that Carver's article explains how psychiatric conditions are created by abnormalities in the neurotransmitter system. In truth, this grossly misleading article explains little. It is largely a work of fiction misrepresented as truth, laced with misinformation and seriously erroneous deductions.

Drew Westen is Research Associate Professor in the Department of Psychology at Boston University. In his 2003 book *Psychology: Brain Behaviour and Culture* Westen wrote:

> Decreased serotonin in the brain is common in severe depression. [35]

As outlined earlier, such claims are erroneous. There is no confirmatory scientific evidence to confirm such claims, claims that misinform the reader. Westen also stated (brackets mine):

> Biological treatments use medication to restore the brain to as normal functioning as possible . . . Most psychotropic medications (a term that includes antidepressants) act at neurotransmitter sites. Some inhibit overactive neurotransmitters or receptors that are overly sensitive and hence lead neurons to fire too frequently. [36]

This passage contains several factual errors. No abnormal brain functioning has been identified in depression that requires restoration to "normal functioning". There are three errors of fact in his last sentence. There is no evidence that neurotransmitters or receptors are overactive, that receptors are overly sensitive, or that neurons fire too frequently. All this misinformation originated from a professor of psychology attached to a highly respected university. This is a testament to how widely accepted the depression brain chemical imbalance delusion has become.

Misinformation about depression regularly originates from highly respectable and apparently credible sources, whose pronouncements are all the more likely to be believed by the general public. *Beating Stress, Anxiety and Depression* is a 2008 book written by Professor Jane Plant and Janet Stephenson. On the back cover Jane Plant is described as having overcome advanced breast cancer, a Professor of Environmental Geochemistry at Imperial College, London, and the recipient of a CBE for services to earth sciences. Janet Stephenson is described as a psychologist working within the National Health Service in Britain, working in drug and alcohol addiction. The authors' desire to help is obvious but as mentioned earlier, a desire to help does not necessarily equate with providing accurate information. [37] According to the authors:

> Some international scientists now base their classification—and treatment—of the different types of depression on imbalances in different groups of neurotransmitters or on the results of functional brain scans. This is a far more scientific approach that lends itself to accurate diagnosis and improved treatment. [38]

Since there are no known imbalances of neurotransmitters, scientists cannot base either their classification or their treatment on known imbalances of transmitters. Some "international scientists" may base their classification and treatment on their theories, but that is an entirely different thing. As I discuss in a future book in detail, functional brain scans play no part in the diagnosis of depression or any other psychiatric diagnosis. For the moment, the following accurate cautionary note—in a psychiatry textbook written five years *after* these claims were made—contradicts these optimistic comments about the results of functional brain scans:

> Brain imagining adds little to the diagnosis of primary psychiatric disorders, and should only be used when there is good evidence of possible neurological problems. With the exception of organic disorders (e.g. the dementias), the sensitivity and specificity of imaging findings for most psychiatric conditions has yet to be established. [39]

The authors of *Beating Stress, Anxiety and Depression* continued:

> Put simply, when levels of important neurotransmitters become depleted or unbalanced, the brain circuits do not work properly. [40]

This may have been "put simply" but it has also been put incorrectly, since no scientific evidence exists to validate this statement. According to the authors:

> Low levels of this neurotransmitter (serotonin) can lead to severe depression. [41]

This assertion is also incorrect. Low levels of brain serotonin have yet to be confirmed in any living human being, therefore it cannot be correctly claimed that low levels can lead to severe depression. The authors continue:

> Only 1 or 2 per cent of the body's serotonin is found in the brain. The rest . . . is kept out of the brain by the blood-brain barrier; otherwise our moods would fluctuate even more than they do. [42]

Here, the authors present a theory as an established fact, which by definition is misinformation. It is true to say that the vast majority of serotonin in the body occurs outside the brain and that serotonin does not cross from the general blood stream into brain tissues. However there is not a shred of scientific evidence to support the conclusion that serotonin crossing from the blood-brain barrier would inevitably result in a tsunami of fluctuating emotions. Such statements are utter conjecture.

Paul Gilbert is a leading British psychology professor and author. First published in 1997, his well-known book *Overcoming Depression: A Self-Help Guide Using Cognitive Behavioural Techniques* is very popular, with over 125,000 copies sold by the publication of the 2009 edition which I read. In this book, Gilbert provides an example of the phenomenon I referred to previously as the subtle seamless shift from theory to fact, a shift that is not logical and should not occur if one's eye is truly on the ball. Professor Gilbert correctly wrote (italics mine):

> In depression, these mood neurotransmitters are *believed* to be depleted and not working properly. [43]

In the same paragraph, the belief has apparently become a fact (italics mine):

> A key question is: why *have* these changes occurred in the brain? [44]

Moving from a possibility—"mood neurotransmitters are *believed* to be depleted and not working properly"—to an established fact—"why *have* these changes occurred in the brain?" in two consecutive sentences is not a logical sequence of thought. The reader may not notice this, and is likely to be misled into thinking that depleted mood neurotransmitters are an established fact in depression. Elsewhere in this 2009 edition of his book, Professor Gilbert wrote:

> Certain brain chemicals are also affected. Generally, there are fewer of these chemicals in the brain when we are depressed, and this is why some people find benefit from drugs that allow them to build up. [45]

This brief passage contains incorrect and misleading assertions. There is no evidence that "there are fewer of these chemicals in the brain when we are depressed". Therefore Gilbert's claim cannot be correctly asserted as a fact when the premise upon which it is built is itself not an established fact. This is a Begging the Question logical fallacy. [46] That this widely respected professor of psychology would be so misinformed regarding brain chemicals and depression and yet certain that he is correct is further evidence of the pervasiveness of the brain chemical depression delusion.

Depression: Cognitive Behaviour Therapy with Children and Young People was published in 2009, written by three psychologists. These authors provide a further example of the illogical subtle seamless shift from theory to fact (italics mine):

> Biochemical *theories*, such as the monoamine hypothesis, describe how underactivity in brain amine systems *causes* depression. [47]

Theories of causation are not in themselves definitive evidence either of fact or causation, as they are presented to be in this passage. This is therefore another Begging the Question logical fallacy. [48] *Tackling Depression: A Practical Guide to Everyday Coping* is a 2010 book written by Irish counselling psychologist Ian Birthistle. According to the author:

> Much research has shown that serotonin abnormalities can have a significant link to depression. [49]

While much research has *sought* to establish serotonin abnormalities, such abnormalities have never been *established* to anything approaching a scientifically acceptable degree. Since the presence of serotonin abnormalities have not been demonstrated to exist in depression, it cannot be correct to state that "much research has shown that serotonin abnormalities can have a significant link to depression".

Psychologist Deborah Serani is the author of the 2012 book *Living with Depression: Why Biology and Biography Matter Along the Path to Hope and Healing*. Serani was herself first diagnosed with depression at the age of nineteen, and has largely remained on medication up to the time of writing this book at the age of fifty. Serani wrote:

> For decades, evidence-based data has shown that many mental illnesses stem from biological issues. Specifically, children and adults with mental illness have difficulties in the areas of neurotransmission—the process by which neurons and the brain communicate. These signaling networks can also show disruptions in the production and/or absorption of brain chemical messengers, called neurotransmitters. [50]

None of the above is true. No "evidence-based data has shown that many mental illnesses stem from biological issues". It has never been reliably demonstrated that "children and adults with mental illnesses have difficulties in the area of neurotransmission". No such "disruptions in the production and/or absorption of brain chemicals" has been "shown". To claim otherwise is clearly misinformation. I am sure that Deborah Serani's intentions were good and that she had no desire to mislead her readers. Such is the nature of a mass delusion; misinformation is passed on through many channels as an inevitable consequence of the mass acceptance of falsehoods as truth.

Psychology Information Online is a popular internet site that provides information on a wide range of issues including depression. According to the website, it is privately owned and provides information about the practice of psychology for the benefit of consumers and psychologists. Most of the material on the site is copyrighted by Donald J. Franklin Ph.D., a licensed psychologist in New Jersey, New York. The challenge facing the public to ascertain the truth about brain chemicals and depression is illustrated on this site's depression webpage. In the following passage, the author rightly questions the repeated claim that chemical imbalances cause depression:

> The chemical imbalances that occur during depression usually disappear when you complete psychotherapy for depression, without taking any medications to correct the imbalance. This suggests that the imbalance is the body's physical response to psychological depression, rather than the other way around. [51]

The author does not appear to realize that the assumption of "chemical imbalances that occur in depression" which "usually disappear when you complete psychotherapy for depression" even without "taking any medications to correct the imbalance" has no scientific foundation. Chemical imbalances have never been demonstrated to occur in depression, and something that cannot be identified as present cannot be correctly claimed to have disappeared.

PSYCHOTHERAPY AND COUNSELLING

Dealing with Depression in 12-Step Recovery is a 1990 book in the Fellow Travelers book series. The author, who in the book identifies himself simply as Jack O., is described on the back cover as "a therapist and 12 step member" who "offers clear and practical techniques for working through depression". The back cover also refers to his "insights", one of which appears under the heading "Biological depression":

> When we speak of biological or clinical depression, we are referring to an imbalance of chemicals in the brain which regulate feelings, thought and behaviour. [52]

Since depression has never been scientifically established to be primarily biological, the heading and term "Biological Depression", one also used commonly by doctors, is itself highly questionable. Since there are no identified brain chemical imbalances in depression, the commonly perceived notion of clinical depression espoused by Jack O in the above passage as "an imbalance of chemicals in the brain" has no basis in fact. In 1996, clinical hypnotherapist Norman McMaster wrote:

> There can be no doubt that chemical imbalance is involved in severe depression, however a first cause is more likely to be stressful life events, which in turn give rise to the chemical imbalance. Correction of the imbalance still leaves the psychological problem of ingrained habit patterns. [53]

Clearly respected within his profession, Norman McMaster is currently listed as an Editorial Consultant of The Australian Society of Clinical Hypnotherapists. Nevertheless, his assertion that "there can be no doubt that chemical imbalance is involved in severe depression" is without foundation scientifically.

The pervasiveness of the depression delusion is illustrated by the fact that many people who question the medical approach to depression have come to accept that biochemical abnormalities are a given, known to occur in depression. The following passage illustrates how difficult it is for those outside the medical and pharmaceutical alliance to ascertain accurate information in this regard. The passage appears on the website of the Portland Psychotherapy Depression Treatment Program in Oregon, U.S.A. This site raises some important questions regarding the dominance of the chemical imbalance idea, yet inadvertently misinforms its readers that chemical imbalances are known to occur in depression. The United States is one of only a few countries where direct-to-consumer advertising of prescribed medications is permitted in the media. Under the heading "Selling the idea of a 'chemical imbalance'", the authors state:

Television and print commercials stating that depression is caused by a "chemical imbalance" have become commonplace . . . this depiction of depression is greatly oversimplified and leaves out many important factors in understanding this problem . . . describing depression as due to a chemical imbalance may be useful in helping a drug company sell more of its products . . . Many others have written about this misconception and advertising technique . . . A number of studies have shown that people with depression often have unusual levels of variety of neurotransmitters in certain parts of the brain. Based on these findings, some people . . . have concluded that lower levels of particular chemicals in the brain "cause" depression. This conclusion is based on an error of logic. Correlation does not mean causation. It also ignores the heaps of research showing that depression is associated with people's behaviour, with their thinking patterns, and with their history. Depression is at least as correlated with these things as it is with brain chemicals. In terms of brain chemicals, the only conclusive thing we can say is that depression is associated with lower levels of certain chemicals in the brain, not that depression is "caused by" the levels of these chemicals. [54]

Their website lists their team of five licensed psychologists and one social worker. The authors are correct in much of what they say in the above passage, with some important exceptions. Like so many others, they mistakenly accept as a fact that "a number of studies have shown that people with depression often have unusual levels of a variety of neurotransmitters in certain parts of their brain". They are also mistaken in being convinced that "depression is associated with lower levels of certain chemicals in the brain" is "the only conclusive thing" that can be said regarding depression and brain chemicals. As I discussed in chapter two, there is no scientific evidence to support such statements. Non-medical people can be forgiven for succumbing to this erroneous conclusion, given how frequently they have heard this claim asserted as truth by members of the medical profession and by the manufacturers of these substances. This reflects just how difficult it is for people to obtain accurate information in the face of the virtually global depression delusion.

The authors of the above passage make a strong case for their position that the biochemical imbalance idea has been overvalued. They are not aware that their case is actually stronger than they realize. Such is the pervasive nature of the depression delusion that many therapists working in mental health who intelligently question the degree of emphasis given to the brain chemical imbalance idea do not question its fundamental veracity.

As psychologist and researcher Irving Kirsch wrote in his 2009 *The Emperor's New Drugs: Exploding the Antidepressant Myth*:

Depression, we are told over and over again, is a brain disease, a chemical imbalance that can be adjusted by antidepressant medication. In an informational brochure issued to inform the public about depression, the U.S. National Institute of Mental Health tells people that "depressive illnesses are disorders of the brain" and adds that "important neurotransmitters—chemicals that brain cells use to communicate—appear to be out of balance". This view is so widespread that it was even proffered by the editors of *PLoS (Public Library of Science) Medicine* in their summary that accompanied our article. "Depression", they wrote, "is a serious medical illness caused by imbalances in the brain chemicals that regulate mood", and they went on to say that antidepressants are supposed to work by correcting these imbalances. The editors wrote their comment on chemical imbalances as if it were an established fact, and this is also how it is presented by drug companies. Actually, it is not. Instead, even its proponents have to admit that it is a controversial hypothesis that has not yet been proven. Not only is the chemical imbalance hypothesis unproven, but I will argue that it is about as close as a theory gets in science to being disproven by the evidence. [55]

Douglas Bloch is a counsellor, teacher and mental health coach. His Healing From Depression website contains some helpful ideas and information. Unfortunately, his site also contains misinformation about brain chemical imbalances and depression:

> In many respects, antidepressants have revolutionized the treatment of depression. By rebalancing the neurotransmitters in the brain, they impact mood at the biochemical level. [56]

Bloch's statement that antidepressants correct neurotransmitter imbalances is not true. Chemical imbalances have not been identified in depression. It is inappropriate to state unequivocally that antidepressants correct imbalances that have not even been identified as occurring. Douglas Bloch is also the author of *Healing from Depression: 12 Weeks to a Better Mood.* [57] The front cover describes the book as "a body, mind and spirit program". According to the author:

> Current theory links the biochemical causes of mood disorders to a deficiency of three of the brain's neurotransmitters—serotonin, norepinephrine, and dopamine in the brain. . . . Antidepressants . . . are believed to limit the reabsorption of these chemicals into the brain's nerve cells . . . This . . . causes a better neural transmission from cell to cell, resulting in an elevation of mood. [58]

Bloch's statement that current theory links neurotransmitter deficiency to depression and other so-called "mood disorders" is correct. However, such comments do not illustrate the very tenuous nature of these links, for which there is no reliable scientific confirming evidence. There is no actual evidence that limiting the reabsorption of neurotransmitters causes better neural transmission, or that such postulated enhancement of neural transmission from cell to cell elevates mood.

Some psychologists and psychotherapists have managed to speak and write effectively about depression without succumbing to the depression delusion. The 2007 book *The Mindful Way through Depression: Freeing Yourself from Chronic Unhappiness* is one such example. The authors have written a good book containing considerable insights into depression without resorting to unproven brain chemical imbalance theories. Serotonin does not appear in the index and is not mentioned anywhere in the book. This book contains thirteen pages under the heading "Anatomy of depression", which includes three pages on depression and the body. The text is cogently presented without resorting to red herrings—discussed in chapter twelve—commonly included by many authors including text and diagrams on brain function, most of whom fail to inform the reader of just how poorly brain function is actually understood. [59]

Notes to Chapter Seven

1. https://www.psychologytoday.com/basics/depression/causes-depression, accessed 03 February 2015.

2. Brent D. Slife, Colin M. Burchfield &. Dawson Hedges, "Hook, Line and Sinker: Psychology's Uncritical Acceptance of Biological Explanation", Invited Address at the 2002 Rocky Mountain Psychological Association, Park City, Utah, U.S.A., http://brentslife.com/article/upload/biologization/Hook,%20line,%20and%20sinker.pdf, accessed 19 August 2014.

3. Robert Plomin, "Environment and Genes: Determinants of Behavior", *American Psychologist*, 44, 105-111, p. 105.

4. See R.N. Williams, "The Biologization of Psychotherapy: Understanding the Nature of influence", in B.D. Slife, R. Williams & S. Barlow, eds, *Critical Issues in Psychotherapy: Translating New Ideas Into Practice*, Thousand Oaks, CA: Sage Publications, 2001, pp 51-67; and A.M. Fisher, "Modern manifestations of materialism: A legacy of the enlightenment discourse", *Journal of Theoretical and Philosophical Psychology*, 1997, 17, 45-55.

5. R. Wright, "Our Cheating Hearts", *Time*, New York: Time-Warner Inc, 15 August 1994.

6. At the time of writing—20 September 2014—Matthew H. Erdelyi's YouTube "What is depression?" video had been watched by 1,059, 348 people, https://www.youtube.com/watch?v=IeZCmqePLzM, accessed 20 September 2014.

7. Rita Atkinson, Richard C Atkinson & Ernest Hilgard, *Introduction to Psychology*, 8th edition, New York: Harcourt Brace Jovanovich, pps 468, 519.

8. Rita Atkinson, Richard C. Atkinson & Ernest Hilgard, *Introduction to Psychology*, 8th edition, New York: Harcourt Brace Jovanovich, p. 468.

9. Rita Atkinson, Richard C. Atkinson & Ernest Hilgard, *Introduction to Psychology*, 8th edition, New York: Harcourt Brace Jovanovich, p. 469.

10. Rita Atkinson, Richard C. Atkinson & Ernest Hilgard, *Introduction to Psychology*, 8th edition, New York: Harcourt Brace Jovanovich, p. 519.

11. Gerald D. Oster & and Janice E. Caro, *Understanding and Treating Depressed Adolescents and their Families*, New York: John Wiley & Sons Ltd, 1990, pps. 39-40.

12. D.F. Klein &P. H. Wender, *Understanding Depression: A Complete Guide To Its Diagnosis And Treatment*, New York: Oxford University Press, 1993, p. 212.

13. Anthony (Tony) Bates, "Depression", in *Nervous Breakdown*, ed. Colm Keane, Dublin: Mercier Press, 1994, p. 33.

14. Tony Bates, *Depression: The Common Sense Approach*, Dublin: Gill & MacMillan Ltd, 1999, p. 32.

15. Tony Bates, *Coming Through Depression*, Dublin, Gill & MacMillan, 2011, p. 33.

16. Tony Bates, *Coming Through Depression*, Dublin, Gill & MacMillan, 2011, p. 33.

17. Joseph Carver, "The 'Chemical Imbalance' in Mental Health Problems", January 2002, http://www.drjoecarver.com/clients/49355/File/Chemical%2520Imbalance.html, accessed 18 March 2014.

18. Joseph Carver, "The 'Chemical Imbalance' in Mental Health Problems", January 2002, http://www.drjoecarver.com/clients/49355/File/Chemical%2520Imbalance.html, accessed 18 March 2014.

19. Joseph Carver, "The 'Chemical Imbalance' in Mental Health Problems", January 2002, http://www.drjoecarver.com/clients/49355/File/Chemical%2520Imbalance.html, accessed 18 March 2014.

20. Joseph Carver, "The 'Chemical Imbalance' in Mental Health Problems", January 2002, http://www.drjoecarver.com/clients/49355/File/Chemical%2520Imbalance.html, accessed 18 March 2014.

21. Joseph Carver, "The 'Chemical Imbalance' in Mental Health Problems", January 2002, http://www.drjoecarver.com/clients/49355/File/Chemical%2520Imbalance.html, accessed 18 March 2014.

22. Joseph Carver, "The 'Chemical Imbalance' in Mental Health Problems", January 2002, http://www.drjoecarver.com/clients/49355/File/Chemical%2520Imbalance.html, accessed 18 March 2014.

23. For information on Begging the Question logical fallacies see note 22 in the Notes to the Introduction.

24. Joseph Carver, "The 'Chemical Imbalance' in Mental Health Problems", January 2002, http://www.drjoecarver.com/clients/49355/File/Chemical%2520Imbalance.html, accessed 18 March 2014.

25. Joseph Carver, "The 'Chemical Imbalance' in Mental Health Problems", January 2002, http://www.drjoecarver.com/clients/49355/File/Chemical%2520Imbalance.html, accessed 18 March 2014.

26. Joseph Carver, "The 'Chemical Imbalance' in Mental Health Problems", January 2002, http://www.drjoecarver.com/clients/49355/File/Chemical%2520Imbalance.html, accessed 18 March 2014.

27. Joseph Carver, "The 'Chemical Imbalance' in Mental Health Problems", January 2002, http://www.drjoecarver.com/clients/49355/File/Chemical%2520Imbalance.html, accessed 18 March 2014.

28. Joseph Carver, "The 'Chemical Imbalance' in Mental Health Problems", January 2002, http://www.drjoecarver.com/clients/49355/File/Chemical%2520Imbalance.html, accessed 18 March 2014.

29. Joseph Carver, "The 'Chemical Imbalance' in Mental Health Problems", January 2002, http://www.drjoecarver.com/clients/49355/File/Chemical%2520Imbalance.html, accessed 18 March 2014.

30. Joseph Carver, "The 'Chemical Imbalance' in Mental Health Problems", January 2002, http://www.drjoecarver.com/clients/49355/File/Chemical%2520Imbalance.html, accessed 18 March 2014.

31. Joseph Carver, "The 'Chemical Imbalance' in Mental Health Problems", January 2002, http://www.drjoecarver.com/clients/49355/File/Chemical%2520Imbalance.html, accessed 18 March 2014.

32. Joseph Carver, "The 'Chemical Imbalance' in Mental Health Problems", January 2002, http://www.drjoecarver.com/clients/49355/File/Chemical%2520Imbalance.html, accessed 18 March 2014.

33. Joseph Carver, "The 'Chemical Imbalance' in Mental Health Problems", January 2002, http://www.drjoecarver.com/clients/49355/File/Chemical%2520Imbalance.html, accessed 18 March 2014.

34. Joseph Carver, "The 'Chemical Imbalance' in Mental Health Problems", January 2002, http://www.drjoecarver.com/clients/49355/File/Chemical%2520Imbalance.html, accessed 18 March 2014.

35. Drew Westen, *Psychology: Brain, Behaviour and Culture*, 3rd edition, New York: John Wiley & Sons Inc., 2003, p. 73.

36. Drew Weston, *Psychology: Brain, Behaviour and Culture*, 3rd edition, New York: John Wiley & Sons Inc., 2003, pps. 578-9.

37. See Gabor Gombos quote, note 2 in the Notes to the Introduction.

38. Jane Plant & Janet Stephenson, *Beating Stress, Anxiety and Depression*, 2008, London: Piatkus

Books, p. 34.

39. David Semple & Roger Smyth, *The Oxford Handbook of Psychiatry*, 3rd edition, Oxford: Oxford University Press, 2013, p. 78-9.

40. Jane Plant & Janet Stephenson, *Beating Stress, Anxiety and Depression*, London: Piatkus Books, 2008, p. 53.

41. Jane Plant & Janet Stephenson, *Beating Stress, Anxiety and Depression*, London: Piatkus Books, 2008, p. 58.

42. Jane Plant & Janet Stephenson, *Beating Stress, Anxiety and Depression*, London: Piatkus Books, 2008, p. 58.

43. Paul Gilbert, *Overcoming Depression: A Self-Help Guide Using Cognitive Behavioural Techniques*, London: Constable & Robinson Ltd, 2009, p. 63.

44. Paul Gilbert, *Overcoming Depression: A Self-Help Guide Using Cognitive Behavioural Techniques*, London: Constable & Robinson Ltd, 2009, p. 63.

45. Paul Gilbert, *Overcoming Depression: A Self-Help Guide Using Cognitive Behavioural Techniques*, London: Constable & Robinson Ltd, 2009, p. 7.

46. For information on Begging the Question logical fallacies see note 22 in the Notes to the Introduction.

47. Chrissie Verduyn, Julia Rogers, & Alison Wood, *Depression: Cognitive Behaviour Therapy with Children and Young People*, Hove: Routledge, 2009.

48. For information on Begging the Question logical fallacies see note 22 in the Notes to the Introduction.

49. Ian Birthistle, Ian, *Tackling Depression: A Practical Guide to Everyday Coping*, Dublin: Kite Books, 2010.

50. Deborah Serani, *Living with Depression: Why Biology and Biography Matter Along the Path to Hope and Healing*, Lanham, Maryland: Rowman & Littlefield, 2012, p. 19.

51. Psychology Information Online website, http://psychologyinfo.com/depression/causes.html, accessed 14 April 2014.

52. Jack O., *Dealing with Depression in 12-Step Recovery*, 1990, Hazleden, 1990, p. 5.

53. Norman McMaster, "Major Depression: A Hypno-Cognitive-Behavioural Intervention", *Australian Journal of Hypnotherapy and Hypnosis*, Vol. 17, No. 1, March 1996, p. 18, https://www.asch. com.au/publications/editorial-consultants, accessed 25 April 2014.

54. "Selling the idea of a 'chemical imbalance'", Portland Psychotherapy Depression Treatment Program http://www.portlanddepressiontreatment.com/is-depression-just-a-chemical-imbalance/, accessed 24 February 2014.

55. Irving Kirsch, *The Emperor's New Drugs: Exploding the Antidepressant Myth*, London; Random House, 2009, p. 81.

56. Douglas Bloch, counsellor, "Natural Remedies for Depression", Healing From Depression website, http://www.healingfromdepression.com/natural-alternatives-to-prozac.htm#, accessed 28 August 2014.

57. Douglas Bloch, *Healing from Depression: 12 Weeks to a Better Mood*, Berkeley: Celestial Arts, 2002.

58. Douglas Bloch, *Healing from Depression: 12 Weeks to a Better Mood*, Berkeley: Celestial Arts, 2002, p. 188.

59. Mark Williams, John Teasdale, Zindel Segal & Jon Kabat-Zinn, *The Mindful Way through Depression: Freeing Yourself from Chronic Unhappiness*, 2007, New York: The Guilford Press.

8. MENTAL HEALTH ORGANIZATIONS, THE MEDIA AND THE GENERAL PUBLIC

Many mental health organizations provide information to the public about mental health matters. It is not surprising that the information provided by many mental health organizations follows the lead of the medical profession and pharmaceutical companies. Whether intentionally or not, incorrect and misleading information about depression and brain chemical imbalances is regularly passed on to the public by many mental health organizations.

The U.S. National Institute of Mental Health is one of the world's most powerful and influential mental health organizations. Regrettably, misinformation originating from this organization regarding brain biochemistry and depression is not uncommon. In an informational brochure issued to inform the public about depression, the U.S. National Institute of Mental Health informed people that "depressive illnesses are disorders of the brain", adding that "important neurotransmitters—chemicals that brain cells use to communicate—appear to be out of balance". [1]

Despite the widespread belief that depression is a disorder of the brain, this hypothesis has not been scientifically verified. It is therefore wrong that such an influential organization would have unequivocally stated that "depressive illnesses are disorders of the brain". It is also incorrect to assert that neurotransmitters "appear to be out of balance". This conveys a level of knowledge far in excess of the scientific evidence. Neurotransmitters do not "appear" to be out of balance at all. It cannot be truthfully said that something "appears" to be there when there is not a shred of reliable evidence to support such apparent appearances.

The following appears on the "Brain Basics" webpage of the National Institute of Mental Health website:

> Neurotransmitters send chemical messages between neurons. Mental illnesses, such as depression, can occur when this process does not work correctly . . . Research shows that people with depression often have lower than normal levels of serotonin. [2]

It is grossly misleading of this U.S. government-backed organization to misinform the public in this way. No scientific evidence confirms that depression "can occur when the process" of chemical messenger transmitters "does not work correctly". No research has even identified a single piece of reliable evidence that chemical messenger transmitters do ever "not work correctly", let alone link this reliably to depression. The National Institute of Mental Health's claim that "research shows that people with depression often have lower levels of serotonin" is therefore a blatant falsehood. This has never been established, and it grossly irresponsible of this organization to misinform the public in this manner.

The American Psychiatric Association's website's "Resources" page lists several organizations that explicitly misinform the public that the brain chemical imbalance notion is an established fact. [3] The National Alliance on Mental Illness (NAMI) is a major influential American mental health association. In a currently available 2009 Depression Factsheet, NAMI assert:

> Whatever the specific causes of depression, scientific research has firmly established that depression is a biological, medical illness. Norepinephrine, serotonin and dopamine are three neurotransmitters thought to be involved with major depression. Scientists believe that if there is a chemical imbalance in these neurotransmitters, then clinical states of depression result. [4]

There are many falsehoods and flaws in this passage. Scientific research has not "firmly established that depression is a biological, medical illness" at all. In fact, as set out repeatedly in this and my next book, scientific research has not identified a single item of reliable evidence that depression is a biological, medical illness.

By 2012 the National Alliance on Mental Illness was less bullish about neurotransmitter involvement. In NAMI's 2012 twenty-six-page booklet on depression titled "Depression", neurotransmitters receive no mention. The principal author was Ken Duckworth, M.D., NAMI Medical Director. Under "causes", "brain chemistry imbalance" is listed as one of several factors that "play significant roles in the development of a depression". No further details are provided about the claimed imbalances anywhere in this document. [5] Yet the National Alliance on Mental Illness continues to promote misinformation about brain chemicals and mental health problems on its website. On a webpage available in the NAMI website in mid-2014, this organization referred to (italics mine):

> The *knowledge* that most mental illnesses are caused by chemical imbalances. [6]

There is no such knowledge.

Nottinghamshire Healthcare is a major British National Health Service trust, employing over 8,800 staff, with a revenue income of £435 million for 2014. [7] I read the "Learn More About Medicines" page on their "Information" webpage to see what information they provided regarding antidepressants. Under the heading "How do SSRIs work?" the following information is provided:

> The brain has many naturally occurring chemical messengers. One of these is called serotonin . . . It is known that this serotonin is not as effective or active as normal in the brain when someone is feeling depressed. The SSRI antidepressants increase the amount of this serotonin chemical messenger in the brain. This can help correct the lack of action of serotonin and help to improve mood. [8]

This brief passage on an official British National Health Service website contains false information. As I discussed in detail in chapter two, there are no identified chemical abnormalities in depression. It is not "known" that either the activity or effectiveness of serotonin is decreased when someone is feeling depressed or diagnosed as having depression. Claims that SSRI antidepressants increase the "lack of action of serotonin" are therefore also false. The Nottinghamshire Healthcare website contains further misinformation on depression and antidepressants. The following appears in a webpage titled "What happens when transmitter activity is low?":

> If a person has too little serotonin and noradrenaline in the part of the brain that controls mood, this will produce too little activity, and that part of the brain becomes slower and less effective . . . there may be many possible reasons for this . . . Stress may cause changes in the body and then the brain, which can then result in reduced levels of serotonin and noradrenaline. [9]

Since low brain levels of either serotonin or noradrenaline have never even been identified in human beings, the premise upon which the first part of this passage is built has no basis in fact. This passage is therefore a Begging the Question logical fallacy.[10] The last line is also incorrect and misleading, since claims of "reduced levels of serotonin and noradrenaline" have no factual or scientific basis. Elsewhere on the Nottinghamshire Healthcare website I came across the following:

> The brain has a very complex structure about which, in all honesty, we know very little. [11]

This admission is accurate. It is regrettable that this fact was not taken into account when making the false claims in relation to brain chemicals and depression on this official National Health Service Trust website.

I reviewed a number of other UK National Health Service Trust websites. Many appear to be linked to a centralised information system. For example, websites of the Leeds Community Healthcare NHS Trust and the Liverpool Community Healthcare NHS Trust—and possibly many other trusts—contain identical pages regarding the cause of depression. [12] No mention is made on this webpage of brain chemical abnormalities as a definite or even a possible cause of depression, a further indicator of the absence of evidence for such claims.

The major British Mental Health Charity MIND officially supported a 1991 mental health book written by Elaine Farrell with the impressive title, *The Complete Guide to Mental Health: The Comprehensive Guide to Choosing Therapy, Counselling and Psychiatric Care.* Unfortunately, the book totally misinformed its readers regarding depression and serotonin:

> When someone is depressed, there is a lowering in the level of serotonin in the brain. [13]

It is regrettable that a book purporting to be the complete guide to mental health and which has MIND's stamp of approval in bold print on the front cover contains such misinformation. That it does so is further evidence of the widespread nature of the depression brain chemical imbalance delusion.

Rethink Mental Illness is another major British mental health association. In 2009 Rethink published a guide to depression. In this guide, Rethink stated that "there is no single known cause for depression". The first listed heading under causes is "biochemical", the first line of which reads:

> It is known that in people experiencing depression there is a change in their brain messaging chemicals. [14]

Rethink also asserted that:

> When an imbalance of brain chemicals occur, it is believed that depression can result. [15]

They added:

> It is also possible that brain chemicals may change because of depression occurring. [16]

It is to their credit that Rethink include the last sentence in the above passage. By considering that depression may cause chemical changes or be caused by them, they avoid the common error of False Cause logical fallacy. [17] Nevertheless Rethink's information is misleading because no imbalance of brain chemicals has been found to occur in people diagnosed with depression in the first instance. Therefore their statement that "it is known that in people experiencing depression there is a change in their brain messaging chemicals" is a falsehood. It is also wrong to state "*when* an imbalance of brain chemicals occur" (italics mine), since it has never been established that any such imbalances occur.

These claims are made as unequivocal facts in this 2009 Rethink publication. As I write this book six years later, the information about depression and brain chemistry on the Rethink website in August 2014 is no longer unequivocal. What Rethink stated as fact in 2009 is apparently now merely a hypothesis:

> Nobody knows exactly what causes depression . . . Scientists think that if you have depression, some of the chemicals in your brain are out of balance. In particular, having lower amounts of a chemical called "serotonin" in your brain may cause depression. [18]

The belated realization that biochemical abnormalities are not actually established in depression is also reflected in the dropping of the heading "Biochemical" in Rethink's 2009 publication, replaced on the website in 2014 by "Your body". Nevertheless, informing the public that scientists think that brain chemicals are out of balance in depression, and that having lower amounts of serotonin may cause depression is likely to be interpreted by many readers as sufficiently credible "evidence" that brain chemical imbalances are known to occur in depression.

In a 2013 article psychiatrist Joanna Moncrieff wrote:

> In 1995, the pharmaceutical industry provided funding for a campaign in the United States organized by the National Alliance for Research on Schizophrenia and Depression, entitled "Depression, a flaw in chemistry not character". This was an offshoot organization formed by the National Alliance on Mental Illness (NAMI), and two other patient advocacy groups in the US, which also receive other financial support from the pharmaceutical industry. Advertisements in the national press and leaflets distributed as part of this campaign asserted that depression had been shown to be due to "an insufficient level of the neurotransmitter serotonin. . . in the frontal lobes of the brain". [19]

This 1995 advertisement, funded by National Alliance for Research on Schizophrenia and Depression, consisted of a large advertisement placed in newspapers nationwide across America. The advertisement was part of this organization's "Depression: A Flaw in Chemistry, not Character" campaign, a phrase placed in big bold print at the head of the advertisement.

There were multiple examples of untruths and misinformation scattered throughout the advertisement. According to the advertisement, "recent medical research has taught us that depression is often biological, caused by a chemical imbalance in the brain". [20] As outlined in detail in this book, no such evidence existed either then or now. This claim is therefore a blatant untruth. The advertisement described depression as a physical disease requiring antidepressants, analogous to diabetics requiring insulin. Presenting the public with just two possible interpretations of depression—that depression is either a flaw in chemistry or a flaw in character—and ignoring other possible ways of understanding depression is a False Dilemma logical fallacy. [21] Presented with just two options, one of which is cleverly pitched as a "flaw in character", it is hardly surprising that people would embrace the second option.

Also in 1995, the American Foundation for Suicide Prevention Research Award was given to psychiatrist J. John Mann:

> For his breakthrough research on serotonin levels as a predictor of suicide risk. Dr. Mann's research has helped to uncover the chemical imbalances that occur in depressed patients, and his work on hormonal abnormalities in suicidal patients has fostered the development of tests that predict suicide risk. His studies of the different tests measuring perturbations in the brain's secretion of the hormone serotonin have contributed substantially to recent advances in the field. [22]

This foundation's gushing praise contains many inaccuracies. Neither in 1995 nor in 2015 could it be correctly stated that "serotonin levels" are a "predictor of suicide risk" or that Dr. Mann or anyone else has managed to "uncover the chemical imbalances that occur in depressed patients". This pattern of misinformation continues to this day, often originating from major mental health associations and consumer groups that have become widely trusted.

Mental Health America is a major mental health organization. This organization describes itself as:

> The leading advocacy organization addressing the full spectrum of mental and substance use conditions and their effects nationwide, works to reform, advocate and enable access to quality behavioural health services for all Americans. [23]

Under the heading "Depression: What you need to know", this organization misinforms anyone who reads their material:

> People with depression typically have too little or too much of certain brain chemicals, called "neurotransmitters". [24]

Formerly known as the Child and Adolescent Bipolar Foundation, the Balanced Mind Parent Network is a major American mental health association that is endorsed by the American Psychiatric Association. [25] According to their website, this organization "guides families raising children with mood disorders to the answers, support and stability they seek". [26] Their website contains an article titled "Fact Sheet: Facts about Teenage Depression", published on 27 November 2009 and currently available on their website. The first heading "Just the Facts" reinforces the message that one will not find any fiction in this factsheet. The lay reader is therefore not likely to realize that the following passage from this "Factsheet" has no basis in fact but rather is entirely a work of fiction:

> Depression is a medical illness caused by a chemical imbalance in the brain . . .
> In depression, these neurons do not function normally, which leads to changes in the person's thoughts, feelings and behaviour. Antidepressant medication work to restore proper chemical balance in the brain. [27]

There are 26 members of the Scientific Advisory Council of the Balanced Mind Parent Network, 21 of whom are professors of psychiatry. [28] Clearly these psychiatrists have no difficulty with such misinformation appearing on the organization's website.

The Depression and Bipolar Support Alliance (DBSA) is a major American mental health organization and consumer group. By including false information about depression and brain chemicals such as the following on its website and public information material, this organization has contributed to the spreading of the depression delusion:

> Depression is a medical illness that can be treated, just like arthritis or diabetes . . . Having an illness of the brain and getting treatment is no reason to be ashamed . . . Depression is caused by a chemical imbalance in the brain. [29]

As was the case with the Balanced Mind Parent Network, The so-called "Facts About Depression" page on the Depression and Bipolar Support Alliance website contains some impressive pieces of fiction including the following:

> People with depression have an imbalance of certain brain chemicals known as neurotransmitters. This imbalance produces serious and persistent physical symptoms. [30] . . . Scientists believe that depression and bipolar disorder are caused by an imbalance of brain chemicals called neurotransmitters. Medications used to treat mood disorders work to correct this imbalance by changing brain chemistry. [31]

The Depression and Bipolar Support Alliance is overseen by a Scientific Advisory Board, 35 out of a total of 47 are professors of psychiatry. [32] There is no indication from the website that any member of this organization's Scientific Advisory Board had any qualms about the organization's misinformation.

Spunout.ie is a popular Irish mental health website for people between the ages of sixteen and twenty-five. The site provides much helpful information for young people about mental health, with over half a million website hits in 2012. [33] Unfortunately, spunout.ie is not immune to the virtually global delusion that brain chemical imbalances are known to occur in depression. The site lists seven causes of depression, including:

> Chemical imbalances in the brain can cause depression. [34]

THE MEDIA AND THE GENERAL PUBLIC

One might expect the media to reflect the public understanding and awareness of various topics, and this is true regarding depression. References to the widespread delusion that biochemical abnormalities occur in depression have appeared regularly in the media over the past thirty years. No doubt influenced by all they have read and heard about depression and neurotransmitters, it is to be expected that well-meaning people who write and speak about depression will make such factual errors. This incorrect message is thus passed on to thousands and sometimes millions of people as established facts. Given the pervasiveness of medical and pharmaceutical claims, it is not surprising that many journalists and media commentators appear to view such claims as fact.

Examples of the depression brain chemical imbalance delusion keep surfacing. As I was finalizing the text for this book in November 2014, in a four-day period I came across three further examples of unequivocal assertions of depression being a chemical imbalance in national media. Such claims reinforce this falsehood in the minds of the many thousands and in some cases millions of people who listen to and read them and respect their words.

ITV's popular programme *Loose Women* on 07 November 2014 featured Sharon Osbourne, Andrea McLean, Nadia Sawalha and Jane Moore. All of these women are well known and respected in Britain and beyond. The discussion turned to antidepressants and Sharon Osbourne's admission that she had taken antidepressants for sixteen years. While Sharon Osbourne's openness about her experiences was certainly welcome, the show inadvertently misinformed its many thousands of listeners regarding brain chemicals.

During the discussion, Nadia Sawalha said, "It's a chemical thing, isn't it?", to which Sharon Osbourne replied, "It is, it's a chemical thing." None of the four women on the panel mentioned that the chemical imbalance notion was an unproven and largely discredited theory, presumably because they did not realize this. In 2013 the ITV "Loose Women" website described Nadia Sawalha as:

One of television's busiest presenters, having never been off our screens for the last 16 years. [35]

Sharon Osbourne is a darling of the British public, known and loved for many things including her marriage to musician Ozzie Osbourne and her appearances as a judge on music talent shows such as Xfactor. When two of the best known and most influential women in Britain inadvertently misinform their listeners because they themselves are misinformed, there is clearly a big problem.

Other comments from Sharon Osbourne pointed to the attraction of the chemical imbalance notion as a publicly acceptable explanation that might reduce stigma, making depression seem like any typical health problem:

When you have a bad leg, you can go to the doctor, bad arm, whatever, but when it's in your head, people go, oh, cray-cray, crazy, we knew she was nuts, and it's not that way at all. [36]

The potential for an untrue explanation for depression to reduce stigma is clearly limited, even if it seems palatable. So many people fail to see that the real stigma is not about what is called "mental illness". Rather, it concerns the widespread rejection in society of emotional pain, overwhelm, distress and vulnerability—including the many ways in which this pain and distress may be experienced and expressed—and ultimately, the rejection of the people who experience and exhibit these experiences and behaviours.

The following day on Irish national radio, author Marian Keyes gave an honest and courageous account of her experience of depression, including being suicidal for long periods. Marian Keyes is an Irish novelist and non-fiction writer. An Irish Book Awards winner, over 26 million copies of her novels have been sold worldwide. Her books have been translated into 32 languages. On 08 November 2014, Marian Keyes was interviewed on Irish national radio by Marian Finucane, one of Ireland's best known and most popular broadcasters. Her interview understandably provoked a major outpouring of support and appreciation from listeners. I do not think that many listeners noticed Marian Keyes' unintentional endorsement of a falsehood—the depression brain chemical imbalance delusion. During the interview, Marian Keyes stated the following about depression with considerable conviction:

> The brain is the most peculiar place where all kinds of minute chemical imbalances can cause the most distorted thinking and no amount of lovely husbands or cars or shoes will alter that. [37]

As Marian Keyes described eloquently during this interview, people in such states experience often indescribable pain and distress. She is correct to say that in that state, no matter how many good things you have in your life or how good your life appears to others, these things often cannot make you feel better. She is incorrect to assume that chemical imbalances are present and that they are the explanation for this apparent contradiction, which when one reflects on such situations more deeply, one finds are not contradictions at all. [38] Marian Keyes can certainly be forgiven for not realising that her own story contradicts rather than supports claims that brain chemical imbalances occur in depression:

> The whole medicine for mental illness is incredibly hit or miss . . . because again the brain is so complicated, it's so delicate . . . it's very hard to get it right . . . I couldn't tell you the number of combinations of different antidepressants and antipsychotics . . . they kept trying new ones, and nothing worked, because it's a strange, mysterious illness. [39]

Marian Keyes' experience—one shared by many—is the polar opposite of what happens in the treatment of an actual chemical imbalance. As I discuss in detail in chapter ten, the treatment of illnesses characterized by a known chemical imbalance is now refined and precise, not "incredibly hit and miss". In conditions where chemical imbalances are known to occur, the choice of treatment is inevitably straightforward. Like is replaced with like. Diabetic patients who need insulin to correct their chemical imbalance are prescribed insulin and nothing else. There is no protracted search for what type of insulin or treatment that might work, or for other treatments apart from insulin. When there is an insulin deficiency, insulin replacement will *always* work, except in very rare circumstances such as the presence of antibodies to insulin. It is a similar story with all conditions known to be characterized by a chemical abnormality.

Just two days after the Marian Keyes interview, a 10 November 2014 *Guardian* article written by the newspaper's political correspondent Juliette Jowit claimed unequivocally:

> The physical basis of mental illness is clear. [40]

Jowit wrote of "firm evidence" for this assertion, and referred principally to British psychiatrist Tim Cantopher to support her claim:

> A psychiatrist, Tim Cantopher, says that if he were to draw fluid from the spinal cord of depressed patients he would find a deficiency of two chemicals: serotonin and noradrenaline. . . "Depressive illness is not a psychological or an emotional state and is not a mental illness. It is a physical illness", Cantopher has written. "This is not a metaphor. It is a fact".

Astonished that a psychiatrist would say something as incorrect as to claim that a lumbar puncture in people who are depressed would regularly reveal low levels of serotonin or noradrenaline, I searched for an original reference. Remarkably, Tim Cantopher did indeed make such claims, in his 2012 book *Depressive Illness: The Curse of the Strong* (brackets his):

> If I were to perform a lumbar puncture on my patients (which, new patients of mine will be pleased to hear, I don't), I would be able to demonstrate in the chemical analysis of the cerebro-spinal fluid (the fluid around the brain and spine), a deficiency of two chemicals. [41]

Over the years, I have become used to seeing misinformation regarding mental health, but I have to admit that I nearly fell of my chair when I read this. As I discuss in the "Serotonin breakdown products and depression" section in chapter two, this is an utterly unfounded claim, and Tim Cantopher either knows or should know this. This is therefore a bizarre claim, one that is bound to seriously mislead the unsuspecting reader, of which there have been many. On the day I searched for Cantopher's book on amazon.co.uk—11 November 2014—this book was ranked number one, two and three in amazon.co.uk's Depression, Mood Disorders, and Mental Diseases and Disorders categories respectively.

Cantopher's statement that he does not perform lumbar punctures on his depressed patients is more revealing than might first appear. Lumbar punctures are regularly carried out when they are clinically indicated, whenever an examination of the cerebro-spinal fluid is likely to be helpful clinically. Given psychiatry's immense desire to legitimize its practices, if lumbar punctures revealed anything remotely like what Cantopher claims, lumbar punctures would be regularly carried out to diagnose depression. The fact that they never are tells its own story.

As journalist Juliette Jowit stated, Dr. Tim Cantopher did indeed write that:

> Depressive illness is not a psychological or an emotional state and is not a mental illness. It is a physical illness. This is not a metaphor. It is a fact. [42]

Perhaps setting out his stall, Cantopher wrote this in the very first paragraph of his 2012 book. Generally in society, when facts are claimed to exist, evidence of their existence is usually required. Not for the first time, it seems that the rules for what constitutes "facts" are quite different for psychiatry than for the rest of society. Just 24 hours after publication, Jowit's article had been shared 8,680 times on Facebook, 274 times on Twitter and 40 on LinkedIn. A case of misinformation going viral.

Every neurologist in the world knows that Dr. Tim Cantopher's claims are blatantly untrue. Every GP and neurologist knows that every condition characterised by abnormalities in the cerebro-spinal fluid falls exclusively within the remit of neurology and neurosurgery, never psychiatry. Yet all these doctors remain silent. The silence of these doctors conveys a message of tacit agreement, giving the public the impression that doctors such as Tim Cantopher must be correct. Doctors are one of the most trusted groups in the world. Most people assume that doctors would not deceive or misinform them and that if they did, their colleagues would step in and correct the situation in the public interest. Unfortunately, this is not always the case. The brotherhood that exists within medicine can be a powerful machine sometimes.

Mary Kenny has had a long and illustrious career as a writer and commentator in Britain and Ireland. Yet some of her writings on depression are way off track as far as accuracy is concerned. In 1998 Mary Kenny wrote:

> Serotonin is the natural chemical which produces the unmistakable feel-good factor; when you are happy, your serotonin is high. And when you are wretched, your serotonin is low. An unhappy event in your life sends your serotonin shooting right down. Prozac was developed as a consequence of the discovery of serotonin levels. Prozac makes people feel good by upping their serotonin levels. [43]

It has not been reliably established scientifically that "when you are happy, your serotonin is high"; that "when you are wretched, your serotonin is low"; that "an unhappy event sends your serotonin shooting right down". Prozac was not "developed as a consequence of the discovery of serotonin levels", since we still cannot even measure serotonin levels, let alone know whether serotonin levels ever do or can become abnormal. Nor is it accurate to state as a fact that Prozac works by upping serotonin levels, since no tests exist to prove this notion. Her first sentence implies that serotonin is a chemical that "produces the unmistakable feel-good factor". Given the miniscule degree to which the complexity of the brain is understood, such conclusions are rather premature, though similar claims have been made by many medical professionals who really should know better.

In June 1999 the popular *Chat* magazine carried an article by their advice columnist who was referred to as a "holistic doctor". According to the article:

> Depression is an unpleasant condition that . . . is caused by an imbalance of certain chemicals in the brain . . . Your GP may recommend antidepressants, which work by correcting the chemical imbalance. [44]

Depression cannot truthfully be claimed to be caused by a chemical brain imbalance that has not even been identified to exist. Nor can antidepressants be truthfully claimed to work by correcting a chemical imbalance that has not been demonstrated to exist.

According to an article on depression in the *Irish Examiner* in 2000, Prozac and similar antidepressant drugs "restore levels of the neurotransmitter serotonin in the brain". In same article, Dr. Robert Daly, then Professor of Psychiatry at University College Cork, was quoted as saying that antidepressants "target a brain chemical deficiency". [45] Neither of these claims is true.

American author Andrew Solomon has stated publicly that he has suffered from depression for much of his life. His 2002 book *The Noonday Demon: An Anatomy of Depression* won the prestigious MIND Annual Book of the Year Award in 2002. This book is a valuable personal memoir, but the author has included much misinformation in relation to serotonin:

Three separate events—decrease in serotonin receptors; rise in cortisol, a stress hormone; and depression—are coincident . . . If you depress a person, levels of serotonin go down . . . The substance of the decade had been serotonin, and the treatments mostly used in depression are ones that raise the functional level of serotonin in the brain. Every time you affect serotonin, you also modify the stress systems and change the cortisol levels in the brain . . . Suicides have low levels of serotonin at certain key locations in the brain. They have excessive numbers of serotonin receptors, which may reflect the brain's attempt to make up for the low levels of serotonin. The level of serotonin seems to be especially low in the areas associated with inhibition, and this deficiency appears to create a powerful freedom to act impulsively on emotion. [46]

There are many incorrect and misleading statements in the above passage. There is no scientific evidence of a decrease in serotonin receptors in depression. It has not been scientifically established that if you "depress a person", whatever that means, "levels of serotonin go down"; or that antidepressants "raise the functional level of serotonin in the brain". Solomon's reference to functional serotonin levels is wishful thinking, as it is totally unproven. The comment, "every time you affect serotonin" is misleading. Serotonin cannot be easily and deliberately "affected" as the author suggests, since there is no way of measuring serotonin levels and how these might be affected in live situations. There is therefore no reliable scientific evidence confirming that brain cortisol levels are directly and continually affected by changing levels of serotonin. People who take their lives have not been scientifically found to have "low levels of serotonin", "excessive numbers of serotonin receptors", or "especially low" serotonin levels in areas of the brain associated with inhibition. Since there is no established deficiency, Solomon's claim that "this deficiency appears to create a powerful freedom to act impulsively on emotion" is erroneous on two counts; there is no deficiency, and the stated effect of the supposed deficiency is consequently also incorrect. That is a lot of factual errors and misleading statements in just a few paragraphs of a prize-winning book that has been highly influential in shaping people's understanding of depression.

While as I discussed in chapter two, medical textbooks contain few and in many cases no references to serotonin, Solomon's book includes 42 references to serotonin in the index, a further 22 index entries for selective serotonin reuptake inhibitors and many references to individual named antidepressant substances. That's pretty striking for a substance whose levels cannot even be measured in the human brain. Solomon's conclusion that serotonin had been "the substance of the decade" is a testament to the success of the propaganda and the extent of the delusion. A solid case could be made for serotonin being the delusion of the decade. Solomon is well read on the subject matter. He is clearly an intelligent writer with a personal interest in matters relating to depression, yet he too has fallen into the depression brain chemical imbalance delusion trap.

The fact that Solomon's book won the 2002 MIND Book of the Year Award while containing such fundamental errors of fact suggests that the judges also subscribed to the depression delusion and were unaware that these assertions had no basis in fact. The author of the otherwise insightful and balanced *New York Times* review of

Solomon's book does not appear to have spotted these falsehoods either. She described his book as "exhaustively researched" and "including an informed discussion on psychotropic drugs, including the ever-popular Prozac". [47]

In his 2003 book *A Day Called Hope*, an excellent description of his experience of and recovery from depression, well known Irish broadcaster Gareth O'Callaghan has understandably accepted much of the prevailing view about serotonin and antidepressants. He can certainly be forgiven for doing so, given how pervasive this falsehood has become:

> Serotonin is often known as "the happy hormone"; it is an essential chemical, manufactured in the brain, that creates feelings of well-being, contentment and balance within us. But in some people the process is faulty, and they need SSRIs to prevent the serotonin they produce from being reabsorbed by the brain and causing a serious lack of balance. [48]

As set out in this book, there is no scientific evidence to support the conclusion that brain serotonin levels are in any way faulty or in "a serious lack of balance". Later in his book, regarding "the loss of the ability to express our deepest feelings", O'Callaghan again made incorrect statements about the degree of knowledge about brain functioning that science has made possible:

> Scientists say there is a rational explanation; they have tracked the precise pathways in the brain along which the neurotransmitters travel with their messages that help us to express our feelings and convert them into thought power so that we can put them into appropriate words. One of these powerful chemical messengers is dopamine. Depression weakens the production plant that oversees the availability of both serotonin and dopamine. [49]

The real level of knowledge of neurotransmitter function is far less than that described here. Scientists have not "tracked the precise pathways of the brain" to anything like the intricate degree described above. It has not been established that neurotransmitters "help us express our feelings and convert them into thought power so that we can put them into appropriate words". Accepting this as an established fact is to accept as fact something that is far beyond what is known about neurotransmitter function. It is not a scientifically established fact that any supposed "production plant" that supposedly "oversees the availability of both serotonin and dopamine" is "weakened" by anything, depression included.

Ronnie O'Sullivan has achieved international success and acclaim as one of the most talented snooker players of all time. In his autobiography, *Ronnie: The Autobiography of Ronnie O'Sullivan*, he outlined his doctor's assessment of his emotional and psychological problems:

> "You suffer from depression" said Dr. Hodges . . . He told me about how we create the chemical serotonin, and how we need it to give us energy and make ourselves feel good. He said if normal people are usually about a level of ten, and

on a bad day they will go down to nine, then I was at a level of three or four. He said there is something that's breaking down the serotonin every time it wants to do its job. "I'm going to put you on these pills that make serotonin and they will make you function like a normal human being again," he told me. It made sense to me . . . "When you get to level two or three, that is suicidal. I think you're on three or three and a half," he told me again just to hammer the point. [50]

None of these assertions about serotonin abnormalities are true. Dr. Hodges could not tell anything about Ronnie O'Sullivan's serotonin levels, either by just looking at him or by carrying out any tests. O'Sullivan clearly believed what his doctor told him.

In the foreword to the 2006 book *Understanding Mental Health*, well known Irish journalist and broadcaster Vincent Browne wrote:

Depression is caused by "the malfunction of chemical transmitters in the brain".[51]

Browne's reference to chemical transmitter malfunction appears to be a quotation from the chapter on depression he was referring to, which was written by Irish psychiatrist Siobhan Barry. I was unable to locate this exact line in Siobhan Barry's chapter. As I mentioned in chapter five, Dr. Siobhan Barry did write:

Irregularities in brain chemistry can involve substances called neurotransmitters and electrolytes. Many of the commonly effective antidepressants act to increase levels of the neurotransmitter serotonin, which suggests that irregularities in this neurotransmitter may be involved in depression. There is also evidence that abnormalities in the neurotransmitter noradrenaline are involved in other types of depression. [52]

It would appear that Vincent Browne wrote that depression is caused by malfunction of chemical transmitters in the brain based either on his reading of Siobhan Barry's chapter, his own long-held interest in mental health or a combination of the two. Whatever the context in which this was written, it is factually incorrect to state that depression is caused by the malfunction of brain chemical neurotransmitters, since no reliable scientific evidence validates this assertion. That Vincent Browne's comment passed his own editing and that of the two editors, both of whom are psychiatrists, suggests that they did not see any problem with it and were therefore happy to leave this inaccurate comment in the book.

According to a 2007 article on depression in the *Pittsburgh Tribune*:

Depression is not a personal deficit, but something that needs to be looked at as a chemical imbalance. [53]

This is flawed logic, a False Dilemma logical fallacy. [54] Only two possible options are considered; depression is either a "personal deficit" or a "chemical imbalance". The former is presented in quite a pejorative fashion, making the only other mentioned possibility appear a great deal more palatable. As I discuss in chapter four and in more detail in later books, depression can be accurately understood using neither of these options; as an expression of woundedness, distress and defense mechanisms.

Author Nicolette Heaton-Harris has written several mental health-related books including one on depression. In her 2008 book *Understanding Depression*, regarding depression and neurotransmitters she wrote:

> These three neurotransmitters (noradrenaline, serotonin and dopamine) will be in short supply if a person is suffering from depression. The synapses are low in these important chemicals, leading to a breakdown in communication and faulty connections of messages, directly causing depressive symptoms. [55]

This is a tidy and complete-looking explanation, but none if it is true.

Ray D'Arcy is a well-known Irish broadcaster. He has been interested in depression for years and has been involved in several national media programmes on depression in Ireland. Unfortunately, genuine interest does not protect one from being misinformed. On his national morning radio show on 06 December 2011, Ray D'Arcy informed his many thousand listeners that:

> Some depressions are caused by a chemical imbalance. [56]

Ray D'Arcy is a well-informed and experienced national broadcaster, yet he is utterly misinformed on this one. This again illustrates how pervasive the depression chemical imbalance delusion has become.

Irish actress Mary McEvoy has spoken publicly about her experience of depression over many years. In her 2011 book *How the Light Gets In: My Journey with Depression*, she described exchanges with her doctor relating to her having a brain chemical imbalance:

> My doctor and I have discussed this at length and we both feel that I am one of those people whose brains can't manufacture enough happy chemicals, such as serotonin. Depression is sometimes a sign that our serotonin levels are low, and when the levels are low, dealing with the normal ups and downs of life becomes very difficult . . . In many cases, serotonin levels can be brought back to normal levels by other means than medication. But some people, myself included, cannot manufacture enough serotonin naturally, so our levels need topping up. [57]

Several issues arise in this passage. Mary McEvoy and her psychiatrist both *felt* that she had a serotonin deficiency. Real chemical abnormalities are never diagnosed in accordance with how either the doctor or the patient *feels*. They are diagnosed through reliable scientific laboratory investigations through which the chemical abnormality is then reliably established. Can you imagine a diabetes specialist diagnosing and treating diabetes because the doctor and patient both *feel* that the patient has a chemical imbalance, without carrying out laboratory tests to establish the diagnosis? McEvoy's statement regarding "being one of those people whose brains cannot manufacture enough happy chemicals" has no basis in fact, since no such group of people has been scientifically and reliably identified. There is no evidence that "depression is sometimes a sign that our serotonin levels are low". Since brain serotonin cannot even be measured and there is no scientific evidence regarding what might constitute normal or low serotonin levels, McEvoy's assertion that "when the levels are low, dealing with the normal ups and downs of life becomes very difficult" is clearly without foundation. Her statements that "In many cases, serotonin levels can be brought back to normal levels by other means by medication" and "some people, myself included, cannot manufacture enough serotonin naturally, so our levels need topping up" are equally unfounded for the same reason.

Mary McEvoy's level of responsibility for this misinformation is considerably lower than, for example, a doctor who might have provided her with incorrect and misleading information about depression and serotonin. Her opinions are probably largely shaped by what she has heard from professionals and other supposedly trustworthy sources. Mary McEvoy is much loved and respected in Ireland. Her words reach many people, most of whom are likely to believe what she says, including what she says about serotonin and depression. She appears regularly in the Irish national media in discussions about depression and mental health. Her book was a best-seller in Ireland. Generally seen as an ordinary, "one of us" sort of person, her words on serotonin will likely be well received and believed by readers. Every reader who does believe what she has written about depression and serotonin has been misinformed and misled, albeit unintentionally. The fact that Mary McEvoy was not deliberately seeking to mislead does not reduce the impact of her words.

Science writer Jonathan Crowe is Editor-in-Chief for Natural, Health & Clinical Sciences in the Higher Education Department at Oxford University Press. A biochemistry graduate and co-author of *Chemistry for the Biosciences*, Crowe manages Oxford University Press' undergraduate textbook publishing programme across the range of science and science-related disciplines. On the Oxford Mental Health Forum blog in March 2012 Jonathan Crowe wrote:

> Studies have found that depressed individuals often have low levels of serotonin in their bodies. Actually, to be precise, these studies have found that levels of the chemicals that are generated when serotonin is naturally broken down by the body are lower than normal in those with depression. And, if the levels of the chemicals that are made from serotonin are low, we can deduce that the levels of serotonin itself are also low. So, if serotonin levels are often found to be abnormally low in those with depression, it would make sense that one way to treat depression would be to return serotonin levels to normal. And this is exactly what some therapeutic strategies try to do. [58]

There are several inaccuracies in this passage. In chapter two I explained that studies of the breakdown products of serotonin have been inconsistent and inconclusive. Crowe's claims in this regard are therefore incorrect and misleading. His unequivocal assertions regarding low serotonin levels are also false and therefore misleading. As outlined earlier, studies have not "found that depressed individuals often have low levels of serotonin in their bodies". As Leo and Lacasse pointed out in 2005:

Not a single peer-reviewed article . . . supports claims of serotonin deficiency in any mental disorder. [59]

Crowe's assertion, "So, if serotonin levels are often found to be abnormally low in those with depression, it would make sense that one way to treat depression would be to return serotonin levels to normal. And this is exactly what some therapeutic strategies try to do" is highly questionable. The first half of the first sentence in this passage is presented as though "serotonin levels are often found to be abnormally low in those with depression". Since serotonin levels are never identified as "abnormally low", this is a Begging the Question logical fallacy. [60] The premise upon which the rest of this passage is based is dependent on the first part being an established fact which it is most certainly not. Logically, this renders the second part null and void.

The *New York Times* has an "In-Depth Report" on depression in the health guide section of its website. In its consideration of the cause of depression, the Report contains the following (italics theirs):

Evidence supports the theory that depression has a biological basis. The basic biologic causes of depression are strongly linked to abnormalities in the delivery of certain key neurotransmitters—chemical messengers in the brain. These neurotransmitters include: *Serotonin* . . . Imbalances in the brain's serotonin levels can trigger depression and other mood disorders. [61]

In truth, there is no evidence that supports the theory that depression has a biological basis. There are no established scientific links between any "basic biologic causes of depression" and "abnormalities in the delivery of certain key neurotransmitters", never mind strong links. The existence of abnormalities in the delivery of certain key neurotransmitters have never been demonstrated. How can there be strong or indeed any links between two things, one of which has never been shown to exist? This is yet another Begging the Question logical fallacy. [62]

It is stated on this *New York Times* depression "In-depth Report" webpage that the content was reviewed on 26 March 2013 by two eminent doctors. [63] The reader might therefore feel reassured that the content is accurate, since these experts allowed this content on the website. Yet when the corresponding diagram on this webpage is included, this brief passage on the website of one of the world's most respected newspapers contains three falsehoods. As outlined previously, evidence does not support the assumption that depression has a biological basis. There are no known "basic biological causes of depression". These to-date imaginary causes of depression are not "strongly linked" to depression in any true scientific sense, only in the minds of those who favour the theory. Since no "imbalances in the brain's serotonin levels" have yet been scientifically identified, it is some stretch of the imagination to assert that unestablished imbalances in the brain's serotonin can trigger depression.

A second logical fallacy—False Cause—is present in the above passage. [64] Even if brain biochemical abnormalities were ever found, something that is increasingly conceded as very unlikely, it would be logically unsound to assume that because two phenomena occur together one causes the other, without adequate evidence. [65]

Michelle L. Devon is a freelance writer and author of several books. In her internet article titled "Depression really is a medical condition", Devon makes many assertions about depression (emphasis hers):

> It is clear . . . that depression can indeed be a medical problem . . . Blood work is often taken from someone who is suspected of having depression . . . Now, if depression were only mental health, and not a true medical problem, why all the medical tests? . . . Depression is not something that has been caused by life circumstances . . . The only way the sadness, the melancholy and withdrawal of a very young child can be explained is through a diagnosis of a medical condition known as depression . . . Now, it's important to note that counselling is suggested for people with depression, NOT because depression is a mental health issue, but because having depression causes additional mental health issues. In other words, patients with depression are not sent to counsellors to cure their depression. Rather, depression patients are sent to a counsellor to deal with the symptoms that depression causes, much like a doctor often sends a cancer patient or a rheumatoid arthritis patient or a multiple sclerosis or lupus patient to a counsellor in order to deal with the issues pertaining to their illnesses. [66]

There is a whole series of misinformation and inaccuracies in this passage including many that I have alluded to earlier. Blood tests are *never* taken in order to diagnose depression. When blood tests are carried out, the purpose is never to diagnose depression using these tests, but to rule out known organic diseases. Depression is often caused by life circumstances. To claim that the only way to explain the great sadness in a young child is by a diagnosis of depression is seriously flawed logic, an example of the False Dilemma logical fallacy. [67] Counselling has helped many people recover fully from depression, not just from the "symptoms that depression causes". Her comment that "if depression were only mental health, and not a true medical problem, why all the medical tests?" is testament to the confusion and lack of clarity caused by psychiatric terminology. Most people, including many doctors, are not at all clear what "mental illness" is or means. This situation is inevitable given the absence of scientific evidence to verify that psychiatric diagnoses are indeed diseases.

LaShon Fryer has been a freelance writer since 2006. She has a Bachelor's Degree in Communications from Temple University and has pursued a Master's Degree in Broadcasting Telecommunications and Mass Media. Here is what she has to say about depression in a web eHow article titled "Chemical Imbalance that Causes Depression":

> If something prevents neurotransmitters from relaying messages to your nerve cells, you will become imbalanced and unable to function correctly. This can often lead to depression . . . When serotonin levels are low, the body functions that serotonin regulates are adversely effected, causing a chemical imbalance that commonly results in depression . . . When norepinephrine levels are low, you can lack focus and feel unmotivated and tired . . . To balance your norepinephrine levels, your physician may prescribe antidepressants or serotonin and norepinephrine reuptake inhibitors. If you have anxiety associated with high levels

of norepinephrine, you will be treated for your anxiety. Numerous triggers, such as divorce or sudden loss of a loved one, can cause a chemical imbalance. [68]

There are many inaccuracies in this passage. There is no known "something" that "prevents neurotransmitters from relaying messages to your nerve cells". Concluding that "You will become imbalanced and unable to function correctly. This can often lead to depression" is a Begging the Question logical fallacy, [69] since the supposed cause—the "something" that prevents messages being relayed—is assumed to be a fact when in truth it is one hundred per cent unverified conjecture. The sentence "When serotonin levels are low, the body functions that serotonin regulates are adversely effected, causing a chemical imbalance that commonly results in depression" contains several errors of fact. Since serotonin levels have never been demonstrated to be low, the two claimed consequences of low serotonin are also Begging the Question logical fallacies. [70] Since the premise—"when serotonin levels are low"—has no scientific validity, it cannot be truthfully claimed that "the body functions that serotonin regulates are adversely affected", or that there is a resulting "chemical imbalance that commonly results in depression".

Similar problems arise from the author's assertion that "When norepinephrine levels are low, you can lack focus and feel unmotivated and tired". This too is a Begging the Question logical fallacy, since the premise upon which the second half of the sentence is built is itself has no scientific verification. [71] There is no evidence that confirms low norepinephrine levels to begin with. While many doctors may inform patients that some antidepressants "balance your norepinephrine levels", these claims are unsubstantiated scientifically. There is no scientific basis to the statement that anxiety is known to be "associated with high levels of norepinephrine" in the brain. While it certainly is true to say that "Numerous triggers, such as divorce or sudden loss of a loved one, can cause" a great deal of distress, grief, loss and depression, no evidence confirms that such very difficult life events "cause a chemical imbalance".

The recurring pattern whereby intelligent, well-educated and well-intentioned people such as Lashon Fryer and many others I have mentioned in this book get the facts about depression so wrong is no coincidence. This phenomenon occurs because of the vacuous and misleading nature of pronouncements about depression by society's appointed experts in the field, not least, by medical doctors. There is no such confusion and inaccuracy in similar writings about diabetes, multiple sclerosis, arthritis or other known biological diseases by non-medical interested parties. The reason for this difference is straightforward. Many facts about the biological nature of these diseases are well understood. There are not many yawning gaps in the biological understanding of these conditions, so the public can make sense of them. In contrast, gaps the size of the Grand Canyon exist in the medical understanding of depression. The biological dots do not and perhaps cannot join. People try to make a logical sequence out of the limited and often misleading information they pick up from supposedly reputable sources, often leading to wildly inaccurate and unsubstantiated conclusions, as we have seen.

The misinformation and lack of clear thinking that regularly characterizes discussions on depression is encapsulated in an article on the eHow Health website with the authoritative-sounding title "Signs and symptoms of Chemical Imbalance of the Brain". The writer remains anonymous. The article has been shared thirty times on Facebook. The article begins:

> Chemical imbalance in the brain is a medical condition which results when there are discrepancies in the levels of chemical compounds in the brain. There are medical conditions which are considered to be signs and symptoms of the chemical imbalance disease in the brain. [72]

None of the above is factually correct. The author added:

> It is also important to point out that there is a lot of controversy within the medical community regarding the cause and effect of brain chemical imbalance. [73]

This sentence erroneously implies that brain chemical imbalances have been identified, and that the only controversy surrounds whether these imbalances are cause or effect. This is a Red Herring logical fallacy since it side-steps the more fundamental question; the fact that no chemical imbalances have been identified at all. [74]

Having correctly stated that "chemical imbalance in the brain is one of the theories which seeks to explain causes of mental illness" and "not everyone agrees that chemical imbalance in the brain causes mental illness", the author reverts to presenting fantasy as an established fact. Directly after discussing depression as a chemical imbalance, the author wrote that "Diabetes is another disease that is often associated with a chemical imbalance". Depression and diabetes are stated to be equally caused by chemical imbalances. In truth, diabetes is *always* associated a chemical imbalance—raised blood glucose—while depression *never* is. This is therefore a Weak Analogy logical fallacy. [75] According to the author:

> When imbalances occur in some neurotransmitters in the brain—such as serotonin, norepinephrine and dopamine—such imbalance could lead to depression.

This claim is without substance. Imbalances that have never been identified to occur cannot be unequivocally claimed to cause depression.

"Testing for chemical imbalance" is another eHow internet article that contains a host of inaccuracies, written by an author who calls themselves Alexis Writing. Erroneous though much of the following is, it does represent an attempt to make sense of the yawning gaps in psychiatry's knowledge and the vacuum of common sense and logic that is characteristic of many medical pronouncements on depression and brain chemical abnormalities:

> Most of the time, tests for chemical imbalance are performed by mental health professionals when there is a change in a person's behaviour. [76]

The truth is that no diagnostic laboratory, radiological or chemical tests of any kind are carried out to identify brain chemical imbalances when there is a change in a person's behaviour or at any other time. One cannot carry out tests that do not exist. According to the author:

> Mental health professionals, such as psychiatrists, are trained to evaluate patients and look for thought, behaviour, mood, perception and speed changes that are indicative of identified mental disorders. These changes, therefore, indicate a chemical imbalance in the brain, or an abnormal level of neurotransmitters (Carver, 2009). These tests, and not a PET scan or other formal diagnostic medical procedure, are the most common way of determining when a chemical imbalance exists. [77]

This is quite a mixed-up passage. Suggesting that changes in "thought, behavior, mood, perception and speed" . . . "indicate a chemical imbalance in the brain or an abnormal level of neurotransmitters" is a remarkable stretch of the imagination. The author continued:

> Medications are prescribed for patients who are observed to have chemical imbalances in order to encourage production of the correct chemical and bring the count back to normal within the body (Carver 2009). [78]

None of the above passage is true. On two occasions this author references Joseph Carver, some of whose fiction writing on chemical imbalances I referred to in chapter seven. This is an example of how misinformation from a supposedly reputable source—Joseph Carver is a psychologist—is interpreted as fact and quoted as such by others. And so the misinformation and the delusion spreads.

The popular Psych Central mental health website has a webpage titled "Depression Myths and Facts Demystified". According to the author, who has a Bachelor's and Master's degree in psychology: [79]

> Chemicals in the brain that control appetite, sleep, mood and cognition may function abnormally in depression. [80]

While commonly presumed to be the case, it has not been scientifically established that brain chemicals control appetite, sleep, mood and cognition. Our primitive understanding of the complexity of the brain cautions us to be careful about coming to any such premature conclusions.

WebMD is a major American health website with a strong psychiatry input. WebMD is described by psychiatrist Daniel Carlat as an "incredibly successful company". [81] Four of the five WebMD Health senior staff and editorial team are medical doctors including the chief medical editor. This site has a range of specialists addressing health topics including psychiatry. According to the WebMD website in December 2013:

Doctors aren't sure what causes depression, but a prominent theory is altered brain structure and chemical function. Chemicals called neurotransmitters become unbalanced. What pushed these chemicals off course? One possibility is the stress of a traumatic event, such as losing a loved one or a job. Other triggers could include certain medications, alcohol or substance abuse, hormonal changes, or even the season. [82]

This passage appears entirely reasonable and balanced at first glance, but not when one looks more closely. Notice the subtle seamless shift from "a prominent *theory*" in the first sentence to statements of apparent facts in the following two sentences; "chemicals called neurotransmitters *become* unbalanced. What *pushed* these chemicals off course?" Neither the two cornerstones of the stated prominent theory—"altered brain structure and chemical function"—have been identified in depression in spite of vigorous attempts to do so over many decades.

On 18 August 2014 I happened to check the WebMD's website "Depression Slideshow". I noticed that the wording in the above passage had been altered since I reviewed it eight months previously. All that remained was the first sentence:

Doctors aren't sure what causes depression, but a prominent theory is altered brain structure and chemical function. [83]

The next four sentences appear to have been quietly removed:

Chemicals called neurotransmitters become unbalanced. What pushed these chemicals off course? One possibility is the stress of a traumatic event, such as losing a loved one or a job. Other triggers could include certain medications, alcohol or substance abuse, hormonal changes, or even the season. [84]

The entire passage appeared verbatim in an 18 December 2010 article titled "Why Aren't More Americans Happy?" on Jeremy Person's website—attributed to the WebMD Depression Slideshow—confirming that my eyes had not been deceiving me.[85] The question arises; why would WebMD remove this wording, which had been on its website for a minimum of three years and probably much longer? [86] Why did WebMD feel the need to remove wording about chemical imbalances that had been previously presented as unequivocal established facts? In my opinion, the most likely reason is that the website owners could no longer defend these indefensible claims and discretely removed the references, perhaps hoping that no one would notice. Predictably, the revised text does contain reference to the medically-prompted notion that depression is fundamentally a biological problem:

One must be biologically prone to develop the disorder. [87]

This is utter misinformation, since biological vulnerability to depression has never been reliably identified to begin with. Maintaining this myth serves to preserve the position of doctors as *the* experts in depression, since doctors are considered society's experts in biological illnesses. In my opinion, that is the reason such false claims are regularly made. Elsewhere on the WebMD site, the long-promoted but unevidenced link between depression and brain chemical imbalances continues to feature. One of the "myths" described on WebMD's "Myths and facts about depression" slideshow is the following:

> Myth: It's Not a Real Illness: Depression is a serious medical condition—and the top cause of disability in American adults. Biological evidence of the illness can be seen on brain scans, which show abnormal activity levels. Key brain chemicals that carry signals between nerves—shown here—also appear to be out of balance in depressed people. [88]

Presented as a set of facts, there are many inaccuracies contained within this passage. As I discuss in this book and subsequent books, it has not been scientifically established that depression is a real medical illness. While it is regularly asserted that depression is a medical condition, depression does not meet the usual required criteria for a medical condition. [89] "Biological evidence of the illness" *cannot* "be seen on brain scans". Since so-called "normal" levels of activity have not been reliably established, talk of abnormal levels is inappropriate. Increased levels of activity occurring in various emotional and psychological states does not equate with "abnormal activity levels". The activity is reflecting what the person is experiencing emotionally and psychologically. Given the complexity of the brain, we have no clue regarding what constitutes normal and abnormal levels, or even if this simplistic concept of normality and abnormality applies to brain chemicals and depression. It cannot therefore be truthfully stated that "brain scans . . . show abnormal activity levels". Nor is there any evidence that "key brain chemicals . . . appear to be out of balance" in depressed people.

Another article on the WebMD website manages to contain a mix of truth, false information and a logical fallacy all in one paragraph:

> Although it is widely believed that a serotonin deficiency plays a role in depression, there is no way to measure its levels in the living brain. Therefore, there have not been any studies proving that brain levels of this or any other neurotransmitter are in short supply when depression or any other mental illness develops. Blood serotonin levels are measurable—and have been shown to be lower in people who suffer from depression—but researchers don't know if blood levels reflect the brain's level of serotonin. Also researchers don't know whether the dip in serotonin causes the depression, or the depression causes the serotonin levels to drop. [90]

This article was written by Colette Bouchez, an award-winning medical journalist with over 20 years' experience. She was the former medical editor of the *New York Daily News* and the author of seven health books for women. [91] Bouchez's article was reviewed by Brunilda Nazario MD to ensure "accuracy, timelessness and credibility".[92]

Readers of this article might reasonably assume that this combination of considerable medical journalistic experience and medical overseeing would ensure accuracy and credibility throughout. Because of the pervasiveness of the depression chemical imbalance delusion, sadly this is not the case. The author's statements regarding the immeasurability of brain serotonin levels are correct. The author's claim that blood serotonin levels can be measured is also correct, but as discussed earlier in this book, blood serotonin levels provide no reliable information regarding brain serotonin levels. It is *not* correct to claim that blood serotonin levels have been found to be lower in people who suffer from depression. Having incorrectly claimed that blood serotonin levels are low in depression, and acknowledged that researchers "don't know if blood levels reflect the brain's level of serotonin", in the next sentence the author spoke of "the dip in serotonin", as though this was an established reality. She then wondered whether this supposed dip "causes the depression, or the depression causes the serotonin levels to drop".

Actually, researchers *are* sure that blood serotonin levels provide no reliable indication of brain serotonin levels, which is why blood serotonin levels are not carried out by doctors in people thought to have depression. Considerations of whether "the dip in serotonin" causes depression or is the result of depression are logically unsound, since the claimed dip in serotonin has never been identified to exist. Such comments are classic Begging the Question logical fallacies. [93]

Beyond Blue is an Australian organization with about 60 staff, described on its website as:

> An independent, not-for-profit organization working to increase awareness of anxiety and depression in Australia and reduce the associated stigma. [94]

As already mentioned, in considerations of depression and brain chemical levels, the subtle seamless shift from theory to fact within a few sentences is regrettably a common phenomenon. An example of this appears in a section the Australian Beyond Blue depression information leaflet, under the heading "Changes in the brain":

> What happens in the brain to cause depression is not fully understood. Evidence suggests that it may be related to the changes in the levels or activity of certain chemicals that carry messages within the brain—particularly serotonin, norepinephrine and dopamine, which are the three main chemicals related to mood and motivation . . . Changes in brain chemistry have been more commonly associated with severe depression, rather than mild or moderate depression. [95]

This passage is misinformed and logically flawed on several levels. The first sentence contains contradictory certainty and uncertainty. How can one be certain that something "happens in the brain to cause depression" when what happens in the brain is "not fully understood" or even identified as occurring? The common practice of exaggerating understanding features in this first sentence. If communicating truthful information were the writers' number one priority, "not fully understood" in the first sentence would have been replaced by "very poorly understood". No "evidence" suggests that depression may be related to changes in brain chemical levels or activity. This has always been just a theory, a hypothesis that fifty years of intense research has failed to verify scientifically. In the final sentence of the above passage, the assertion that "changes in brain chemistry have been more commonly associated with severe depression, rather than mild or moderate depression" is without foundation, yet it is presented as a fact.

Such misinformation should not appear in material made available to the public by professionals or organizations to whom the public look for accurate and honest information. Regrettably, regarding depression and brain chemicals, this is a common practice.

On its twitter account page, Brainphysics.com is described as "a growing mental health community" whose goal is:

> To bring people together around mental health-related issues. Depression, anxiety, OCD. [96]

Despite an extensive search, I was unable to identify who funds or runs Brainphysics' sophisticated website. On their "How Prozac works" webpage, the Brainphysics.com website claims:

> Too little serotonin may be associated with disorders like major depression, obsessive-compulsive disorder and other anxiety disorders. Prozac may help to correct this by increasing the brain's supply of serotonin. [97]

"Too little serotonin" has never been identified as occurring in the brain. It is a major leap of faith to assume that Prozac can "correct" a deficiency that has not been identified to exist.

The fact that there are no evidenced biological abnormalities often results in and is revealed in inconsistencies and contradictions that regularly surface. One such inconsistency occurs on the Brainphysics.com website. While the "How Prozac works" webpage asserts in considerable detail that biochemical abnormalities are central to depression, the site's "Major Depressive Disorder" page does not even mention brain chemicals as a possible cause of depression. [98]

The eMedTV website appears professional and sophisticated, run by Clinaero, which is described on the website as a privately held software and services company focusing on clinical trials and health information. Clinaero uses revenue from advertising and clinical trial products to fund eMedTV. According to eMedTV's "Paxil CR" webpage, this drug (brackets theirs):

> Works by helping to keep the levels of a certain chemical in the brain (serotonin) balanced . . . Serotonin is one of several chemicals used to send messages from one nerve cell to another. As a message travels down a nerve, it causes the end of the cell to release serotonin. The serotonin enters the gap between the first nerve cell and the one next to it. When enough serotonin reaches the second nerve cell, it activates receptors on the cell and the message continues on its way. The first cell then quickly absorbs any serotonin that remains in the gap between cells. This is called "reuptake". Normally, this process works without any problems. When

the level of serotonin becomes unbalanced, however, it can cause a variety of conditions, including depression. Paxil CR helps to block the reuptake of serotonin so that more serotonin remains in the space between the brain's nerve cells. This gives the serotonin a better chance of activating the receptors on the next nerve cell. [99]

The unequivocal assertion that Paxil CR works "by helping to keep the levels of a certain chemical in the brain balanced" is a falsehood, since there is no evidence to support this claim. The statement that "when the level of serotonin becomes unbalanced, however, it can cause a variety of conditions, including depression" is misleading, since levels of serotonin have never been identified to be unbalanced. The claim that increasing the amount of serotonin "gives the serotonin a better chance of activating the receptors in the next nerve cell" is a major assumption. There is no evidence of a problem in activating the receptors to begin with. Since there is no evidence that these levels were low, the addition of extra serotonin is likely to create rather than alleviate a chemical imbalance.

The eMedTV website also has a series of videos about depression. The following is from the site's "What causes depression?" video:

You might have heard that depression is caused by an imbalance of certain chemicals in the brain called neurotransmitters. These neurotransmitters allow brain cells to communicate with each other by sending and receiving messages. These are the same chemicals that many of the current depression medications affect. Since these medicines are useful in treating depression, it can be assumed that neurotransmitters have an impact on depression. What is not known is whether a chemical imbalance plays a part in causing depression or if the imbalance occurs as a result of a person being depressed. [100]

Many problems arise in this passage. The erroneous notion that depression is caused by brain chemical imbalances is supported in the first sentence above. This passage contains one major leap of faith, a very dubious deduction; "Since these medicines are useful in treating depression, it can be assumed that neurotransmitters have an impact on depression". Given the currently unfathomable complexity of the human brain, this is a highly misleading assertion, although people watching this video may not pick this up. This sloppy logic is typical of psychiatric and drug company thinking over the past thirty years. It is highly flawed. Neurotransmitter problems have never been identified in depression. It is highly unscientific to assume that, because substances that interfere with neurotransmitter function sometimes help people who are depressed, neurotransmitters problems routinely occur in depression. Because morphine eases pain does not mean that the person had a pre-existing morphine or opiate deficiency. According to their website:

Through eMedTV, Clinaero is committed to providing accurate and credible health information to consumers, both in written and multimedia format. Our mission is to offer the most comprehensive health information resource on the

Web, which combined with knowledge from their healthcare providers, will allow people to make better informed and more confident healthcare decisions. [101]

Unfortunately, as outlined above, Clinaero is in fact providing some inaccurate information that is contributing to the maintenance of the widespread depression delusion that abnormal brain biochemistry has been established to occur in depression.

The depression brain chemical imbalance delusion makes its presence felt on the popular KidsHealth website:

> Depression involves the balance of naturally occurring chemicals in the brain. These chemicals, called neurotransmitters, affect mood. Many things can affect the brain's production of neurotransmitters—including daylight and seasons, a change in the social environment, life events, and certain medical conditions. [102]

Misinformation is unfortunately present here. It is not scientifically established that "depression involves the balance of naturally occurring chemicals in the brain". This is theory misrepresented as a fact, as is the third sentence. There is no reliable scientific evidence that verifies claims that "many things can affect the brain's production of neurotransmitters".

The depression brain chemical imbalance delusion is also alive and well on the well-known depression-guide website:

> Like any disease, there is not a single cause for a depression. Depression is a combination of biological, genetic and psychological factors. At the biological level, depression results from abnormal levels of certain neurotransmitters in the brain. This can be caused by changing levels of hormones, explaining why many people first experience depression during puberty . . . Depression is not a state a mind. It is related to physical changes in the brain, and related to a chemical imbalance in the brain that carries signals in your brain and nerves. These chemicals are called neurotransmitters. [103]

This passage contains many inaccuracies and much misinformation. The sentence "At the biological level, depression results from abnormal levels of certain neurotransmitters in the brain" is utterly untrue. Since this sentence is untrue, so inevitably is the subsequent one, which is consequently a Begging the Question logical fallacy; [104] "This can be caused by changing levels of hormones, explaining why many people first experience depression during puberty". I find it shocking that a website purporting to guide people about depression presents such misinformation and in the process grossly underestimates the role of emotional and psychological aspects including those associated with adolescence. The assertion that depression "is related to physical changes in the brain, and related to a chemical imbalance in the brain that carries signals in your brain and nerves" is theory misrepresented as fact, a theory for which there is not a shred of supporting direct scientific evidence.

According to the Cnsdiseases website:

> The internal balance of several natural chemicals in our brains influences how we feel emotionally and physically . . . Disturbances in your brain's chemistry can lead to the symptoms of depression . . . Prescription antidepressant medications reverse this process by replenishing depleted chemical messengers in the brain. [105]

This brief passage contains two falsehoods. Disturbances in brain chemistry that are associated with depression have never been identified. It cannot therefore be rightly claimed that "disturbances in your brain's chemistry can lead to the symptoms of depression". Secondly, it cannot be stated as a fact that "prescription antidepressant medications reverse this process by replenishing depleted chemical messengers in the brain". No such "process" has been identified that needs reversing, and no deficit of chemical messengers has ever been demonstrated that requires "replenishing". The Cnsdiseases website makes further unsubstantiated claims:

> Today scientists know that many people suffering from mental illnesses have imbalances in the ways their brains metabolize certain chemicals called neurotransmitters. Too much or too little of these chemicals may result in depression, anxiety or other emotional or physical disorders. This knowledge has allowed pharmaceutical company researchers to develop medicines that can alter the way in which the brain produces, stores and releases neurotransmitter chemicals, thereby alleviating the symptoms of some mental illnesses. [106]

Scientists do not "know" that people diagnosed with mental illnesses "have imbalances in . . . chemicals called neurotransmitters". Since it cannot be established what anyone's brain chemical levels are, claims of "too much or too little of these chemicals" are scientifically unsubstantiated as are claims that depression results from these imagined abnormalities.

The passage, "This knowledge has allowed pharmaceutical company researchers to develop medicines that can alter the way in which the brain produces, stores and releases neurotransmitter chemicals, thereby alleviating the symptoms of some mental illnesses" is very problematic, another Begging the Question logical fallacy. [107] This passage relies on the first part—"this knowledge"—being true, but it is not true. This is not knowledge; it is unverified conjecture. Therefore, the rest of this passage has to be logically flawed since it is grounded upon a false premise. In fact, it happened the other way around. The drugs came first, and the neurotransmitter hypotheses were created as an attempt to scientifically validate the drugs and justify their use. The 2013 *Oxford Handbook of Psychiatry* acknowledged that drugs and drug research have been "hypothesis creating" rather than "hypothesis driven". [108]

According to the 2004 book *The Complete Book of Men's Health: Everything a Man Needs to Know*:

> Research suggests that serious depression may be caused by an imbalance of the brain's chemical messengers, the neurotransmitters. [109]

As I mentioned earlier, it is the researchers that suggest this, not the research itself.

Men and Depression: What to Do When the Man You Care About is Depressed is a 2002 book written by Theresa Francis-Cheung and Robin Grey. Theresa Francis-Cheung is a respected health writer. Robin Grey is an accredited psychotherapist with the British Association of Counselling and has worked for the mental health association MIND. According to the authors:

> Imbalances in certain brain chemicals called neurotransmitters—especially serotonin, dopamine and norepinephrine—are thought to be linked with depression. Antidepressant medication attempts to regulate these imbalances. [110]

These two sentences contain an example of a common trend we have seen; slipping subtly and seamlessly from theory to fact. The first sentence mentions that chemical imbalances are *thought* to occur in depression. In the next sentence it is stated that antidepressants *regulate* these imbalances, which now appear to be definite entities.

Sophie Tighe is a Senior Reporter at Yahoo Lifestyle UK. On 12 August 2014, she wrote an article on Yahoo Lifestyle UK about the death of actor Robin Williams in which she claimed:

> Depression, in various forms, has been classified as a mental disorder since 1952 by the *Diagnostic and Statistical Manual of Mental Disorders (DSM)* as a chemical imbalance in the brain that can be triggered by genetic vulnerability, stress, medication and medical issues. [111]

Just seven hours after publication, this article had already been shared 472 times on Facebook. Every reader of Sophie Tighe's article has been misinformed. The *Diagnostic and Statistical Manual of Mental Disorders* does not classify depression as a chemical imbalance in the brain at all. There is no reference within the *DSM-5* to serotonin or any other supposed chemical imbalances in relation to depression. In the *DSM-5* it is admitted regarding depression that:

> No laboratory test has yielded results of sufficient sensitivity and specificity to be used as a diagnostic tool for this disorder. [112]

It would appear that, like many others, this senior Yahoo reporter has come to believe the much-repeated falsehood that chemical imbalances are synonymous with depression.

Described as a "science journalist" on Ireland's East Coast FM radio website, Sean Duke provided yet another example of the depression brain chemical imbalance delusion on the radio station's "The Morning Show with Declan Meehan" on 24 July 2014:

> Serotonin is linked to emotions in the brain, and when you don't have enough serotonin, you become depressed. [113]

Sean Duke's curriculum vitae is impressive—Bachelor's degree in Science, Master's degree in Science and Environmental Reporting; former editor of *Technology Ireland* magazine; work shop leader with the Innovation Academy, a project involving three Irish universities that is designed to "develop a new kind of PhD graduate"; [114] a regular media science contributor to the *Sunday Times* Irish edition and Irish regional and national radio programmes. [115] That a respected and informed science enthusiast such as Sean Duke could be so wrong regarding serotonin and the brain is testament to the degree of penetration of this delusion within the developed world.

BUPA is a major international healthcare group, serving over 22 million customers in over 190 countries. Depression is discussed in some detail on the BUPA UK website, including a section on the causes of depression. There is no reference to brain chemical levels in any of the eleven listed causes of depression, the majority of which point to the psycho-social causes such as relationship breakdown, divorce, bereavement, poverty, abuse and neglect, poor parent-child relationships in early life and isolation from friends and family. [116] Later on the same webpage however, BUPA include the following:

> Selective serotonin reuptake inhibitors (SSRIs) . . . increase the level of serotonin in your brain, lifting your depression. [117]

The apparent simplicity and certainty of this assertion conveys the impression that by increasing serotonin brain levels, depression is lifted. This is problematic on several fronts. This claim does not acknowledge the unfathomable complexity of the brain or the absence of evidence of pre-existing low serotonin levels. It is also a False Cause logical fallacy and a Begging the Question logical fallacy. The "lifting" of depression is attributed to raised serotonin levels, when in truth it is not known if SSRIs actually cause a sustained raise in brain serotonin levels to occur at all.

NOTES TO CHAPTER EIGHT

1.   See Irving Kirsch, *The Emperor's New Drugs: Exploding the Antidepressant Myth*, London: The Bodley Head, Random House, 2009, p. 81.
2.   The National Institute of Mental Health website, "Brain Basics" webpage, http://www. nimh. nih. gov/health/educational-resources/brain-basics/brain-basics. shtml#Working-Brain, accessed 24 February 2014.
3.   These include the National Alliance on Mental Illness (NAMI); the Child and Adolescent Bipolar Foundation, now known as The Balanced Mind Parent Network; The Depression and Bipolar Support Alliance (DBSA); Mental Health America (MHA).
4.   National Alliance on Mental Illness, Depression Factsheet, 2009, http://www.nami.org/content/ NavigationMenu/Mental_Illnesses/Depression/NAMI_Depression_ FactSheet_2009.pdf accessed 28 March 2014.

5. National Alliance on Mental Illness, "Depression", 2012, http://www.nami.org/Template. cfm? Section=Depression&template=contentmanagement/contentdisplay.cfm&ContentID=67727, accessed 26 February 2014.

6. National Institute on Mental Illness website, http://www.nami.org/Content/NavigationMenu /Hearts_and_Minds/8NamiConfrontingStigmas.PDF.pdf, accessed 15 June 2014.

7. Nottinghamshire Healthcare, NHS trust, http://www.nottinghamshirehealthcare. nhs.uk /about us/, accessed 24 August 2014.

8. Nottinghamshire Healthcare website, "How do SSRIs work?", http://www.choiceandmedication .org/nottinghamshirehealthcare/class/9/, accessed 24 August 2014.

9. Nottinghamshire Healthcare NHS Trust website, "What happens when transmitter activity is low?", http://www.choiceandmedication.org/nottinghamshirehealthcare/questions/1170/, accessed 24 August 2014.

10. For information on Begging the Question logical fallacies see note 22 in the Notes to the Introduction.

11. Nottinghamshire Healthcare NHS Trust website, "How do medicines work in the brain?", http://www.choiceandmedication.org/nottinghamshirehealthcare/questions/1164/, accessed 24 August 2014.

12. Identical pages for "Clinical Depression-Causes" appear on many NHS Trust websites, including the Leeds Community Healthcare NHS Trust and the Liverpool Community Healthcare NHS Trust, http://www.nhs.uk/Conditions/Depression/Pages/Causes.aspx, accessed 25 August 2014.

13. Elaine Farrell, *The Complete Guide to Mental Health: The Comprehensive Guide to Choosing Therapy, Counselling and Psychiatric Care*, London: Vermilion, 1991, p. 20.

14. Rethink Mental Illness, "Depression", 2009, updated January 2010, http://www.vetlife.org.uk/ sites/default/files/resource-files/Rethink%20Guide%20to%20Depression.pdf, accessed 17 August 2014.

15. Rethink Mental Illness, "Depression", 2009, updated January 2010, http://www.vetlife. org.uk/ sites/default/files/resource-files/Rethink%20Guide%20to%20Depression.pdf, accessed 17 August 2014.

16. Rethink Mental Illness, "Depression", 2009, updated January 2010, http://www.vetlife. org.uk /sites/default/files/resource-files/Rethink%20Guide%20to%20Depression.pdf, accessed 17 August 2014.

17. For information on False Cause logical fallacies see note 42 in the Notes to Chapter Five.

18. Rethink Mental Illness website, "Depression–Causes", http://www.rethink.org/diagnosis-treatment/conditions/depression/causes, accessed 18 August 2014.

19. Joanna Moncrieff, "Is Psychiatry for Sale?: An Examination of the Influence of the Pharmaceutical Industry on Academic and Practical Psychiatry", June 2013, http://www.critpsy-net.freeuk. com/pharmaceuticalindustry.htm, accessed 05 March 2014, advertisement reproduced in Elliot S. Valenstein, *Blaming the Brain: The Truth About Drugs and Mental Health*, New York: The Free Press, 1998, chap 6, p. 178-181.

20. Elliot S. Valenstein, *Blaming the Brain: The Truth About Drugs and Mental Health*, New York: The Free Press, 1998, p. 177.

21. For information on False Dilemma logical fallacies see note 38 in the Notes to Chapter Five.

22. Vera Hassner Sharav, "Depression-serotonin: How did so many smart people get it so wrong?", Alliance for Human Research Protection website, 19 November 2005, http://www.ahrp.org/ cms/content/view/67/55/, accessed 12 May 2014.

23. Mental Health America website, http://www.mentalhealthamerica.net/who-we-are, accessed 15 June 2014.

24. Mental Health America, "Depression: What you need to know", http://www.mentalhealth america.net/conditions/depression#depression, accessed 15 June 2014.

25. The Child and Adolescent Bipolar Foundation is listed on the American Psychiatric Association website's "Resources" webpage, http://www.psychiatry.org/mental-health/links-for-more-information, accessed 15 June 2013.

26. The Balanced Mind Parent Network website, formerly known as the Child and Adolescent Bipolar Foundation, the http://www.thebalancedmind.org/about-us, accessed 15 June 2014.

27. The Balanced Mind Parent Network website, "Fact Sheet: Facts about Teenage Depression", 27 November 2009, http://www.thebalancedmind.org/learn/library/facts-about-teenage-depression, accessed 15 June 2014.

28. The Balanced Mind Parent Network Scientific Advisory Council membership, http://www.the balancedmind.org/about/staff/cabf-scientific-advisory-council, accessed 15 June 2014.

29. Depression and Bipolar Support Alliance website, "Coping with Mood Changes Later in Life", http://www.dbsalliance.org/site/PageServer? pagename=education_brochures_coping_mood changes, accessed 14 June 2014.

30. Depression and Bipolar Support Alliance website, "Facts about depression", http://www.dbsalliance.org/site/PageServer?pagename=press_facts_depression, accessed 15 June 2014.

31. Depression and Bipolar Support Alliance website, "Technological Alternative Treatments", http://www.dbsalliance.org/site/PageServer?pagename=wellness_depression_emerging_technolog ies, accessed 17 August 2014.

32. Depression and Bipolar Support Alliance Scientific Advisory Panel, http://www.dbsalliance.org /site/PageServer?pagename=DBSA_board_scientific, accessed 15 June 2014.

33. Spunout.ie, 2012 web statistics, http://spunout.ie/about, accessed 15 September 2014.

34. "Dealing with depression", spunout.ie website, http://spunout.ie/health/article/dealing-with-depression?gclid=CjwKEAjwnNqgBRDdgOitrZPj6yYSJACM86tD8pt 7L46m HPb KseLlUoZC 8fdJbvPFcDgnq_z5Wq1_3hoCLhTw_wcB, accessed 15 September 2014.

35. Nadia Sawalha, ITV *Loose Women* panelist, 01 November 2013, http://www.itv.com/loosewomen/presenters/nadia-sawalha, accessed 11 November 2014.

36. ITV, *Loose Women*, 07 November 2014, https://www.itv.com/itvplayer/loose-women, accessed 10 November 2014.

37. Author Marian Keyes, interviewed on the Marian Finucane Show, RTE Radio One, 08 November 2014, http://www.rte.ie/radio1/podcast/podcast_marianfinucane.xml, Marian Keyes, accessed 08 November 2014.

38. In my next book, *Depression: Its True Nature,* I will set out in detail an explanation of the experiences and behaviours that fall within the current definition of depression. Emotional and psychological shutdown explains the experience described here by Marian Keyes. This shutdown is a defense mechanism that many of us employ to minimize contact with our deeper pain. The price we pay for this defense mechanism is the inability to feel happiness and joy, as well as the raw pain and sorrow that we seeking to distance ourselves from by withdrawing and shutting down. This is a price we are willing to pay, as minimizing contact with our deeper pain is then our number one priority.

39. Author Marian Keyes, interviewed on the Marian Finucane Show, RTE Radio One, 08 November 2014, http://www.rte.ie/radio1/podcast/podcast_marianfinucane.xml, accessed 08 November 2014.

40. Juliette Jowit, "NHS can no longer act as if minds don't matter", *Guardian,* 10.11.2014, http://www.theguardian.com/commentisfree/2014/nov/10/nhs-mental-illness-health-services?utm _source=twitterfeed&utm_medium=twitter&commentpage=2, accessed 11.11.2014.

41. Tim Cantopher, *Depressive Illness: The Curse of the Strong,* 3rd edition, Sheldon Press, 2012, p.1.

42. Tim Cantopher, *Depressive Illness: The Curse of the Strong,* 3rd edition, Sheldon Press, 2012, p.1.

43. Mary Kenny, *Irish Independent,* December 1998, quoted by Terry Lynch, *Beyond Prozac: Healing Mental Distress,* Ross-on-Wye: PCCS Books, 2004. p. 27.

44. S. Brewer, Holistic Doctor, *Chat* magazine, June 1999.

45. Linda McGrory, *Irish Examiner,* 14 August 2000.

46. Andrew Solomon, *The Noonday Demon: An Anatomy of Depression,* London: Vintage, 2002, pps. 57, 253.

47. Joyce Carol Oates, "I'm Not O.k., You're Not O.K.", *New York Times,* 24 June 2001, https://www.nytimes.com/books/01/06/24/reviews/010624.24oatest.html, accessed 28 June 2014.

48. Gareth O'Callaghan, *A Day Called Hope: A Personal Journey Beyond Depression,* London: Hodder & Stoughton, 2003, p. 89.

49. Gareth O'Callaghan, *A Day Called Hope: A Personal Journey Beyond Depression,* London: Hodder & Stoughton, 2003.

50. Ronnie O'Sullivan, with Simon Hattenstone, *Ronnie: The Autobiography of Ronnie O'Sullivan,* London: Orion, 2003, p. 175.

51. Vincent Browne, in foreword to *Understanding Mental Health,* eds. Siobhan Barry and Abbie Lane, Dublin: Blackhall Publishing, 2006, p. x.
52. Siobhan Barry, *Understanding Mental Health,* Dublin: Blackhall Publishing, 2006, p. 58.
53. Noelle Creamer, *The Pittsburgh Tribune Review,* 04 April 2007.
54. For information on False Dilemma logical fallacies see note 38 in the Notes to Chapter Five.
55. Nicolette Heaton-Harris, *Understanding Depression,* Brighton: Emerald Guides, 2008, p. 23.
56. Ray D'Arcy speaking on The Ray D'Arcy Show, Today FM (an Irish national radio channel), 06 December 2011.
57. Mary McEvoy, *How the Light Gets In: My Journey with Depression,* Dublin: Hachette Books, 2011, pps. 135-6.
58. Jonathan Crowe, science writer, "Why do antidepressants take so long to work?", Oxford Mental Health Forum blog, 18 March 2012, http://www.oxfordmhf.org.uk/blog/2012/03/why-do-antidepressants-take-so-long-to-work/, accessed 20 February 2014.
59. J.R. Lacasse & J. Leo, "Serotonin and Depression: A Disconnect between the Advertisements and the Scientific Literature", *PLoS Med* 2(12), 2005: e392 doi:10.1371/journal.pmed.0020392, accessed 28 February 2014.
60. For information on Begging the Question logical fallacies see note 22 in the Notes to the Introduction.
61. *New York Times* "Major Depression In-depth Report", http://www.nytimes.com/health/guides/disease/major-depression/causes.html, accessed 24 January 2014.
62. For information on Begging the Question logical fallacies see note 22 in the notes to the Introduction.
63. Harvey Simon, Editor-in-Chief, Associate Professor of Medicine, Harvard Medical School, Physician at the Massachusetts General Hospital, & Dr. David Zieve, M.D., M.H.A., Medical Director, A.D.A.M. Inc.
64. For information on False Cause logical fallacies see note 42 in the Notes to Chapter Five.
65. *New York Times* "Major Depression In-depth Report", http:// voices. yahoo.com/depression-really-medical-condition-77858.html?cat=5, http://www.nytimes.com/health/guides /disease/major-depression/causes.html, accessed 24 February 2014.
66. Michelle L. Devon, "Depression really is a medical condition", 21 September 2006, accessed 12 November 2013; also available on Alternative Healthy Living website, http://alternativehealthlifestyle. com/?p=547, accessed 17 August 2014.
67. For information on False Dilemma logical fallacies see note 38 in the Notes to Chapter Five.
68. Lashon Fryer, eHow Contributor, "Chemical Imbalance that Causes Depression", eHow website, http://www.ehow.com/how-does_5641768_chemical-imbalance-causes-depression.html, accessed 10 December 2013.
69. For information on Begging the Question logical fallacies see note 22 in the Notes to the Introduction.
70. For information on Begging the Question logical fallacies see note 22 in the Notes to the Introduction.
71. For information on Begging the Question logical fallacies see note 22 in the Notes to the introduction.
72. An eHow contributor, "Signs and symptoms of Chemical Imbalance of the Brain", http:// www. ehow.com/about_5366233_signs-symptoms-chemical-imbalance-brain.html, accessed 16 December 2013.
73. An eHow contributor, "Signs and symptoms of Chemical Imbalance of the Brain", http:// www. ehow.com/about_5366233_signs-symptoms-chemical-imbalance-brain.html, accessed 16 December 2013.
74. For information on Red Herring logical fallacies see note 23 in the Notes to the Introduction.
75. For information on Weak Analogy logical fallacies see note 69 in the Notes to Chapter Five.
76. Alexis Writing, eHow Contributor, "Testing for Chemical Imbalance", http://www.ehow. com/way_5516127_testing-chemical-imbalance.html, accessed 29 March 2014.
77. Alexis Writing, eHow Contributor, "Testing for Chemical Imbalance", http://www.ehow. com/way_5516127_testing-chemical-imbalance.html, accessed 29 March 2014.
78. Alexis Writing, eHow Contributor, "Testing for Chemical Imbalance", http://www.ehow. com/way_5516127_testing-chemical-imbalance.html, accessed 29 March 2014.

79. About Margarita Tartakovsky, http://margaritatartakovsky.com/about/, accessed 18 August 2014.

80. Margarita Tartakovsky, "Depression Myths and Facts Demystified", Psych Central website, 30 January 2013, http://psychcentral.com/lib/depression-myths-and-facts-demystified/0003777, accessed 10 March 2014.

81. Daniel Carlat's description of WebMD, http://carlatpsychiatry.blogspot.ie/2010/02/ webmds-big-lie.html, accessed 02 January 2014.

82. WebMD website, "Depression Overview Slideshow", http://www.webmd.com/depression/ss/ slideshow-depression-overview, accessed 31 December 2013.

83. WebMD website, "Depression Overview Slideshow", http://www.webmd.com/depression/ss/ slideshow-depression-overview, (slide number 8), accessed 18 August 2014.

84. WebMD website, "Depression Overview Slideshow, http://www.webmd.com/depression/ss/ slideshow-depression-overview, (slide number 8), accessed 18 August 2014.

85. In Jeremy Person, "Why Aren't More Americans Happy?" 18 December 2010, http://www.jeremyperson.com/category/cookingfooddrink/page/3/, accessed 18 August 2014.

86. This inaccurate wording was definitely on the site between 18 December 2010 (see previous note) and 31 December 2013 when I first read it, and probably for longer.

87. WebMD website, "Depression Overview Slideshow", http://www.webmd.com/depression/ss/ slideshow-depression-overview, slide no. 8, accessed 18 August 2014.

88. WebMD website, "Slideshow: Myths and Facts About Depression", http://www.webmd. com/ depression/ss/slideshow-depression-myths, slide no. 2, accessed 18 August 2014.

89. Depression does not meet generally accepted medical definitions of disease. This topic is beyond the scope of this book. I discuss in in detail in my next book, which will be published about twelve months after this book.

90. Colette Bouchez, "Serotonin: 9 Questions and Answers", Depression Health Center, WebMD website, http://www.webmd.com/depression/features/serotonin, accessed 16 September 2014. The site states that this article has been reviewed by Brunilda Nazario, MD.

91. Colette Bouchez Biography, WebMD website, http://www.webmd.com/colette-bouchez, accessed 16 September 2014.

92. Brunilda Nazario MD Biography, WebMD website, http://www.webmd.com/brunilda-nazario, accessed 16 September 2014.

93. For information on Begging the Question logical fallacies see note 22 in the Notes to the Introduction.

94. Beyondblue website, "About Us", http://www.beyondblue.org.au/about-us, accessed 26 December 2013.

95. Beyondblue website, "What causes depression?", http://www.beyondblue.org.au/the-facts/depression/what-causes-depression, accessed 18 August 2014.

96. https://twitter.com/BrainPhysics1, accessed 10 May 2014.

97. http://www.brainphysics.com/howprozacworks.php, accessed 11 May 2014.

98. http://www.brainphysics.com/major-depression.php, accessed 11 May 2014.

99. Paxil CR webpage, eMedTV website, http://depression.emedtv.com/paxil-cr/paxil-cr. html, accessed 11 May 2014.

100. "What causes depression?" video, eMedTV website, http://depression.emedtv.com/depression -video/causes-of-depression-video.html, accessed 11 May 2014.

101. "About eMedTV", http://www.emedtv.com/about.html, accessed 11 May 2014.

102. Kidshealth website, Depression: "Why do people get depressed?", http://kidshealth.org/ teen/your_mind/mental_health/depression.html#, accessed 15 April 2014.

103. Depression-guide.com website, "What are the Causes of Depression—factors play a role in depression?", http://www.depression-guide.com/depression-causes.htm, accessed 14 April 2014.

104. For information on Begging the Question logical fallacies see note 22 in the notes to the Introduction.

105. cnsdiseases.com website, "What you should know about antidepressants", http://cnsdiseases.com/what-you-should-know-about-antidepressants, accessed 30 December 2013.

106. cnsdiseases.com website, "'Chemical imbalances' and psychiatric drug action", http://cnsdiseases.com/chemical-imbalances-and-psychiatric-drug-action, accessed 30 December 2013.

107. For information on Begging the Question logical fallacies see note 22 in the Notes to the Introduction.
108. David Semple & Roger Smyth, *The Oxford Handbook of Psychiatry,* 3rd edition, Oxford University Press: Oxford, 2013, p. 30.
109. *The Complete Book of Men's Health: Everything a Man Needs to Know*, London: Mitchell Beazley, 2004, p. 179.
110. Theresa Francis-Cheung & Robin Grey, *Men and Depression: What to Do When the Man You Care About is Depressed*, London, Thorsons, 2002, p. 211.
111. Sophie Tighe, "Robin Williams Death: Depression Is A Real Illness and Its Killing People", 12 August 2014, https://uk.lifestyle.yahoo.com/blogs/icymi/robin-williams-death--depression-is-a-real-illness-and-it-s-killing-people-115213458.html, accessed 12 August 2014.
112. American Psychiatric Association, *The Diagnostic And Statistical Manual Of Mental Disorders,* 5th edition, *(DSM-5)*, Washington: American Psychiatric Publishing, 2013, p. 165.
113. "The Morning Show with Declan Meehan", Thursday 24 July 2014, East Coast FM, http://www.eastcoast/on-air/morningshow/listen-back, accessed 28 July 2014. Sean Duke is described as a "science journalist" on the Show's website.
114. The Innovation Academy, http://www.innovationacademy.ie/, accessed 19 September 2014.
115. "About Sean" webpage, http://seanduke.com/about/, accessed 19 September 2014.
116. "Depression", BUPA website, http://www.bupa.co.uk/B550_1/individuals/health-information/directory/d/hi-depression, accessed 15 September 2014.
117. "Depression", BUPA website, http://www.bupa.co.uk/B550_1/individuals/health-information/directory/d/hi-depression, accessed 15 September 2014.

9. THE NUTRITION INDUSTRY

Given the widespread public acceptance of the existence of brain chemical imbalances in depression, it is not surprising that the depression brain chemical imbalance delusion has spread to aspects of the nutrition industry.

Patrick Holford is known internationally as a leading authority on nutrition. His website describes Holford as:

> A leading spokesman on nutrition in the media, specializing in the field of mental health. He is the author of 36 books, translated into over 30 languages and selling millions of copies worldwide . . . His educational website attracts half a million visits a year. [1]

In his 2003 book *Optimum Nutrition for the Mind*, Patrick Holford has a lot to say about brain chemicals and depression, serotonin in particular:

> Serotonin deficiency is one of the most common findings in people with mental health problems . . . What has been learnt about serotonin in the last few years is that there are six main reasons for deficiency, in addition to a lack of tryptophan:
> Not enough oestrogen [2] (women).
> Not enough testosterone (men).
> Not enough light.
> Not enough exercise.
> Too much stress, especially in women.
> Not enough co-factor vitamin and minerals.
> If you are suffering from low mood, feel tense and irritable, are low in energy, tend to comfort eat, have sleeping problems and a reduced interest in sex, and the above apply to you, the chances are that you are low in serotonin . . . low oestrogen means low serotonin and low moods . . . Light stimulates oestrogen and most of us don't get enough of it . . . certainly not enough to maximize serotonin production . . . Stress also rapidly reduces serotonin levels . . . Physical exercise improves stress response, and therefore reduces stress-induced depletion of serotonin. [3]

In these passages, Patrick Holford presented a picture of serotonin deficiency and its causes that appears comprehensive and complete. The reader is likely to be impressed and convinced, but a closer examination of this information reveals many problems.

The fundamental flaw in Patrick Holford's claims regarding serotonin and depression is identical to that of both the medical profession and the pharmaceutical industry; *brain serotonin deficiency has never been established to exist.* Far from being "one of the most common findings in people with mental health problems", serotonin deficiency is never a *finding* at all. Rather, it is an *assumption* that cannot be confirmed, a major Begging the Question logical fallacy. [4]

In the above passage, Patrick Holford named seven "main reasons for deficiency" of brain serotonin—deficiencies of tryptophan, oestrogen, testosterone, light, exercise, co-factor vitamins and minerals, and an excess of stress. Let us look at how these claims stack up.

The WebMD website contains a webpage titled "Estrogen and women's emotions". According to this article:

> Exactly how estrogen affects emotion is much less straightforward. Is it too much estrogen? Not enough? It turns out estrogen's emotional effects are nearly as mysterious as moods themselves . . . Normal estrogen levels vary widely . . . Large differences are typical in a woman on different days, or between two women on the same day of their cycles. The actual measured level of estrogen doesn't predict emotional disturbances. [5]

WebMD does state that estrogen raises serotonin levels—a dubious claim in itself, since brain serotonin levels cannot actually be directly measured. The WebMD site cautions the reader from extrapolating anything from this statement:

> What these effects mean in an individual woman is impossible to predict. Estrogen's actions are too complex for researchers to understand fully. As an example, despite estrogen's apparently positive effects on the brain, many women's moods improve after menopause, when estrogen levels are very low. [6]

In the above passage, Patrick Holford also asserted that serotonin deficiency is caused by insufficient levels of testosterone in men, not enough light, not enough exercise and too much stress. While it is true that all of these situations can affect mood, no reliable scientific evidence has ever established that this affect is due to serotonin deficiency. This reality is confirmed by the medical literature. An article published a year after the publication of Holford's book in which he makes these assertions addressed the link between low testosterone and depression. Written by a psychiatry professor, the article included considerable detail regarding links between testosterone levels and depression, including the biochemical effects of testosterone deficiency on the brain. [7] Serotonin is not mentioned anywhere in this article. Testosterone deficiency is a chemical imbalance, and is therefore treated with hormone replacement when necessary, not with serotonin-related products. Testosterone is not even mentioned in the extensive index to the 2013 psychiatry textbook, the *Oxford Handbook of Psychiatry*. This book does not claim that serotonin deficiency is an establish fact, and contains no reference to testosterone or oestrogen deficiency as a cause of serotonin deficiency. The WebMD site contains extensive information on testosterone, including a detailed commentary on the effects of testosterone deficiency. There is no mention of serotonin deficiency within this information as being caused by testosterone deficiency. Of the many references I reviewed while writing this book that erroneously promoted serotonin deficiency as a common cause of depression, none mentioned testosterone or oestrogen deficiency as a definite or even a possible cause of serotonin deficiency.

In practice, demonstrable testosterone deficiency as a cause of depression is rare. Of the millions of people diagnosed with depression annually, only a tiny fraction are caused by a testosterone deficiency verifiable by tests. In this group, no link to serotonin levels is ever established. Testosterone deficiency as a cause of depression is so rare that, in the category of illness this deficiency belongs to, the endocrine and metabolic causes of depression, six conditions are named in the *Oxford Handbook of Psychiatry*; testosterone deficiency is not mentioned, nor is oestrogen deficiency. [8] When testosterone deficiency has been established as a cause of depression, it is part of a much wider picture of testosterone deficiency with many obvious biological features. It falls within the category of organic causes of depression, not the much larger group for which brain chemical imbalances have been wrongly promoted as an established fact.

While exercise and reducing stress are both known to be beneficial for emotional and mental health, no scientific evidence confirms that this benefit is due to correction of decreased serotonin levels. Nor does mainstream scientific research support claims that low levels of co-factor vitamin and mineral levels balance serotonin levels. Whatever benefit these compounds may have, claims that they effect benefit by balancing serotonin levels are without foundation.

In the above passage in which Patrick Holford lists seven causes of serotonin deficiency, the first mentioned is a "lack of tryptophan". Tryptophan is an essential amino acid. Amino acids are described as "essential" if they are required for good health but cannot be synthesised by the body. External sources of the amino acid are required. Tryptophan is a precursor of the B vitamin niacin, supplying up to half of our niacin daily intake. A principle function of tryptophan therefore is to contribute to the production of niacin. Tryptophan is an integral part of dietary protein. It is in almost all protein foods especially meat, poultry, fish, nuts and enriched and wholegrain products. It is stable when heated, so little is lost in cooking. [9] To ascertain whether recognised textbooks on nutrition concurred with Patrick Holford's claims, I reviewed five textbooks on nutrition in the University of Limerick library.

Modern Nutrition in Health and Disease is a comprehensive 2006 nutrition textbook of 2,069 pages. This book contains a comprehensive 42-page index, in which there are just two entries for depression (the index contains 40 references to diabetes). One entry refers to depression and cancer, and the other to depression and obesity. There is no mention of any established or even possible link between depression and tryptophan deficiency in this book. According to the authors, tryptophan:

Had been promoted by the health food industry to treat insomnia, depression, premenstrual syndrome, and overweight, although it had not proven safe and effective for these purposes. [10]

Under the heading "Deficiencies and Manifestations", pellagra is the only condition mentioned as being caused by niacin deficiency. [11] Hartnup syndrome, an extremely rare genetically inherited condition characterized by an inability to synthesize niacin from tryptophan, is also mentioned, as a cause of pellagra-like symptoms. Major textbooks that refer to extremely rare conditions like Hartnup syndrome would also routinely refer to more common conditions such as depression, if the evidence justified doing so. The fact that depression is not mentioned in this major textbook as the result of tryptophan or niacin deficiency therefore speaks volumes. Under the heading "Who is at risk of (Niacin) deficiency?" the authors wrote, "Those in economically deprived areas", where the diet contains insufficient protein sources. [12]

This book contains a chapter titled "Nutrition in disorders of the nervous system". If any reliable evidence existed that linked depression to tryptophan or niacin deficiency, it would have featured in this chapter. Depression as a stand-alone entity caused by tryptophan or niacin deficiency received no mention in this chapter or elsewhere in this book. The only illness due to such deficiencies is pellagra, a very striking condition characterised by dramatic obvious biological phenomena including a dramatic form of dermatitis, skin pigmentation, cracking and peeling, an obviously inflamed tongue in addition to clearly biological neurological features. [13]

Essentials of Human Nutrition is a 2007 textbook on nutrition. This book contains ten index entries for niacin and just two for tryptophan. None of these entries contain any reference to depression. There is no mention of depression at all in the index, which one might expect if there were established links between tryptophan, niacin and depression. This book is also very clear regarding the existence of just one disease that is caused by niacin deficiency, and it is not depression (brackets theirs):

> There is one deficiency disease, *pellagra* (the name means "sour skin" in Italian). The skin is inflamed where it is exposed to sunlight, resembling severe sunburn . . . the skin lesions progress to pigmentation, cracking and peeling . . . Pellagra is rare in developed countries. [14]

The 2013 textbook *Discovering Nutrition* concurs:

> Pellagra is the disease of severe niacin deficiency. The word *pellagra* means "rough skin" in Italian and describes the dermatitis—a rough, darkened rash—that occurs where the victim's skin is exposed to sunlight . . . deficiency devastates the entire body. The hallmarks of pellagra are "the four Ds": dermatitis, diarrhoea, dementia and ultimately, death . . . Today, pellagra has virtually disappeared in industrialized countries. [15]

This book contains two references to depression in the index, none of which refer to tryptophan deficiency in depression.

A similar picture occurs in the 2008 textbook *Nutrition: A Health Promotion Approach*. This book contains just two references to tryptophan in the index, none of which refer to depression. There is no mention of depression in the book's index. Again, pellagra is the only condition referred to regarding niacin deficiency. Under the heading "Niacin – vitamin B3, Key Facts" is written: "Effects of deficiency: Pellagra".[16]

The position of these nutrition textbooks is consistent and very clear. All of these books share the equating of niacin deficiency with pellagra. None refer to other states such as depression in which a tryptophan or niacin deficiency has been identified.

For their laudable adherence to common sense and scientific realities, perhaps the last word on this should go to the authors of the 2013 textbook *Understanding Nutrition*:

> Recommendations (for tryptophan) have led to widespread public use . . . enthusiastic popular reports preceded careful scientific experiments and health recommendations . . . Several nutrient interventions to relieve depression have been studied, but evidence of effectiveness is inconclusive. A balanced healthy diet may be the best nutritional approach to reducing symptoms of depression and improving quality of life. [17]

In his 2003 book *Optimum Nutrition for the Mind*, Patrick Holford wrote about a serotonin blood test, "A neurotransmitter Screening Test". His words are infused with certainty and apparent scientific credibility. Under the dubious heading "Serotonin Imbalance", Holford listed 10 scenarios characteristic of serotonin deficiency, which probably cover at least half the general population:

> Depression, especially post-menopausal; anxiety; aggressive or suicidal thoughts; violent or impulsive behaviour; mood swings, especially premenstrual tension; obsessive or compulsive tendencies; alcohol or drug use; sensitive to pain (low pain threshold); craves sweet foods; sleeping problems. [18]

According to Patrick Holford:

> If you score five or more (in the above list) you may be low in serotonin. [19]

Holford does not explain why five or more means serotonin deficiency while four of less does not. He then informs his many readers about a reliable blood test for brain serotonin levels, something that will come as news to even the most enthusiastic medical supporters of the brain chemical imbalance notion:

> A Neurotransmitter Screening Test can help you confirm this. Your nutritionist can arrange this blood test for you. If you're low, there are specific nutrients, including the amino acids tryptophan or 5-hydroxytryptophan (5-HTP) which can help restore normal mental health. [20]

Curious to know whether some great discovery had somehow passed me by, I checked Patrick Holford's website for further information about this serotonin test. Sure enough, his website contains a 2013 article titled "Biochemical tests for Brain Chemistry Imbalances". In this article Holford wrote that when people come to his clinics for help, they generally "take some initial tests for brain chemistry imbalance". He continued (brackets his):

> The most common laboratory biochemical/nutritional tests that we use are listed here. These tests are often not performed in routine medical screening. Neurotransmitter tests measure blood platelet levels of dopamine, noradrenaline,

adrenaline, serotonin and acetylcholine. These levels are a good indicator of levels found in the fluid in the brain (the cerebrospinal fluid-CSF), thus indicating excesses, deficiencies and imbalances in neurotransmitters. This test is also available through doctors and nutritional therapists. [21]

If measuring blood platelet levels of serotonin really was "a good indicator of levels found in the fluid in the brain" as Holford claims, this test would be routinely carried out by GPs and psychiatrists who have been searching for a reliable depression diagnostic test for fifty years. Even doctors such as the aforementioned American family physician Greg Castello, whose convictions regarding serotonin deficiency bear little relation to the facts, have publicly acknowledged the absence of any reliable way of measuring brain serotonin. [22] The truth is that, as expressed in an article published in 2011 in *Current Psychiatry*, tests evaluating the serotonin levels of platelets:

> Are of questionable value, since peripheral processes may not be an accurate reflection of the corresponding processes in the CNS. In research focusing on this question contradictory results were obtained. [23]

Nowhere in mainstream medicine are blood serotonin level tests considered an accurate and reliable reflection of brain serotonin levels. As I discussed toward the end of the "What the textbooks say" section of chapter two, blood tests for serotonin levels are only carried out to diagnose one condition—carcinoid tumour, a very rare tumour of the intestine.

First published in 1998, *Potatoes Not Prozac* has been a highly successful book. Author Kathleen DesMaisons wrote in 2012 that:

> Since its first publication in 1998, hundreds of thousands of copies have been sold, and I have heard from people from all over the world. [24]

Sugar sensitivity as a cause of emotional distress and mood swings is a core theme in *Potatoes Not Prozac*. The author links sugar sensitivity to low levels of serotonin in the brain. On many occasions in the book, she makes unequivocal statements about serotonin. Here are some examples:

> You have a body . . . with a low level of . . . a brain chemical called serotonin. [25]

Regarding a woman she described as a compulsive eater, who often talks of losing weight but whose resolve evaporates when bread appears on the table in a restaurant, the author is prepared to conclude:

> Diane has low levels of serotonin. [26]

The author made many further unequivocal claims about serotonin:

The effect of low serotonin levels has been widely talked about in the last few years; books about Prozac and several "food and mood" books have examined the value of raising serotonin levels. [27]

When your serotonin is low, you may feel depressed, act impulsively and have intense cravings for alcohol, sweets or carbohydrates. [28]

If your serotonin gets too low, your brain will open up more receptors so it can get more hits . . . if you are sugar sensitive and have naturally low levels of serotonin, then you also have more serotonin receptors. [29]

People with low serotonin have low impulse control. It is almost impossible for them to "just say no" because there is such a short time period between the urge to do something and doing it. This is why the warm cookies on the kitchen table hop into your mouth before you even know what has happened. This is why no matter how many times you vow to stick to your diet, you are not able to. The insufficient serotonin level in your brain isn't giving you the time you need to make good decisions. [30]

Being "too busy" can also reflect an unfocussed and scattered mind, which is one of the symptoms of low serotonin. [31]

If you find yourself feeling impulsive and irritable, flying off the handle, you are experiencing low serotonin. [32]

The scientific evidence for the impact of serotonin on mood and behaviour is well documented. Lowered levels of serotonin are associated with obesity, carbohydrate craving, depression, impulsivity and violence. Lowered levels of serotonin are associated with alcoholism. Persons who have Post Traumatic Stress Disorder show decreased levels of serotonin. [33]

Regarding antidepressants, according to author Kathleen DesMaisons:

The scientists who developed antidepressants focused on creating drugs that would cause the original low number of serotonin molecules released by a depressed person's brain cells to remain in the space between cells for a longer time, thus allowing these molecules to hit the serotonin receptors more than once . . . in effect, your brain is getting the most out of the serotonin you have. . . . The good thing about drugs like Prozac is that they do increase your serotonin level and improve the problem moods and behaviour associated with low serotonin.[34]

Many people appear to have been helped by this book. However, as far as notions of brain chemical balances are concerned, the author has unintentionally misinformed her hundreds of thousands of readers, conveying an illusion of understanding and certainty regarding brain chemical imbalances that has no basis in science or reliable evidence.

Since low brain serotonin levels have never even been established to exist, the author's many assertions of low serotonin in depression are groundless. Her many claims that are built upon the premise of low serotonin are therefore without foundation. They are all Begging the Question logical fallacies. [35] Her claimed links between low serotonin and a wide range of feelings and behaviours are therefore unjustified. Her assertion that low serotonin levels cause obesity will be news to medical specialists in obesity and endocrinology. All of Desmaison's statements are examples of a common human tendency to create elaborate theories that one would like to be true but have no basis in fact. These theories are generally mesmerizingly attractive, often becoming accepted as fact despite any reliable supporting evidence, theories described by psychiatrist Daniel Carlat in 2010 as "ingenious but unproven". [36]

Aforementioned counsellor, teacher and mental health coach Douglas Bloch provides an example of how misinformation spreads by quoting the words of a supposed expert. On his website, Bloch refers to Kathleen DesMaisons and her book, and presents her assertions on serotonin as though they were established facts:

> In her book *Potatoes Not Prozac*, Kathleen DesMaisons, Ph.D., an addiction and nutrition expert, claims that many people who are prone to addictive disorders, as well as to depression, are also sugar sensitive-i.e., they have a special body chemistry that reacts in extreme ways to sugar and refined carbohydrates. The reaction throws off not only the blood sugar levels, but also the levels of serotonin and beta-endorphins (nature's pain killers) in the brain. This in turn causes an inability to concentrate; creates feelings of exhaustion, hopelessness and despair; and contributes to confusion, irritability, and low self-esteem—i.e., symptoms of clinical depression! [37]

Bloch makes a similar claim in his 2002 book *Healing From Depression: 12 Weeks to a Better Mood*:

> The reaction (to sugar and refined carbohydrates) throws off . . . the levels of serotonin. [38]

Claims that brain serotonin levels are "thrown off" by sensitivity to sugar are without foundation scientifically, since brain serotonin levels cannot even be measured. No scientific evidence verifies claims that sugar or refined carbohydrates "throw off levels of serotonin". Such is the widespread acceptance of the notion of serotonin deficiency that people easily slip into ideas regarding serotonin and assume their ideas are plausible. Because these theories originate from trusted medical doctors, the public trust in them, assume they are true and pass them on to others.

NOTES TO CHAPTER NINE

1. Patrick Holford's website, "Patrick's Bio", https://www.patrickholford.com/patricks-bio, accessed 15 November 2014.
2. Oestrogen is spelt "estrogen" in some countries.
3. Patrick Holford, *Optimum Nutrition for the Mind*, London: Judy Piatkus Ltd., 2003, pps. 165, 110-11.
4. For information about Begging the Question logical fallacies see note 22 in the Notes to the Introduction.
5. WebMD website, "Estrogen and women's emotions", http://www.webmd.com/women/guide/estrogen-and-womens-emotions, accessed 15 November 2014.
6. WebMD website, "Estrogen and women's emotions", http://www.webmd.com/women/ guide/estrogen-and-womens-emotions, accessed 15 November 2014.
7. Thomas D. Geracioti Jr. MD, Professor and vice chair of psychiatry, University of Cincinnati College of Medicine, "Persistent depression? Low libido? Androgen decline may be to blame", Vol 3, No. 5/May 2004, http://www.currentpsychiatry.com/home/article/persistent-depression-low-libido-androgen-decline-may-be-to-blame/8bbc025c6a0656c3e152c83- 14c87f82.html, accessed 16 November 2014.
8. David Semple & Roger Smyth, "Presentations of organic illness", in the *Oxford Handbook of Psychiatry*, 3rd edition, Oxford: Oxford University Press, 2013, p. 130.
9. Paul Insel et al, *Discovering Nutrition*, 4th edition, Burlington: Jones & Bartlett Learning, 2013, p. 367.
10. Maurice E. Shils et al, eds., *Modern Nutrition in Health and Disease*, 10th edition, Baltimore: Lippincott, Williams & Wilkins, 2006, p. 1959.
11. Maurice E. Shils et al, eds., *Modern Nutrition in Health and Disease*, 10th edition, Baltimore: Lippincott, Williams & Wilkins, 2006, p. 448.
12. Maurice E. Shils et al, eds., *Modern Nutrition in Health and Disease*, 10th edition, Baltimore: Lippincott, Williams & Wilkins, 2006, p. 600.
13. Maurice E. Shils et al, eds., *Modern Nutrition in Health and Disease*, 10th edition, Baltimore: Lippincott, Williams & Wilkins, 2006, p. 1371.
14. Jim Mann & A. Stewart Truswell, eds., *Essentials of Human Nutrition*, 3rd edition, Oxford: Oxford University Press, 2007, p. 188-90.
15. Paul Insel et al, *Discovering Nutrition*, 4th edition, Burlington: Jones & Bartlett Learning, 2013,p.367-8.
16. Geoffrey P. Webb, *Nutrition: A Health Promotion Approach*, 3rd edition, London: Hodder Arnold, 2008, p. 345.
17. Ellie Whitney & Sharon Rady Rolfes, *Understanding Nutrition*, 13th edition, Wadsworth Cengage Learning, 2013, pps 197, 559.
18. Patrick Holford, *Optimum Nutrition for the Mind*, London: Judy Piatkus Ltd., 2003, p. 165.
19. Patrick Holford, *Optimum Nutrition for the Mind*, London: Judy Piatkus Ltd., 2003, p. 165.
20. Patrick Holford, *Optimum Nutrition for the Mind*, London: Judy Piatkus Ltd., 2003, p. 165.
21. Patrick Holford website, "Biochemical tests for Brain Chemistry Imbalances", 09 April 2013, https://www.patrickholford.com/advice/biochemical-tests-brain-chemistry-imbalances, accessed 15 November 2014.
22. See note 116 in Chapter Five and associated text regarding Dr. Greg Castello.
23. Anniek K. D. Visser, "Measuring serotonin synthesis: from conventional methods to PET tracers and their (pre)clinical implications", *Eur J Nucl Med Mol Imaging*. Mar 2011; 38(3): 576-591. Published online 27.11.2010. doi: 10.1007/s00259-010-1663-2, accessed 16.11.14.
24. DesMaisons, Kathleen, Google Books, 2012, http://books.google.ie/books?id= VnWck7-kOCWAC&pg=PT34&lpg=PT34&dq=Potatoes+not+prozac+copies+sold+kathleen+desmaisons&source=bl&ots=APsu_oCFPB&sig=CRyRPCm7znRXqNDf6sYZnYIqIcU-&hl=en&sa=X&ei=K20NVMnmMvSg7Aatt4HQDw&ved=0CDsQ6AEwBA#v=onepage&q=Potatoes%20not%20prozac%20copies%20sold%20kathleen%20desmaisons&f= false, accessed 29 December 2014.
25. Kathleen DesMaisons, *Potatoes Not Prozac*, London:Simon & Schuster, 1999, p. 37-8. First published in 1998.

26. Kathleen DesMaisons, *Potatoes Not Prozac,* London:Simon & Schuster, 1999, pps. 59-60. First published in 1998.
27. Kathleen DesMaisons, *Potatoes Not Prozac,* London:Simon & Schuster, 1999, pps 39-40. First published in 1998.
28. Kathleen DesMaisons, *Potatoes Not Prozac,* London:Simon & Schuster, 1999, p. 41. First published in 1998.
29. Kathleen DesMaisons, *Potatoes Not Prozac,* London:Simon & Schuster, 1999, p. 63. First published in 1998.
30. Kathleen DesMaisons, *Potatoes Not Prozac,* London:Simon & Schuster, 1999, p. 65. First published in 1998.
31. Kathleen DesMaisons, *Potatoes Not Prozac,* London:Simon & Schuster, 1999, p. 151. First published in 1998.
32. Kathleen DesMaisons, *Potatoes Not Prozac,* London:Simon & Schuster, 1999, p. 191-2. First published in 1998.
33. Kathleen DesMaisons, *Potatoes Not Prozac,* London:Simon & Schuster, 1999, p. 201. First published in 1998.
34. Kathleen DesMaisons, *Potatoes Not Prozac,* London:Simon & Schuster, 1999, p. 66-7. First published in 1998.
35. For information on Begging the Question logical fallacies see note 22 in the notes to the Introduction.
36. Daniel Carlat, *Unhinged: The Trouble with Psychiatry—a Doctor's Revelations about a Profession in Crisis,* London: Free Press, 2010, p. 78.
37. Douglas Bloch, "Natural Remedies for Depression", http://www.healingfromdepression. com/natural-alternatives-to-prozac.htm, accessed 18 September 2014.
38. Douglas Bloch, *Healing from Depression: 12 Weeks to a Better Mood,* Berkeley: Celestial Arts, 2002, p. 177.

10. Depression is a Disease Just Like Diabetes, Right?

According to conventional wisdom, depression is a biological illness like diabetes, multiple sclerosis, arthritis or any other disease. For decades, many doctors and several drug companies have compared depression to these diseases, to diabetes in particular. This practice has escalated since the arrival of the SSRI antidepressant substances in the late 1980s.

The website of the U.S. National Alliance on Mental Illness contains the following comparison between depression and long-term medical illnesses:

> Just as diabetes is a disorder of the pancreas, mental illnesses are medical conditions that often result in a diminished capacity for coping with the ordinary demands of life. [1]

This statement by one of America's most influential mental health organizations is a Weak Analogy logical fallacy. [2] A Weak Analogy logical fallacy occurs when comparisons are made without enough similarity to justify such comparison. Stating that diminished capacity for coping with the "ordinary demands of life" is somehow an appropriate comparison to a known biological disorder of pancreatic function is strikingly flawed logic. The second part of this sentence bears no relation to the first part. A valid comparison to diabetes being a disorder of the pancreas would be to refer to examples of known biological disorders of the brain such as multiple sclerosis, dementia or epilepsy. A comparison with depression is not appropriate since unlike diabetes, depression is not a known biological disease.

A 1996 leaflet produced by a consortium known as America's Pharmaceutical Research Companies summarized the prevailing and propagandized version of what is called "depression" presented within the disease-centred framework:

> What many people fail to realize, however, is that mental illnesses are medical illnesses like diabetes, high blood pressure or heart disease . . . Today scientists know that many people suffering from mental illnesses have imbalances in the way their brains metabolize certain chemicals called neurotransmitters. Too much or too little of these chemicals may result in depression, anxiety or other emotional and physical disorders. This knowledge has allowed pharmaceutical company researchers to develop medicines that can alter the way in which the brain produces, stores and releases neurotransmitter chemicals, thereby alleviating the symptoms of some mental illnesses. [3]

The truth is that scientists did not "know" that people have chemical imbalances in 1996, nor do they know this now. There is no scientific evidence to support the claim that "too much or too little of these chemicals may result in depression, anxiety, or other emotional or physical disorders". This is gross misinformation.

On a discussion about depression on 12 August 2014 on British national television—ITV's *This Morning* programme—well known British GP Dr. Dawn Harper stated:

> I use the analogy . . . if I said to you today, "You're diabetic, I'm really sorry, you've got to take insulin", you wouldn't like the idea but you wouldn't argue with me about taking insulin because you know that's what you need to make you better. If you are clinically depressed, and you need antidepressant medication, that's no different. [4]

Many doctors including Dawn Harper have managed to convince themselves that depression and diabetes are "no different". This is a deluded conclusion for which no hard verifying evidence exists, one arrived at through the great desire of the medical profession for what is called "depression" to be widely seen as a disease. As I discuss later in this chapter, from a disease and a chemical perspective, there is a world of difference between depression and diabetes. Dr. Dawn Harper and many other GPs are apparently unaware of these major and pretty obvious differences. Any such comparison is scientifically untenable and constitutes a Weak Analogy logical fallacy. [5]

Irish general practitioner Dr. Muiris Houston has been medical correspondent with the *Irish Times* for many years. In 2001, the year he was named Irish Medical Journalist of the Year, Dr. Houston wrote:

> Depression, in my view, is no different from diabetes. In one you take insulin and in the other you take Prozac or some other antidepressant. Both substances are simply designed to replace natural chemicals missing from the body. [6]

This is a misrepresentation of the facts. Dr. Houston has never ordered or performed a brain serotonin level test for depression. He can't have, because no such tests exist. Being a conscientious GP, I'm sure that none of his diabetic patients are diagnosed without the proper diagnostic blood tests being carried out. The disease status of diabetes is well established, whereas it remains entirely unestablished in relation to depression. It has never been scientifically established that antidepressants "replace natural chemicals missing from the body". Muiris Houston's direct and strong comparison between the two is therefore erroneous and misleading, a Weak Analogy logical fallacy. [7]

The fact that many other doctors make similar comparisons does not alter the facts of the situation. Telling people that they have a brain chemical imbalance and comparing depression to diabetes as a chemical imbalance disease is at best a mixed metaphor. It is akin to comparing apples with oranges while the public think that apples are being compared to apples.

Alan Wade is a GP in Scotland and Medical Director of CPS Clinical Research Centre. In a national Irish newspaper in 2002 Wade referred to (italics mine):

> The *fact* that depressive illnesses have a physical cause just like diabetes or any other disease. [8]

This is a falsehood, a Weak Analogy logical fallacy, [9] since no such fact has been scientifically established.

In his 2010 book *Flagging the Problem: A New Approach to Mental Health*, Irish GP Harry Barry felt it appropriate to inform his readers that:

> Just as diabetes is an illness caused by biological abnormalities in our pancreas, depression, anxiety and addiction are illnesses caused at least in part by biological abnormalities of the brain. [10]

Barry makes this claim as if it were an established fact, but there is no credible scientific evidence to validate any such claims of biological brain abnormalities relating to depression. By inappropriately comparing diabetes to depression, Drs. Harper, Barry, Wade, Houston and many others have articulated misinformation, a Weak Analogy logical fallacy, [11] also known as a False Analogy logical fallacy.

In recent years it has become increasing difficult to justify comparing depression to diabetes against the rising tide of exposure of the inappropriateness of the brain chemical deficiency notion. Nevertheless this seed has by now been well planted in the public mind. This comparison continues to be made in doctors' offices as a means of legitimizing the antidepressant prescription and persuading people to take antidepressants. Although largely responsible for it, the medical profession and the pharmaceutical industry have done little to correct this public misunderstanding. In the following passages I compare depression to diabetes, not in the superficial and misleading manner that many doctors, drug companies and mental health organizations have done during the past thirty years, but in a real and factual way.

Every final year medical student knows or should know what the normal blood sugar range is and at what point blood sugar levels become abnormal, leading directly to a diagnosis of diabetes. No doctor anywhere in the world knows what the normal brain serotonin level is or whether deficiencies of brain serotonin can even occur. Brain serotonin levels cannot be measured. No tests exist for brain serotonin levels. Every person with diabetes can easily find out what their blood sugar level is at any time. Monitoring of blood sugar levels several times a day is the cornerstone of the treatment of diabetes, the pivot around which decisions regarding diagnosis, treatment and dosages revolve. Since brain serotonin levels cannot be measured, the monitoring of serotonin levels in people diagnosed with depression cannot happen. Since the normal range for serotonin levels remains a mystery, any understanding of an assumed point at which serotonin levels might become abnormal is inevitably unknown. The very idea of abnormal brain chemical levels is entirely speculative. The assumption of a significant link between serotonin levels and depression has not been scientifically established.

Despite all their talk about serotonin and other brain chemicals, neither the medical profession nor the pharmaceutical industry ever mention specific figures that depict the normal and abnormal range of brain serotonin, something that is commonplace regarding known chemical imbalance illnesses such as diabetes and hypothyroidism. Since brain serotonin levels cannot be measured, people never have their brain serotonin levels checked. A diagnosis of depression is always made in the absence of laboratory serotonin results that confirm the diagnosis, a practice that would be considered medically negligent if adopted in relation to diabetes. Millions of people worldwide have been told by their doctors that low brain serotonin is responsible for the depression diagnosis the doctor has just made. Apparently, doctors can tell this just by looking at and listening to the person for a few minutes. No wonder that many people believe psychiatrists to be neurotransmitter wizards, as psychiatrist Daniel Carlat wrote in his 2010 book *Unhinged: The Trouble with Psychiatry—A Doctor's Revelations about a Profession in Crisis*:

> Patients often view psychiatrists as wizards of neurotransmitters, who can choose just the right medication for whatever chemical imbalance is at play. This exaggerated conception of our abilities has been encouraged by drug companies, by psychiatrists ourselves, and by our patients' understandable hopes for cures. [12]

People diagnosed with depression never have any other diagnostic tests such as brain scans carried out either, except to rule out real organic diseases. Antidepressants are always prescribed without any knowledge of the person's serotonin levels. The biochemical reaction to the prescribed substance can never be measured either. There is therefore no way of knowing whether the drug is having the assumed chemical effect, that is, raising brain serotonin levels. In diabetes, repeatedly assessing the biological reaction to treatment by closely monitoring blood glucose levels is standard practice, especially at times such as the commencement of treatment, significant treatment changes or when their diabetes is out of control and requires meticulous management. In contrast, even people taking antidepressants for years have never have their serotonin levels checked.

Once a person is diagnosed with diabetes and insulin treatment is commenced, lifelong treatment is the norm. Because real chemical imbalances are generally irreversible, people with diabetes do not subsequently reach a point where they can come off their diabetes medication. As a medical doctor, I would never reduce a person's diabetic or thyroid medication, unless there were very clear reasons to do so based primarily on the patient's laboratory tests. Doing so would inevitably lead to a recurrence of the biochemical deficiency which would have predictable and serious consequences. No responsible doctor would contemplate doing such a thing. An insulin-dependent diabetic who decides to stop taking insulin is guaranteed to soon be in big trouble, slipping into a diabetic coma within days, from which death within days is inevitable unless they receive insulin. Many people who discontinue antidepressants have few if any ongoing problems. If these people had a biochemical serotonin deficiency to begin with it, what happened to it? Did it miraculously disappear on the day the drug was stopped? Was it ever there to begin with? We will never know since brain serotonin levels cannot be measured, but the features of this scenario bear little resemblance to the predictable consequences of stopping replacement therapy for a biochemical deficiency situation.

Real chemical imbalances respond to treatment in a scientifically predictable manner. A dose of insulin temporarily corrects the diabetes chemical imbalance. As the day progresses, the injected insulin is progressively used up. At some point within 24 hours, the total amount that has been injected has been consumed within the body. The person is effectively back to square one. Their biochemical deficiency—of insulin—has fully recurred, as it will every single day. The biological need for treatment therefore recurs, day after day, for life. This is never the case in depression, where there is no established pre-existing underlying chemical imbalance.

The notion that depression is just like diabetes and antidepressants are similar treatments to insulin is a myth. Most patients with depression have heard this falsehood over and over again, from their doctors, pharmacists, in publications and in the media. When a person with diabetes is given insulin, they are given a chemical that they lack, a straightforward like-for-like chemical replacement. Since we have never been able to demonstrate that a patient with depression lacks something that people who are not depressed do not lack, it is clearly misleading and wrong to use this analogy.

Danish physician and medical researcher Dr. Peter Gotzsche is co-founder of the highly respected Cochrane Collaboration. The author of over 300 research papers, including more than 70 publications in the five most prestigious medical journals, [13] his scientific works have been cited over 150,000 times. He is Leader of the Nordic Cochrane Centre in Denmark, Professor of Clinical Research Design and Analysis at the University of Copenhagen, and a member of the Council for Evidence-based Psychiatry. In a 2014 article titled "Psychiatry Gone Astray", Gotzsche wrote:

> At the Nordic Cochrane Centre, we have researched antidepressants for several years and I have long wondered why leading professors of psychiatry base their practice on a number of erroneous myths. Many psychiatrists are well aware that the myths do not hold and have told me so, but they don't dare deviate from their official positions because of career concerns. [14]

Gotzsche wrote that as a specialist in internal medicine he did not risk ruining his career by incurring the wrath of professors of psychiatry. He continued:

> Myth 1: Your disease is caused by a chemical imbalance in the brain:
> Most patients are told this but it is completely wrong. We have no idea about which interplay of psychosocial conditions, biochemical processes, receptors and neural pathways that lead to mental disorders, and the theories that patients with depression lack serotonin and that patients with schizophrenia have too much dopamine have long been refuted. [15]

In a 2013 interview available on the internet, Peter Gotzsche said:

> The hypothesis about serotonin is stone dead. The good studies that have been made could not say that depressed patients were different from normal patients. What these drugs do is, they do not correct a chemical imbalance. That is another lie psychiatrists love; that you have a chemical imbalance, like a diabetic that lacks insulin, so now we are going to correct your chemical imbalance. It is a lie. [16]

Comparing depression to diabetes has been an effective marketing strategy for psychiatry, general practice and the drug industry on several fronts. Diabetes is known to be a serious disease with proven biological features, yet considerable optimism pertains regarding its understanding and treatment. The biological disease status of diabetes has been well known for many decades. Diabetes research has consistently led to an ever more sophisticated understanding of diabetes and to progressive refinement of its management and treatment. Diabetic specialists are well respected by their medical colleagues for the precision of their understanding and treatment of diabetes. Diabetes has a magic bullet treatment—insulin, which corrects raised blood glucose, the known chemical imbalance in diabetes. Diabetes is a lifelong condition. When well managed, patients generally do well. When not well managed, there are complications. All of these characteristics make diabetes a very attractive target for comparison with depression for mental health doctors and drug companies. The power of making such an analogy is its potential to persuade people to transfer the feeling of certainty they have about one subject—diabetes, to another—depression. The fact that depression and diabetes have far more differences than similarities is generally missed or bypassed. The reality that this comparison is like comparing apples to oranges from a disease perspective seemed to slip by most people including many doctors.

It is to be expected that members of the general public will pick up medical comparisons of depression with diabetes and run with them. Having heard doctors and other enthusiasts proclaim that depression and diabetes are very similar conditions, it is not surprising that other mental health professionals and members of the public have become convinced.

Men and Depression: What to Do When the Man You Care About is Depressed is a 2002 book written by health writer Theresa Francis-Cheung and psychotherapist Robin Grey. Regarding antidepressants, according to the authors:

Taking them is no more a sign of weakness than taking insulin for diabetes. [17]

The clear implication of this assertion is that taking antidepressants to correct brain chemical imbalances is just like taking insulin to correct blood sugar imbalances in diabetes. As we have seen, this claim is a Begging the Question logical fallacy [18] and a Weak Analogy logical fallacy. [19] In their apparent reassurance to the reader that taking antidepressants is not "a sign of weakness", the authors also resort to a False Dilemma logical fallacy, whether intentionally or not. [20]

The website of the Cable News Network channel (CNN) contains a 2004 article titled "Depression: a common, but treatable disease". The article quotes a Molly Canfield, who according to the article has experienced depression for twenty years:

It is like a diabetic, who is considering insulin. You wouldn't ask them to go without their insulin. People who have antidepressants and can benefit from them; it plugs in that part of you that's not there. [21]

Unlike diabetes, there is no scientific evidence of any chemical "part" of the person "that's not there" in depression.

I mentioned author and freelance writer Michelle L. Devon earlier. In her 2006 article titled "Depression really is a medical condition" she made a direct comparison between diabetes and depression:

> Diabetes is a disease that is caused by a problem with the pancreas, having to do with a hormone called insulin . . . Depression is a disease that is caused by a problem with the function of the brain—neurotransmitters—having to do with hormones and chemical regulation, most notably serotonin. [22]

Without intending to, Michelle L. Devon is articulating a Weak Analogy logical fallacy in this passage. [23] Her comments about diabetes are correct, but what she says about depression has no basis in fact.

In her book 2011 book *How the Light Gets In*, the comparison Irish actress Mary McEvoy made between depression and diabetes appears reasonable:

> Depressed people who need to take medication should not be ashamed of taking the chemical route. Nobody says don't take your insulin if you are diabetic. Nobody says don't take painkillers if you are in chronic pain, or aspirin to thin your blood if you have a heart condition. [24]

Mary McEvoy can certainly be forgiven for not knowing this, but her analogy is a weak one. It is true that no one says "don't take your insulin" if you are diabetic. That is because everyone understands that people with diabetes have a chemical imbalance provable by blood tests that requires treatment to balance blood sugar levels, the benefit of which is also routinely verified with blood tests. These facts are there for everyone to see. People with a heart condition who take aspirin also have had their physical illness diagnosed with clinical investigations such as coronary angiography. No one is diagnosed with a heart condition without the diagnosis being confirmed by such tests. People in chronic pain are usually advised by their doctors to do everything possible to minimize their need for painkillers. Their doctors will advise them of the risks associated with long-term ingestion of such painkillers. Usually, unlike depression, the biological source of the chronic pain will have been identified and found to be largely uncorrectable before doctors sanction long-term daily use of painkillers. McEvoy makes an interesting comparison between chronic physical and emotional pain. The question arises, are antidepressants emotional painkillers? This important question is beyond the remit of this book. I will address it fully in a future publication.

It is for similar reasons that doctors frequently feel the need to justify and defend their approach to depression but not to diabetes, multiple sclerosis, heart and other known physical diseases. The dots join up in diseases known to have an identified physical component. The gaps of knowledge are not large enough to create doubt in people's mind. There is a steady chain of linkage that doctors and the public can understand. The dots do not join in depression. The gaps in knowledge and evidence are enormous. Drug companies and many doctors do what they can to paper over the yawning gaps with various strategies including deception, distortion, exaggeration, minimization, omission and on occasion, lying. These strategies satisfy most people, who assume that doctors would not deceive or mislead them.

This ties in with a key difference between physical illnesses and what doctors call mental illnesses. We know that physical illnesses are real illnesses because the evidence is irrefutable. If we are being guided by truth as all doctors should be, we cannot say with any degree of certainty that mental illnesses exist as part of reality. All we can say with any certainty is that what doctors call mental illnesses are based on one form of *interpretation* of people's experiences and behavior. The experiences, thoughts, feelings and behavior are very real. The medical interpretation may or may not be.

Within the disease-centred paradigm that pertains in all medical specialties, the nature of a disease is known, to varying degrees depending on the illness, independent of the action of any drug. An established physical basis for the disease or pathology needing treatment is known. From this bank of knowledge emerge theories and research regarding treatments. People with diabetes have a disease involving damage to groups of cells in their pancreas called the Islets of Langerhans. These cells produce insulin. When these cells are diseased as they are in diabetes, insulin production is diminished or absent. Insulin controls blood sugar levels, so their blood sugar level rises accordingly. People with multiple sclerosis have a specific biological disease process occurring within their nervous system. This disease process has been identifiable for several decades through the use of brain scans that are always used to confirm the diagnosis. People with arthritis have a known biological disease process occurring within them. The biological inflammatory process that occurs in arthritis is well understood by doctors, by joint specialists in particular. Any experienced rheumatologist or pathologist could easily present a comprehensive hour-long lecture on the biology of arthritis, with comprehensive supporting evidence including x-rays, scans, abnormal biochemical findings and microscopic detailed photographs of the pathological disease process that is at the heart of arthritis.

NOTES TO CHAPTER TEN

1.   U.S. National Alliance on Mental Illness website, http://www.nami.org/Template.cfm?Section
     =Depression&Template=/ContentManagement/ContentDisplay.cfm&ContentID= 89096,
     accessed 24 November 2013.
2.   For information on Weak Analogy logical fallacies see note 64 in the Notes to Chapter Five.
3.   In Elliot S. Valenstein, *Blaming the Brain: The Truth About Drugs and Mental Health,* New York: The
     Free Press, 1998, pps. 180-182.

4.   Dawn Harper, medical expert on ITV's *This Morning*, during a discussion on depression on 12 August 2014.

5.   For information on Weak Analogy logical fallacies see note 69 in the Notes to Chapter Five.

6.   Muiris Houston, medical correspondent, *Irish Times,* 17 December 2001.

7.   For information on Weak Analogy logical fallacies see note 69 in the Notes to Chapter Five.

8.   Alan Wade, CPS Clinical Centre, Clydebank, Scotland, quoted in *The Examiner,* 07 December 2002.

9.   For information on Weak Analogy logical fallacies see note 69 in the Notes to Chapter Five.

10.   Harry Barry, *Flagging the Problem: A New Approach to Mental Health*, Dublin: Liberties Press, 2010.

11.   For information on Weak Analogy logical fallacies see note 69 in the Notes to Chapter Five.

12.   Daniel Carlat, *Unhinged: The Trouble with Psychiatry—a Doctor's Revelations about a Profession in Crisis,* London: Free Press, 2010.

13.   *British Medical Journal, Lancet, JAMA, Annals of Internal Medicine* & *New England Journal of Medicine.*

14.   Peter Gotzsche, "Psychiatry Gone Astray", 21 January 2014, Rxisk website, http://davidhealy.org/psychiatry-gone-astray/, accessed 26 January 2014.

15.   Peter Gotzsche, "Psychiatry Gone Astray", 21 January 2014, Rxisk website, http://davidhealy.org/psychiatry-gone-astray/, accessed 26 January 2014.

16.   "Interview with Peter Gotzsche", http://truthman30.wordpress.com/2013/11/23/petergotzsche/, accessed 02 February 2014.

17.   Theresa Francis-Cheung & Robin Grey*, Men and Depression: What to Do When the Man You Care About is Depressed,* London, Thorsons, 2002, p. 211.

18.   For information about Begging the Question logical fallacies see note 22 in the Notes to the Introduction.

19.   For information on Weak Analogy logical fallacies see note 69 in the Notes to Chapter Five.

20.   For information on False Dilemma logical fallacies see note 38 in the Notes to Chapter Five.

21.   CNN website, "Depression: a common, but treatable disease", http://edition.cnn.com/2004/HEALTH/01/15/depression/index.html?iref=allsearch, 09 February 2004, accessed 03 October 2014.

22.   Michelle L. Devon, "Depression really is a medical condition",21 September 2006, http://voices.yahoo.com/depression-really-medical-condition-77858.html?cat=5, accessed 12 November 2013; also available on Alternative Healthy Living website, http://alternativehealthlifestyle.com/?p=547, accessed 17 August 2014.

23.   For information on Weak Analogy logical fallacies see note 69 in the Notes to Chapter Five.

24.   Mary McEvoy, *How the Light Gets In: My Journey with Depression*, Hachette Books Ireland: Dublin, 2011, p. 265.

11. THE PROLONGED PROMOTION OF A LONG-DISCREDITED THEORY

In this chapter I discuss how the long-discredited brain chemical imbalance theory of depression came to be so widely accepted as an established fact. The brain chemical imbalance theory of depression was effectively discredited long before the much-heralded arrival of Prozac in 1988. According to psychiatrist and historian Edward Shorter:

> As popular culture was turning toward neurotransmitters as the explanation of what ailed everybody, academic culture was turning away from them. [1]

Why then has this misinformation been widely promoted and believed to this day, twenty-seven years later? Edward Shorter's simplistic statement is not the full story. To this day, many doctors have been among the most enthusiastic promoters of the chemical imbalance notion, often presenting it as an established fact, several decades after the hypothesis had been discredited. The few who shouted "stop" were largely ignored, dismissed or ridiculed.

A PERFECT STORM: WHY THIS FALSEHOOD SURVIVED AND PROSPERED

How can it be that the depression brain chemical imbalance notion has become so embedded within the minds of the public when there has never been any confirming evidence? To understand this, we need to look at each of the main groups involved. It turns out that each of these groups has had a vested interested in believing and promoting this falsehood. The prolonged and widespread promotion of this long-discredited theory has occurred because those who promoted it have benefitted enormously and continue to do so. As neuroscientist Elliot Valenstein wrote in his 1998 book *Blaming the Brain:*

> The chemical theories of mental disorders are widely promoted as though they were firmly established scientific facts. The theory has been so widely accepted because a number of groups, each with its own agenda, have promoted this idea, not infrequently by exaggerating and distorting what is known about mental disorders and the effectiveness and safety of the drugs used to treat them . . . a theory that is wrong is considered preferable to admitting our ignorance. [2]

Who are these groups, each with their own agenda, who have a vested interest in promoting the widespread acceptance of an idea for which there is no scientific basis? They include the pharmaceutical industry, the medical profession, some allied mental health professionals, mental health organizations, some people diagnosed with depression and their families and many mental health organizations.

The vested interest of the pharmaceutical industry is perhaps the most obvious. Antidepressants have added several hundred billion dollars over the past twenty-seven years to the combined turnover of the drug companies that produce these substances. Persuading doctors and the public that brain chemical imbalances occur in depression was pivotal in cultivating the widespread acceptance of antidepressants as a treatment as legitimate as insulin for diabetes.

The public acceptance of the depression brain chemical imbalance notion as a fact has also been enormously helpful to psychiatry on several levels. By promoting this concept as a fact or a likely reality for half a century, many psychiatrists have persuaded themselves and the public that they are real doctors treating real diseases. The brain chemical imbalance fallacy being publicly accepted as truth has elevated the status of psychiatry, perhaps more than any other idea over the past fifty years. GPs too have benefitted greatly. The public acceptance of the depression delusion has facilitated GPs in the creation of a tidy and supposedly scientific rationale for dealing with human distress. Though bogus, this rationale is misrepresented as being consistent with the medical perspective of disease.

This delusion benefits some allied health professionals, in particular, those whose status is increased as a consequence of its widespread acceptance. Such groups include some branches of psychology and counselling, especially those for whom the biological brain chemical imbalance notion is consistent with their training and modus operandi.

The vested interests of some individuals and groups are less obvious but are there nevertheless. Some people who experience great distress or who exhibit behaviour consistent with the psychiatric diagnostic system may feel relieved to be told that their problem is a brain chemical imbalance. Some find this idea attractive as it apparently removes responsibility from them for both their situation and its alleviation. As I discuss in chapter sixteen, this can be a double-edged sword. Family members—including mental health groups comprised largely of family members—may see a brain chemical imbalance notion as a welcome relief, enabling them to avoid any consideration that the person's life experiences had a significant impact. Delegating the problem to the person's brain helps to minimize the self-questioning and guilt that may otherwise arise. International best-selling author Marian Keyes' comments in a national Irish radio interview in November 2014 illustrate the major attraction of seeing depression as an illness, a brain problem. She began by reflecting upon what she perceived as the current stigmatizing position:

> If you get depression, you are in some way culpable . . . you did something yourself, you made this happen, and I still think there's that massive stigma . . . you are the one to blame . . . if we fully accept that depression is an illness—and it is—then it's as mysterious as any other illness. [3]

Marian Keyes does not take into account the fact that many illnesses are not nearly as "mysterious" as depression. The causes of many illnesses are known, to varying degrees. For the majority of illnesses and conditions including those whose cause has not yet been identified, the biological pathological processes have been reliably identified in considerable detail. This is true regarding the three conditions she mentioned in the radio show as being comparable to depression—cancer, emphysema and a fractured leg. None of this is true for depression. The diagnosis of cancer, emphysema and a fractured leg is *always* confirmed by specific physical findings and investigations. A diagnosis of depression is *never* confirmed by either specific physical findings or reliable investigations, since there are none.

Similar reasons account for the long-held enthusiasm for brain chemical imbalances in depression that has been championed by many mental health organizations over the past four decades. Many of these organizations have a strong input from family members, loved ones and friends of people experiencing the features of what we call depression. It is understandable that these groups would support the views of doctors who proclaim that biological research will one day provide all the answers. For many, it has been easier to frame the problem as a brain abnormality— most commonly, a brain chemical imbalance—than to risk opening to anything that might hint at blame or shame, either toward the person or themselves. Some of this is unconscious. Many people become involved in mental health organizations with a genuine desire to help. Focusing attention and research on a supposed brain chemical abnormality is more comfortable. It is otherwise detached from life, existence and relationships. It appears clinical. The experience is normalized, though incorrectly so, as an illness. Claimed brain abnormalities become something acceptable to fight against, to campaign for, to fix. The problem is, they have never been demonstrated to exist.

Other subtle but significant pay-offs have occurred as a consequence of the widespread acceptance of the depression brain chemical imbalance delusion. In many developed Westernized countries there has long been a fear of and resistance to public expressions of distress and of distress-linked behaviours. The brain chemical imbalance delusion has become a tidy way of sanitizing such situations about which many of us feel very uncomfortable. Having sanitized them, we can sweep them under the more acceptable carpet of disease conveniently provided by the medical profession and the pharmaceutical industry. Western societies generally find this approach a great deal more palatable. These pay-offs are experienced across a wide range of society, up to government level. The legitimization of psychiatric practice provided by the brain chemical imbalance delusion has facilitated the handing over by governments of many problems and challenges faced by a significant percentage of the population to the medical profession. This is done under the guise of supposedly legitimate medical illness rather than considering and addressing their distress and experiences as understandable reactions to life within their society.

The consequence of all this is ironic though entirely predictable. Providing societies with an apparently trustworthy rationale for avoiding the reality of human distress has resulted in increasingly costly mental health services within which recovery is a far rarer outcome that it should be. Since the core issues are repeatedly side-stepped, they are not addressed or recognized within these mental health systems. It is not surprising that the costs of such systems keep increasing with little hard evidence that these systems are providing value for money in terms of recovery.

Charles Medawar and Anita Hardon are the authors of the 2004 book *Medicines out of Control?: Antidepressants and the Conspiracy of Goodwill*. Medawar was then executive director of Social Audit UK and a specialist in medicines policy, drug safety issues and matters of corporate, governmental and professional accountability. Anita Hardon was then Professor in Anthropology of Care and Health at the University of Amsterdam and was chair of the Health Action International (Europe) foundation board. In their book Medawar and Hardon wrote about the "inflamed belief" in drug treatment for depression that occurred in the 1990s in the wake of the arrival of the new wave of antidepressants, of which Prozac was the flagship product:

> Brave new talk about the biological basis of depression helped to set the scene. The welcome rumour that depression was actually a deficiency state—and that normal mood could be restored by boosting levels . . . The message was that depressed people needed antidepressants just as some diabetics needed insulin . . . Serotonin deficiency theories were . . . widely promoted and sincerely believed. The widespread acceptance of these ideas had little to do with the facts, but they were easy on the mind. The Pharmas primed and pumped out this message and it was widely received as welcome news. The notion that depression resulted from some simple lack or imbalance of brain serotonin was both persuasive and misleading, a fine example of the Conspiracy of Goodwill.
> The notion of "chemical imbalance" . . . was something of a placebo for everyone. It made psychiatry more credible, scientific and potent; it helped doctors to persuade their patients to accept treatment, and it helped the Pharmas to sell their SSRIs. The "serotonin hypothesis" made depression seem more "normal" by reducing the "stigma" of mental illness. Talk of "disease" and the notion of chemical deficiency relieved patients of blame and responsibility and of the feeling they might be failures who had brought misery on themselves . . . the idea that SSRIs worked by correcting a serotonin deficiency underwrote the notion of drug effectiveness. [4]

A perfect storm was thus created. The public have become so accustomed to hearing that brain chemical imbalances are a standard feature of depression that most people rank this notion above all other possible ways of understanding depression. The primacy of the brain biochemical imbalance idea is now solidly rooted in the collective public mind. This widespread public acceptance has greatly increased the status of doctors as *the* perceived experts in emotional and mental health. This notion has been pivotal in persuading people that depression is a medical illness and therefore falls primarily within the territory of medicine rather than other disciplines.

This dominant position makes it much easier for doctors to move seamlessly from one delusion to others when the existing one is becoming increasingly difficult to defend. As I discuss in chapter fifteen, the process of replacing the brain chemical imbalance delusion with newer ones has already begun. Startling though it may appear, the continuing dominance of the medical profession and their pharmaceutical allies in mental health is dependent on continuing to delude the public and perhaps themselves regarding the nature of depression and other psychiatric diagnoses. This is why other possible ways of understanding mental health problems are either resisted or ignored by the medical profession and the pharmaceutical industry, apart for ideas they benefit from such as genetics, which I address in my next book on depression.

A candid 2010 admission by American psychiatrist Daniel Carlat revealed that misinforming people about brain chemical imbalances may have far more to do with saving face for the doctor than with benefitting patients:

> It gives us something to say when patients ask how the drugs work . . . No doctor wants to admit ignorance about the very problems he or she is trained to manage.[5]

Andrew Scull is listed as Distinguished Professor on the University of California San Diego Department of Sociology webpage. [6] In a 2010 article in a prestigious medical journal, Scull described brain chemical abnormality notions as "biobabble" that was a "priceless" marketing tool:

> In 1990 the Society for Neuroscience persuaded the U.S. Congress to designate the 1990s as the Decade of the Brain. The US National Institute of Mental Health proclaimed the 1990s "The decade of the brain". A simplistic biological reductionism has increasingly ruled the psychiatric roost. Patients and their families learned to attribute mental illness to faulty brain biochemistry, defects of dopamine, or a shortage of serotonin. It is biobabble as deeply misleading as the psychobabble it replaced but as marketing copy it was priceless. Meantime, the psychiatric profession was seduced and bought off with boatloads of research funding. Where once shrinks had been the most marginal of medical men, existing in the twilight zone in the margins of medical respectability, now they were the darlings of medical school deans, the millions upon millions of grants and indirect cost recoveries helping to finance the expansion of the medical-industrial complex. [7]

It will be interesting to see whether this pattern of grants by drug companies will continue now that many drug companies have reversed their long-established lavish financial support for psychiatry and psychiatric research.

Andrew Scull is not alone. Many others both inside and outside psychiatry have reached similar conclusions regarding the marketing and strategic importance of the biochemical deficiency delusion. According to neuroscientist Elliot Valenstein in his 1998 book *Blaming the Brain*, the biochemical theory is held on to principally because it is "useful for promoting drug treatment". [8] In her 2004 *New York Review of Books* article titled "The Truth about the Drug Companies", physician and pathologist Dr. Marcia Angell, former editor-in-chief of the *New England Journal of Medicine* chastised the pharmaceutical industry:

> Primarily a marketing machine to sell drugs of dubious benefit, this industry uses its wealth and power to co-opt every institution that might stand in its way, including the U.S. Congress, the FDA, academic medical centers, and the medical profession itself. [9]

In a 2009 *New York Review of Books* article titled "Drug Companies and Doctors: A Story of Corruption", Dr. Angell again criticized the pharmaceutical industry, adding that the medical profession is "even more culpable" (brackets mine):

> It is easy to fault drug companies for this situation, and they certainly deserve a great deal of blame. Apologists might argue that the pharmaceutical industry is merely trying to do its primary job—furthering the interest of its investors. Physicians, medical schools and professional organizations have no such excuse, since their only fiduciary responsibility is to patients. As reprehensible as many (pharmaceutical) industry practices are, I believe the behavior of much of the medical profession is even more culpable. [10]

In their 2005 book *Depression: An Emotion not a Disease*, Irish psychiatrist Michael Corry and GP and psychotherapist Aine Tubridy wrote:

> The pharmaceutical industry has hijacked science, reversed cause and effect, and idealizes the neurochemical model of illness for profit purposes, a marketing triumph. [11]

In a 2006 article psychiatrist Joanna Moncrieff and Professor of Social Work David Cohen set out just how much is at stake for drug companies and the medical profession in maintaining the biochemical deficiency notion, defunct though it may be:

> The idea that antidepressant drugs target a specific biological state that produces depression strongly justifies the disease model of depression and its medical treatment. Therefore, abandoning the disease-centred model of antidepressant action squarely challenges the notion of depression as a biologically based medical disease. [12]

American psychiatrist David Burns wrote about the notion of the brain chemical imbalance in his 2006 book, *When Panic Attacks: The New Drug-Free Therapy That Can Change Your Life*:

> This theory is fuelled more by drug company marketing than by solid scientific proof. Billions of dollars of annual profits from the sale of antidepressant and anti-anxiety medications are at stake, so drug companies spend vast amounts of money promoting the chemical imbalance theory. They also fund a large part of the budget of the American Psychiatric Association and underwrite an enormous amount of research and education at medical schools. Academic research should be all about getting at the truth. Drug company research is all about selling new products. If I tell you that your depression or your panic attacks result from a chemical imbalance in the brain, then I'm telling you something that cannot be proven, because there is no test for a chemical imbalance in the human brain. [13]

Dr. Catherine DeAngelis, physician and former editor of the prestigious *Journal of the American Medical Association*, wrote in a journal editorial in April 2008:

> The influence that the pharmaceutical companies, the for-profits, are having on every aspect of medicine . . . is so blatant you'd have to be deaf, dumb and blind not to see it. We have just allowed them to take over, and it is our fault, the whole medical community. [14]

Ben Goldacre is a British physician, academic and science writer. He became a member of the Royal College of Psychiatrists in 2005 and a research fellow at the Institute of Psychiatry in London in 2008. In a 2008 *Guardian* article titled "Bad Science: Depression—the facts and the fables", Goldacre wrote:

> In popular culture the depression/serotonin story is proven and absolute, because it was never about research, or theory, it was about marketing, and journalists who pride themselves on never pushing pills or the hegemony will still blindly push the model until the cows come home. [15]

Psychology professor and author Richard Bentall wrote the following in his 2009 book *Doctoring the Mind: Why Psychiatric Treatments Fail*:

> Direct support for the serotonin hypothesis has remained elusive to this day. Nonetheless, the chemical imbalance theory of depression continues to be enthusiastically promoted in drug advertisements and by the popular press. Perhaps it is because the idea is so easy to understand, but also because this type of explanation for mental illness serves the interests of biologically-orientated psychiatrists and drug companies very well. [16]

Psychologist and researcher Irving Kirsch, whose research identified that antidepressants are just slightly more effective than active placebos, wrote in his 2009 book *The Emperor's New Drugs: Exploding the Antidepressant Myth*:

> The theory may be wrong, but it certainly helps to sell antidepressant drugs. [17]

American psychiatrist Daniel Carlat stated in a 2010 radio interview regarding the depression chemical imbalance notion:

> It becomes a very useful marketing line for drug companies, and then it becomes a reasonable thing for us to say to patients to give them more confidence in the treatment that they're getting from us. But it may not be true. [18]

In this passage, Carlat claimed that because the biochemical imbalance notion became "a very useful marketing line for drug companies", it then became a "reasonable thing for us to say to patients". To suggest that drug companies using this notion made it "a reasonable thing" for doctors to do is dubious logic indeed.

In a 2012 article titled "Chemical Imbalances and Other Black Unicorns" published on the Mad in America website, resident psychiatrist Vivek Datta wrote:

> Make no mistake. There is only one reason why we have "learned" that mental disorders are caused by chemical imbalances. To sell more drugs. There is one main reason too, why doctors tell their patients their problems are due to chemical imbalances. To convince people to take more drugs. [19]

Dr. Datta provides an insightful commentary regarding the biochemical imbalance idea presented by doctors to their patients:

> When a physician prescribes an antidepressant, he cannot help but also prescribe an idea. He may not wish to provide the idea, indeed, he is often not aware that he is prescribing the idea, but the physician nevertheless is prescribing the idea. The idea is that the problem is a chemical one, with a chemical solution. [20]

Dr. Datta is correct. It is no coincidence that the idea which many doctors have been selling about depression—that chemical imbalances are known to occur in depression—is one that fits well with the general medical perception of health problems as fundamentally biological. It is therefore an idea with which doctors feel very comfortable.

Most people want a rationale regarding why they should take medication. The chemical imbalance rationale is the one usually handed down by the doctor. This explains why many people continue to be told of the biochemical abnormality notion in the privacy of the doctor's office, and why 71.5 per cent of respondents to a 2007 survey carried out by the www.anxietycentre.com website said that their doctor or mental health professional told them that their depression or anxiety was caused by a brain chemical imbalance. Over 90 per cent of respondents said that their doctor or mental health professional wanted to prescribe medication for their anxiety or depression. [21]

In a January 2013 article on his website entitled "The Antidepressant Era: The Movie", psychiatrist David Healy of the University of Wales referred to the notion that antidepressants balance serotonin levels as "a marketing myth" that "had nothing to do with science". [22] Dr. Healy first wrote this in his doctoral thesis in 1985, two years *before* the launch of Prozac. In his 2013 book *How Everyone Became Depressed*, psychiatrist and historian Edward Shorter wrote:

> Today, these theories are widely disbelieved. Shortages of the standard monoamine transmitters and receptors turned out to have little role in depressive illness except in pharmaceutical advertising and in the explanations that doctors give to patients. [23]

Shorter's statement that brain chemical imbalance theories are "today widely disbelieved" may come as news to many people. In 2014, American psychiatrist and author Stuart Shipko wrote:

Most people are surprised to learn that depression is not caused by a "chemical imbalance" related to serotonin or other neurotransmitter. Actually, the chemical imbalance concept was originally a marketing strategy. [24]

According to John Sommers-Flanagan, Professor of Counselor Education at the University of Montana:

Chemical imbalance is a term that's used as a marketing ploy as opposed to anything that there is scientific evidence to support. [25]

According to Shane Ellison, former research chemist with Eli Lilly:

You are selling drugs to people under false premises under a disease that's been invented. So how do you measure efficacy among a disease that doesn't even exist? [26]

The groups that benefit from the wide public acceptance of the brain chemical imbalance delusion rarely acknowledge the real reasons in public, preferring instead to come up with more publicly acceptable ones, which I discuss in the rest of this chapter.

ANTIDEPRESSANTS WORK, THEREFORE BRAIN CHEMICAL IMBALANCES MUST EXIST

Many doctors and members of the public have convinced themselves that because antidepressants help some people feel better, they must have had a chemical imbalance to begin with. British psychiatrist Alec Coppen was widely regarded as one of the pioneers of biological psychiatry and psychopharmacology. In 1967 Coppen wrote:

One of the most cogent reasons for believing that there is a biochemical basis for depression or mania is the astonishing success of physical methods of treatment of these conditions. [27]

Several problems arise here. Few people would attribute the relieving of their headache by paracetamol to a brain paracetamol deficiency. Also, to claim as "astonishing" the "success" of psychiatric medication is quite an exaggeration, since it is now scientifically established that antidepressants are little more effective than placebo. [28]

A USEFUL METAPHOR OR JUST PLAIN LYING?

Dr. Steven Reidbord is a board-certified psychiatrist with a full-time office practice in San Francisco. Dr. Reidbord has an internet blog titled "Reidbord's Reflections". On 29 April 2012 he published an article on his blog titled "Chemical imbalance-Sloppy thinking in psychiatry 1" in which he wrote:

At best, "chemical imbalance" is shorthand for a presumed brain abnormality that no one has yet proven. At worst, it is disingenuous hand-waving aimed to add medical legitimacy to the field of psychiatry . . . Why is "chemical imbalance" so often advanced as a pseudo-explanation for mental illness? . . . Suffering a "chemical imbalance" implies that proper medication will correct a pre-existing, permanent organic abnormality. The problem here is that the end (patient cooperation) does not justify the means (lying) . . . "Chemical imbalance" gives some psychiatrists the bona fides they crave, but at the price of intellectual laziness and sloppy thinking. This serves no one. Psychiatry must embrace uncertainty, and not seek false security in empty phrases. [29]

On NBC's *Today* programme on 27 June 2005, then president of the American Psychiatric Association Steven Sharfstein was asked about the fact that there are no established brain chemical imbalances that can be balanced using psychiatric drugs. His response was unequivocal:

Well, that's total nonsense. It belies the last 20 years of incredible breakthroughs in neuroscience and our understanding of how the brain works. [30]

Just two weeks later in an 11 July 2005 *People* magazine article, Sharfstein admitted that psychiatrists have no way of testing for a chemical imbalance:

We do not have a clean-cut lab test. [31]

The use of exaggerated superlatives by proponents of psychiatry regarding advancements—such Sharfstein's description of breakthroughs as "incredible"—are not uncommon. There are many other examples of such unwarranted superlatives in this book. I believe they are used in an effort to over-compensate for the lack of any meaningful progress, in an attempt to persuade the public to continue to place their trust in psychiatry and the medical approach to depression.

In recent years many doctors have admitted they tell patients that depression is caused by a brain chemical imbalance not because they believe it themselves, but because it is a useful metaphor that provides some sort of rationale for prescribing and taking antidepressants. To this day, in the privacy of the doctor's office, people are regularly told that they are being prescribed antidepressants because they have a brain chemical deficiency, serotonin being the most frequently cited culprit. As psychiatrist Joanna Moncrieff wrote in 2009:

Even when they acknowledge that there is no evidence for a "chemical imbalance", many psychiatrists believe that the term is still justified and appropriate, thereby demonstrating a deep underlying commitment to the idea. Wayne Goodman, a prominent United States psychiatrist commenting on an article highlighting the fact that there was no established link between serotonin abnormality and depression, still maintained that the term was "a reasonable shorthand for expressing that this is a chemically or brain based problem and that medications help to normalize function". [32]

This is an example of holding on to a fixed idea in the absence of supporting evidence and the presence of considerable conflicting evidence, a hallmark of delusional thinking which I discuss in detail in chapter thirteen. Joanna Moncrieff was correct to refer to Wayne Goodman as a prominent psychiatrist. In 2005 Goodman was Chair of the U.S. Food and Drugs Administration's Psychopharmacologic Advisory Committee. In a 2005 *New Scientist* interview, Goodman admitted the "chemical imbalance" story was merely "a useful metaphor". [33]

For whom is it most useful? It is extremely useful for drug companies, for whom this misinformation has persuaded millions of people to consume their products. It is also very useful for doctors who prescribe these substances, providing a means of persuading their patients that doctors know what they are doing, and deceiving them into believing that there is actually some reliable science behind the diagnosis and the drugs.

In Wayne Goodman's comments quoted by Joanna Moncrieff three paragraphs ago, Goodman wrongly stated that depression "is" rather than "might be" a "chemically or brain based problem". In doing so, this prominent US Food and Drugs Administration official committed a Begging the Question logical fallacy. [34]

Is it appropriate to describe unsubstantiated claims of brain biochemical abnormalities as a metaphor at all? The Merriam-Webster dictionary defines a metaphor as:

A figure of speech in which a word or phrase literally denoting one kind of object or idea is used in place of another to suggest a likeness or analogy between them. [35]

This practice does not satisfy the definition of a metaphor. Telling people that they have a chemical imbalance cannot be a proper metaphor when stated as a fact and without an appropriate comparison being applied. This practice is in fact a mixed metaphor, which "combines different images or ideas in a way which is foolish or illogical", "a figure of speech combining inconsistent or incongruous metaphors". [36]

It is usually pretty obvious when a true metaphor is being employed. If someone says that they are drowning in the amount of paperwork they have to get through, people generally realize that the person is not actually drowning, that a metaphor is being employed for descriptive purposes. When a doctor tells a person that they have a brain chemical imbalance causing their depression and that antidepressants will correct this imbalance, the person is not likely to know that the doctor may be speaking metaphorically. The imbalance of information and power puts the patient at a disadvantage. The patient is likely to believe that they do actually have a chemical imbalance in their brain. It is a bit rich to dress up this deceit as merely an innocent metaphor.

Claiming that the chemical imbalance fictional story is a "useful metaphor" is neither logical nor accurate. I would expect a senior American drug regulatory authority figure such as Wayne Goodman to know that. Trivializing the significance of so doing, as just an innocent and "useful metaphor" might help the users of such statements feel more comfortable about what they are doing. The fact remains that telling anyone in any setting that depression is caused by a chemical imbalance is misleading and constitutes false information.

In a 2010 NPR radio interview, American psychiatrist Daniel Carlat explained how helpful this "metaphor" could be for a doctor. In the interview, Carlat addressed the issue of how antidepressants work in a complex and convoluted manner, as a response to the following statement by show host Dave Davies:

> And it can be reassuring if you're prescribing a medication to tell someone, well, there's really a biological origin to your difficulty here, and we can treat it by treating the biology. [37]

Carlat replied:

> Right, which is exactly why I still tell patients that at times. [38]

So, telling patients untruths is justified on the dubious basis that doctors are actually reassuring them by so doing? I am not convinced that this level of logic would pass a thorough evaluation by a medical ethics committee. Carlat continued:

> What we don't know is how the medications actually work in the brain. So whereas it's not uncommon—and I still do this, actually, when a patient asks me about these medications, I'll often say something like, well, the way Zoloft works is it increases the levels of serotonin in your brain, in your synapses, the neurons, and presumably the reason you're depressed or anxious is that you have some sort of deficiency. And I say this not because I believe it, because I know that the evidence isn't really there for us to understand the mechanism. I think I say that because patients want to know something, and they want to know that we as physicians have some basic understanding of what we're doing when we're prescribing medications. And they certainly don't want to hear that a psychiatrist essentially has no idea how these medications work. [39]

Many concerns arise here. Carlat admitted that doctors do not know what antidepressants do in the brain. This is worrying, but at least it is the truth. He tells his patients that "presumably the reason you're depressed is that you have some sort of deficiency". This is a major assumption, since any such deficiency cannot be and therefore never is verified by any means in any patient. He truthfully acknowledged the alarming fact that he tells patients this although he doesn't personally believe it: "I say this not because I believe it, because I know that the evidence isn't really there for us to understand the mechanism". He does not seem to have a problem telling patients something as the truth that he believes and knows is not the truth. In my opinion this does not seem like a particularly ethical way to work, but Dr. Carlat is merely articulating what has been accepted practice for over twenty-five years.

Carlat then explained why he tells people something he does not himself believe. Apparently he does so for the patient's sake: "I think I say that because patients want to know something, and they want to know that we as physicians have some basic understanding of what we're doing when we're prescribing medications. And they certainly don't want to hear that a psychiatrist essentially has no idea how these medications work". [40]

It seems that Dr. Carlat justifies misinforming his patients on the grounds that the patients expect him to "have some basic understanding". Faking a basic understanding, pretending that doctors know what they are doing here, is apparently an acceptable practice, a better one than being truthful. The real reason is far more likely to be self-preservation. Telling this untruth to their patients rescues doctors from having to admit that they actually haven't a clue about either what is really going on in that person's brain or what effect the substance they are recommending will have within their brain.

According to a 2012 Mad in America website article by Professor of Neuroanatomy Jonathan Leo and Professor of Social Work Jeffrey Lacasse titled "Psychiatry's Grand Confession":

> The psychiatric profession has finally come clean and confessed on a national media that there is no evidence to support the serotonin theory of depression. Today, on NPR's Morning Edition there is a segment about the chemical imbalance theory, and virtually all the psychiatrists who were interviewed acknowledged that there was never any evidence in support of the idea that low serotonin causes depression. But then, amazingly, they go on to say that it is perfectly fine to tell patients that serotonin imbalance causes depression even though they know it isn't the case. [41]

I reviewed this 2012 NPR radio show, for which a full transcript by Alix Spiegel is available. [42] Titled "When it comes to depression, serotonin isn't the whole story", Spiegel begins the transcript with her own personal story from the 1980s, a story that mirrors the experience of millions of people who have visited a GP or psychiatrist in distress over the past thirty years:

> When I was 17, I got so depressed that what felt like an enormous black hole appeared in my chest. Everywhere I went, the black hole went too. So to address the black-hole issue, my parents took me to a psychiatrist at Johns Hopkins Hospital. She did an evaluation and then told me this story; "The problem with you", she explained, "is that you have a chemical imbalance. It's biological, just like diabetes, but it's in your brain. This chemical in your brain called serotonin is too, too low. There's not enough of it, and that's what's causing the chemical imbalance. We need to give you medication to correct that". Then she gave me a prescription for Prozac. [43]

Apparently by just listening to and observing her, the psychiatrist was able to somehow see into her brain and miraculously identify a brain chemical abnormality without performing any tests. No wonder many people think that psychiatrists are neurotransmitter wizards, as psychiatrist Daniel Carlat has remarked. [44] Given the extraordinary complexity of the brain as discussed earlier, this is either a remarkable feat of superhuman proportions or an utter fabrication. Perhaps, like FDA official Wayne Goodman and psychiatrist Daniel Carlat, this psychiatrist was just using a "useful metaphor", omitting to communicate this to her patient and family, who were likely convinced that a real chemical imbalance had been identified.

One of the psychiatrists on this NPR radio show in January 2012 was Alan Frazer, Professor of Pharmacology and Psychiatry and Chair of Pharmacology at the University of Pennsylvania. According to the show's transcript:

> Frazer said that by framing the problem as a deficiency—something that needed to be returned to normal—patients felt more comfortable taking the drug; "If there was this biological reason for them being depressed, some deficiency that the drug was correcting", Frazer says, then taking a drug was okay. "They had a chemical imbalance and the drug was correcting that imbalance". In fact, he says, the story enables many people to come out of the closet about being depressed, which he views as a good thing. [45]

Several major concerns arise in the above passage. "Framing the problem as a deficiency, something that needed to be returned to normal" when no such deficiency has been shown to exist is pure fiction, but the patient is not told that they are being spun a yarn. Having people feeling "more comfortable about taking the drug" is only appropriate if the information is accurate and the rationale does not involve mass public deception. Conveying information in such a way that patients will believe "they had a chemical imbalance and the drug was correcting that imbalance" is tantamount to a regular intentional misinforming of patients, the kind that might result in a doctor facing severe questioning and possibly sanctions from medical regulatory bodies if it were done in any other area of medicine.

In my opinion, the willingness of these doctors to misinform their patients is quite shocking. Dressing this misinformation up as a "useful metaphor" is not credible, but it may enable them to sleep easier at night. It is probably fair to deduce that many other doctors—possibly the majority of psychiatrists and GPs—share the views expressed by those doctors.

Without spinning people the yarn that they have a chemical imbalance which their drugs can correct, doctors would have a pretty difficult time convincing people to take these drugs and convincing the general public that they are practicing real medicine and working in a scientifically valid way. Not many people would swallow these pills if they knew that the only thing doctors know for sure is that these drugs interfere with the reuptake of brain neurotransmitters, without any scientific evidence that this interference is appropriate or necessary. As psychiatrist Daniel Carlat said in the previously quoted interview, people certainly don't want to hear that a psychiatrist or any prescribing doctor has no idea how these medications work, even—perhaps especially—if this is the truth. The chemical imbalance deception solves this problem for doctors. It sounds so convincing and scientific. I know of no situation in life where a falsehood such as the chemical imbalance story has become accepted worldwide simply because this mass deception benefitted only the recipients of the misinformation. In what other area of medicine would such shabby and unscientific standards be considered professional and acceptable?

WE DO IT FOR THE PATIENTS' SAKE

The delusional notion that doctors misinform people about brain chemical imbalances and depression for the patient's sake is well established in medicine. *Psychiatry* is a 2003 psychiatry textbook in which several leading psychiatrists contributed chapters. In one chapter psychiatrist Robert Freedman, Professor and Chairman of the Department of Psychiatry at the University of Colorado wrote:

> At some time in the course of their illness, most patients and families need some explanation of what happened and why. Sometimes the explanation is as simplistic as "a brain chemical imbalance", while other patients may request brain images so that they can see the possible psychopathology or genetic analyses to calculate genetic risk. [46]

Dr. Freedman does not mention that (a) there are no known chemical imbalances, (b) since no psychopathology (i.e. abnormal biology) has been identified in depression, brain imaging techniques can play no part in identifying what has not yet been identified, and (c) genetic analyses are never used to diagnose psychiatric illnesses because no genetic abnormalities have been reliably identified.

Perceived expert on bipolar disorder, psychiatrist Ronald Fieve wrote the following in 1989 regarding bipolar disorder. His comments apply equally to depression:

> It is reassuring for new patients to learn that there is a biochemical basis for an illness they thought for years resulted from unconscious conflicts in their personalities, deeply rooted since childhood . . . Their learning of the biochemical cause of their illness seems to result in a marked diminution of guilt in patients and families about behaviour during attacks. [47]

This passage by a renowned psychiatrist is an example of grossly flawed logic. There is no established biological basis for depression or bipolar disorder, yet this psychiatrist sees nothing wrong with misinforming people that something exists that has not been demonstrated to exist, claiming it to be in the patient's interest to do so.

Psychiatrist Ronald Pies is Clinical Professor of Psychiatry at Tufts University and Lecturer on Psychiatry at Harvard Medical School. In a 2011 Psych Central website article titled "Doctor, Is My Mood Disorder Due to a Chemical Imbalance?" Ronald Pies claims that doctors who tell patients they have a chemical imbalance do so primarily to make the patient feel better:

Of course, there certainly are psychiatrists, and other physicians, who have used the term "chemical imbalance" when explaining psychiatric illness to a patient, or when prescribing medication for depression or anxiety. Why? Many patients who suffer from severe depression or anxiety or psychosis tend to blame themselves for the problem. They have often been told by family members that they are "weak-willed" or "just making excuses" when they get sick, and that they would be fine if they just picked themselves up by the proverbial bootstraps. They are often made to feel guilty for using a medication to help them with their mood swings or depressive bouts. So, some doctors believe they will help the patient feel less blameworthy by telling them, "You have a chemical imbalance causing your problem". [48]

As I discussed in chapter four, depression can be understood without resorting to either fictional chemical imbalance notions or blaming the patient. While Dr. Pies does criticize his medical colleagues who do quote the chemical imbalance notion to patients, he sympathizes with their position and stops well short of accusing them of misinforming their patients:

It's easy to think you are doing the patient a favour by providing this kind of "explanation", but often, this isn't the case. Most of the time, the doctor knows that the "chemical imbalance" business is a vast oversimplification. My impression is that most psychiatrists who use this expression feel uncomfortable and a little embarrassed when they say so. It's a kind of bumper-sticker phrase that saves time, and allows the physician to write out the prescription while feeling that the patient has been "educated". If you are thinking that this is a little lazy on the doctor's part, you are right. But to be fair, remember that the doctor is often scrambling to see those other twenty depressed patients in her waiting room. I'm not offering this as an excuse—just an observation. [49]

What Pies refers to as a "vast oversimplification" is in fact a distortion of truth and therefore misinformation. What he calls "a little lazy" is actually deception. If psychiatrists and GPs "feel uncomfortable and a little embarrassed" telling their patients what is effectively a lie, they generally hide these feelings well. Perhaps their discomfort and embarrassment might lead them to question this practice, but it doesn't seem to. Pies admitted:

Those of us in academia should have done more to correct these beliefs and practices. [50]

Given the enormous consequences of this widespread misleading of the public, that is quite an understatement. Pies also acknowledged:

What we don't know, and shouldn't claim to know, is what the proper "balance" is for any given individual's brain chemistry. [51]

Murtagh's General Practice, a major 2011 medical textbook for trainee GPs also claimed that it is in the patient's interest to tell people they diagnose with depression that they have a brain chemical abnormality:

> The "missing chemical" theory really helps patients and family come to terms with an illness that tends to have socially embarrassing connotations. It also helps compliance with therapy when antidepressant medication is prescribed. [52]

Apparently, the fact that there is no reliable basis for the missing chemical theory and that the patient is in effect being misled is not important. Also, what is described in the above passage as "the 'missing chemical' theory" magically becomes a known fact elsewhere in the same book—"an important chemical is present in smaller amounts".[53]

I don't buy the idea that doctors do this for the patient's benefit. Patients are generally reasonable people. People naturally want to know why they should take a recommended medication. They do not expect their doctor to understand everything about their illnesses. Once they know enough to get some handle on their problem, they are usually satisfied. For the majority of illnesses this doesn't pose any problem, since the doctor generally knows plenty about the biological basis of most illnesses and their treatment. Regarding depression, doctors and drug companies have had a great deal to gain by regularly using this falsehood. It gets doctors off the hook.

THE DRUG COMPANIES ARE TO BLAME

You know there's a problem when people who have been directly involved in something for years start pointing fingers at other bedfellows as the cause of the trouble. Many doctors now blame the drug industry for the mass promotion of the brain chemical imbalance misinformation, conveniently forgetting the major role played by psychiatrists and GPs in promoting the depression chemical imbalance delusion.

Dr. Mark Graff, chair of the Committee of Public Affairs for the American Psychiatric Association was questioned on CBS Studio 2 on 10 July 2005 about the notion of biochemical brain abnormalities. Dr. Graff stated:

> Chemical imbalance . . . it's a shorthand term really, it's probably drug industry derived . . . we don't have tests . . . I agree . . . there aren't any bold tests. [54]

It is also worrying that an official of the American Psychiatrist Association would deem it appropriate to refer to this misinformation as "shorthand". Psychiatrist Ronald Pies also seems to think that the biochemical imbalance notion is the creation of drug companies, along with a few poorly-trained psychiatrists and some "mendacious" antipsychiatry people:

> I am not one who easily loses his temper, but I confess to experiencing markedly increased limbic activity when I hear someone proclaim, "Psychiatrists think all mental disorders are due to a chemical imbalance!" I don't believe I have ever

heard a knowledgeable, well-trained psychiatrist make such a preposterous claim, except perhaps to mock it. On the other hand, the "chemical imbalance" has been tossed around a great deal by opponents of psychiatry, who mendaciously attribute the phrase to psychiatrists themselves. And yes—the "chemical imbalance" image has been vigorously promoted by some pharmaceutical companies, often to the detriment of our patients' understanding. In truth, the "chemical imbalance" notion was always a kind of urban legend—never a theory seriously propounded by well-informed psychiatrists. [55]

If these "well-informed psychiatrists" knew this to be misinformation, they kept pretty quiet about it. Did they not have a responsibility to correct this misinformation? Why did they not carry out their duty to correct their colleagues and to accurately inform the general public? With the possible exception of Ronald Pies' own comments just referred to, I have yet to see or hear any mainstream psychiatrist mock the brain chemical imbalance concept. I am not sure whether or not Dr. Pies would consider each of the many psychiatrists named in this book who have publicly promoted the depression brain chemical imbalance as a known fact as being excluded from the group of "knowledgeable, well-trained psychiatrists" to which he refers.

In attempting to shoot the messenger—those "mendacious" opponents of psychiatry he refers to—Pies actually acknowledged that the biochemical imbalance notion has always been a "little white lie". Yet he still managed to criticize those who questioned psychiatry for repeatedly propagating this lie for several decades:

> In the narrative of the antipsychiatry movement, a monolithic entity called "psychiatry" has deliberately misled the public as to the causes of mental illness, by failing to debunk the chemical imbalance hypothesis. Indeed, this narrative insists that, by promoting this little white lie, psychiatry betrayed the public trust and made it seem as if psychiatrists had magic bullets for psychiatric disorders. [56]

In a 2014 article published on the Mad in America website, Philip Hickey Ph.D. expressed his reaction to Pies' comments (italics and brackets his):

> Note the euphemism "little white lie". Great big black whopper would have been more accurate. And it *was* a betrayal of the public trust; and it *did* create the impression that psychiatrists had magic bullets for depression and other human problems; and it did induce people, who might not otherwise have done so, to take psychiatric drugs; and Big Pharma *was*, and still *is*, in cahoots with psychiatry (69% of the *DMS-5* Task Force had financial links to pharma!). [57]

In this article, Hickey also challenged psychiatrist Ronald Pies' claim that the brain chemical imbalance notion was not promoted by mainstream psychiatry (italics his):

> The fact is that psychiatry, at both the organized and individual level, *did* promote, in characteristically dogmatic fashion, the notion that depression and other significant problems of thinking, feeling, and/or behaving are *caused* by chemical

imbalances in the brain. Nor was this an innocent error. *They promoted this fiction even though they knew it was false*, because it suited their purposes and the purposes of their pharmaceutical allies. This falsehood was vigorously promoted by psychiatrists and by pharma, and tragically has been accepted as fact by two generations in western countries and increasingly in other parts of the world. [58]

ASSUMING THAT WHAT THE EXPERTS SAY IS OBJECTIVE AND TRUSTWORTHY

People with no direct involvement in or knowledge of the medical approach to depression may understandably assume that what they have heard about brain chemical abnormalities are scientifically established facts. In December 2006 the *New York Times* published an article by Michael Kimmelman about Joseph Schildkraut, one of the originators of the brain chemical imbalance theory of depression, titled "The Creative Mind Reader". Kimmelman wrote:

> A groundbreaking paper he published in 1965 suggested that naturally occurring chemical substances in the brain must account for mood swings, which pharmaceuticals could correct, a hypothesis that proved to be right. [59]

According to his biography on the APB Speakers International website, Michael Kimmelman, in addition to being an accomplished pianist, is a best-selling award-winning author and "chief art critic of the *New York Times* and a contributor to the *New York Review of Books* . . . A Pulitzer Prize finalist". [60] Clearly an intelligent and talented man, Kimmelman is grossly misinformed in this matter, given that he believed that Schildkraut's hypothesis "proved to be right". Alarm bells should sound regarding any widely held belief when such generally well-informed, well-intentioned and influential people can be so misinformed. Michael Kimmelman is not unusual in this. Fifty years on, the discredited belief that antidepressants have a specific effect on a biological process in the brain remains the main justification for the widespread public presumption that depression is caused by a brain chemical abnormality. It is a flimsy foundation upon which to build a paradigm and a way of working. But for those with a vested interest, this belief—which supports what doctors and drug companies want to believe and want the public to believe—is a lot better than no foundation, a nightmare scenario that might give rise to many awkward questions.

Professor of Neuroanatomy Jonathan Leo PhD and Lecturer in Social Work Jeffrey Lacasse contacted the author of this *New York Times* article following its publication. They requested a citation from Michael Kimmelman to verify his claim that Schildkraut had been correct, and subsequently wrote:

> Emails to the author requesting a citation to support his statement went unanswered. [61]

Most people have heard about the chemical imbalance notion from a range of sources so many times that they have come to assume it to be a known fact or so close to a fact as makes no difference. In the public mind, the primary group that render credibility to the chemical imbalance idea are medical doctors, one of the most trusted groups in society. Most people are unaware that when it comes to mental health most doctors are (a) biased and (b) ignorant. They are biased toward the ideas they most favour. They have prematurely become convinced that psychiatric diagnoses such as depression are primarily organic disorders. Many doctors are also ignorant; they do not possess sufficient understanding of human emotionality and psychology to properly address the problems and challenges faced by the people who attend them, the significance of which seems to almost routinely pass over their heads. This has been my experience for over ten years in dealing with people from all over Ireland and beyond, people who have attended medical and psychiatric services for emotional and mental health problems. I know from the many contacts I have around the world that the situation is similar in countries where psychiatry reigns as the primary authority in mental health.

BIOLOGY IS KING

No reliable evidence exists of any biological basis to, or of characteristic biological features in, depression. This reality does not prevent many doctors from concluding and asserting that depression is a biological illness. This approach could be paraphrased as follows:

> We don't know what causes depression, and we don't have any evidence confirming a biological nature for depression. But we are fully convinced that whatever the cause and whatever is wrong, it is definitely biological.

Many doctors go even further with this notion. According to Irish GP Dr. Harry Barry in his 2007 book *Flagging the Problem*, even talk therapies such as counselling and psychotherapy "probably work biologically". [62] Barry is not alone within the medical fraternity in holding such views. Speaking at a 1986 American Psychiatric Association meeting, psychiatrist P. Mohl claimed:

> Psychotherapy is a biological treatment that acts through biological mechanisms on biological problems . . . Medication, dream interpretation, and empathy become simply different ways to alter different neurotransmitters . . . Modern developments in basic neuroscience are uncovering the underlying medical nature of psychotherapy. [63]

Since none of these assertions are verified by reliable scientific evidence, it is more accurate to ascribe these claims to wishful thinking than to trustworthy results of scientific endeavour. Because they are over-committed to biology, many doctors really want to believe that biology is at the heart of most if not all considerations regarding depression. To maintain their position as *the* experts on depression, they want and need the public to believe this also.

This reality is illustrated in the comments and writings of many psychiatrists. American psychiatrist Dr. Daniel Carlat expressed this way of thinking in his 2010 book *Unhinged: The Trouble with Psychiatry—a Doctor's Revelations about a Profession in Crisis*:

> How could mental illness not be, ultimately, biological? All thoughts and emotions come from the brain, and so disordered thoughts and emotions must come from a disordered brain . . . Depression must be caused by something that has gone wrong in the brain. [64]

Such thinking is logically flawed, the product of the limited and deluded thinking that has infused psychiatry over the past century. I will address the issue of "how could mental illness not be, ultimately, biological" in detail in future books, as it does not fall within the remit of this book. I and many others, who have been willing to look beyond the narrow limited scope of the flawed biologically-dominated medical view, have come to understand that psychiatric diagnoses including depression are far more accurately understood when a more holistic understanding is employed, as I discussed in chapter four. Such an approach takes proper account of realities often ignored or underestimated within the predominantly biological model such as the accumulation of emotional woundedness experienced in life, emotional and psychological distress, and a wide range of defence mechanisms and self-protection strategies including selfhood reduction [65] that are created in response to the individual's life experiences. Taking such an expanded approach to psychiatric diagnoses including depression, it is eminently possible to see the major limitations of biological interpretations and solutions. We humans are complex sentient beings. Psychiatry's obsession with reducing human beings to their biology—often doing so with considerable distortion and exaggeration of the facts—reveals far more about psychiatry's priorities and understanding than about how human beings function and what they need.

The words of American psychologist Abraham Maslow help to clarify what is happening here. Maslow referred to the common human tendency to become over-reliant on a familiar tool as "The Law of the instrument". In 1964 Maslow stated:

> I call it *the law of the instrument*, and it may be formulated as follows; give a small boy a hammer, and he will find that everything he encounters needs pounding. [66]

In 1966 Maslow wrote:

> I suppose it is tempting, if the only tool you have is a hammer, to treat everything as if it were a nail. [67]

Since the adoption by psychiatry of the notion that depression and other psychiatric diagnoses are primarily biological in origin and nature, biology has increasingly become psychiatry's main and often their only hammer, brain chemical imbalances in particular. In 2010, psychiatrist Daniel Carlat acknowledged:

> We psychiatrists spend our days splitting our patients into two: one is a repository of neurotransmitters, and the other is a person with relationships, a job and aspirations. We treat the neurotransmitters, and we refer the person to somebody else. [68]

Not having an extensive understanding and corresponding vocabulary to describe and understand what is called depression except in largely incorrect biological terms, most doctors do not possess the necessary range of responses to their patients' needs. There is much more to the holistic understanding of depression and other psychiatric diagnoses that the relative merits of medication and psychotherapy. Daniel Carlat's comments above relating to psychiatry and therapy are relevant examples of Maslow's *Law of the Instrument*. His comments are quite honest, but they could be more so. Psychiatrists do not "treat the neurotransmitters". They may have convinced themselves and wish to convince their patients that they are doing so, but their convictions lack any corroborative objective evidence. Since brain neurotransmitter levels cannot be and therefore never are measured, and there is no direct evidence of any neurotransmitter abnormality to begin with, claims that psychiatrists treat neurotransmitters are without foundation. Also, Carlat's comment suggests that psychiatrists regularly send their patients "to somebody else", meaning a therapist. This is often not the case at all. Many psychiatrists recommend to their patients that there is little point in them attending therapy, that medication is the preferred and the only treatment that can work for them.

COLLEGIALITY BEFORE TRUTH

Most major textbooks of general medicine contain detailed sections on each specialty of medicine including psychiatry. One such example is *Davidson's Principles and Practice of Medicine*, published in 2010. [69] The presence of thirty-two copies of this textbook in the University of Limerick library in December 2014 illustrates its importance. A psychiatry section is included within this comprehensive textbook of 1,376 pages. In this section which is written by psychiatrists, the following appears under the heading "Brain Structure and Function":

> Brain structure is normal in most psychiatric disorders. The function of the brain is commonly altered, however, with for example, changes in neurotransmitters such as dopamine, noradrenaline (norepinephrine) and 5-hydroxytryptamine, (5-HT, serotonin), and differences in activity of specific areas of the brain, as seen on functional brain scans. [70]

Notice how this passage is presented as if its contents were established scientific facts, which as I have discussed in this book, they most certainly are not. I would expect practicing psychiatrists such as the authors to be aware of the facts. And the facts are that there is no reliable scientific evidence of any changes in neurotransmitter function in any psychiatric disorder. Such assertions presented as established facts therefore amount to misinformation. There is no reliable evidence to confirm that "the function of the brain is commonly altered", yet the authors presented this as if it is an established fact. The authors specifically mention dopamine, noradrenaline and serotonin, despite that fact that no such abnormalities have ever been reliably identified. They assert that "differences in activity in specific areas of the brain, as seen on functional brain scans" provide satisfactory evidence of "altered brain function". This latter claim is a False Cause logical fallacy, [71] since the authors are erroneously claiming that the presence of changes in activity prove something that activity alone without known parameters of normality and abnormality cannot prove; altered brain function.

Immediately struck by the misinformation in this highly regarded medical textbook, I contacted the publishing company and wrote to the book's commissioning editor. I wrote a comprehensive five-page letter in which I set out why this wording was inaccurate and therefore should not be included in such a highly respected and influential medical textbook. Amongst other points, I wrote:

> This statement is presented as though it were an established fact. I am not aware of any reliable scientific evidence of the existence of established altered function of the brain with changes in neurotransmitters. I have been very interested in mental health for over ten years. Regarding depression, based on my extensive reading and research, it is my understanding that the correct scientific position on this is that there is no scientifically established evidence of any altered brain neurotransmitter function, serotonin included. I have not encountered any evidence of established pre-existing abnormalities in serotonin or any other neurotransmitter.
>
> The following is, I believe, an accurate representation of the facts of the matter. Taking depression as an example, the idea that there might be neurotransmitter abnormalities is encapsulated in the monoamine theory of depression, which includes the serotonin hypothesis. This hypothesis derives not from observations of "the function of the brain" being "commonly altered" or "changes in neurotransmitters", but from observations that drugs increase synapse levels of serotonin, quite a different scenario. From this observation it was deduced that abnormalities of serotonin levels *may* be present in depression. The status of this idea remains a hypothesis. It has not been scientifically demonstrated to be a fact in spite of almost fifty years of intensive research. And as is clear from many of the commentaries included later in this letter, many experienced people in the field believe that there is a considerable degree of evidence confirming the incorrectness of the serotonin hypothesis and monoamine theory.

These were just two of the passages from my letter to the commissioning editor. The commentaries I refer to in the last sentence above are all included in this book. The commissioning editor passed on my letter to the authors of the psychiatry chapter. The authors replied through the commissioning editor:

> We can definitely defend this statement. In fact, it is a fact that pre-synaptic dopamine neurotransmission is upregulated in schizophrenia and is not due to treatment. The evidence is less clear for other conditions but still suggestive—more research is needed—but is enough to justify our general statement. [72]

This reply from the psychiatry chapter authors was very unsatisfactory, for reasons I set out in my second letter to the book's commissioning editor in January 2014:

Unfortunately, for several reasons, the author's response does not contain anything approaching adequate alleviation of my concerns, for reasons that I will set out in this letter... In my original letter, I used serotonin and depression as an example to illustrate the inaccuracy of this passage. In his/her response, the author did not address this issue in relation to depression or serotonin at all. Nor did the author provide any specific reference to noradrenaline, the third neurotransmitter specifically mentioned in the above passage.

Whilst the clear impression from the above passage is that it is referring to psychiatric diagnoses in general, the only psychiatric diagnosis specifically referred to in the author's response is schizophrenia. With regard to all other psychiatric conditions, the author states in their response that: "The evidence is less clear for other conditions but still suggestive—more research is needed—but is enough to justify our general statement".

I beg to differ. As a percentage of total psychiatric diagnoses made, including those made by general practitioners, schizophrenia is a diagnosis made in a small minority of cases. Put another way, of every 1,000 psychiatric diagnoses made, a diagnosis of schizophrenia would be made in a small minority, perhaps 10-50 out of every 1000 diagnoses made. The exact figure does not matter. The point is that a diagnosis of schizophrenia is made in only a small minority of the totality of psychiatric diagnoses made. Therefore, even if altered brain function were reliably established in schizophrenia (and I will address this issue later in this letter), the use of the term "commonly" would not be appropriate. The Dictionary.com website defines "common" as "pertaining or belonging to an entire community, nation or culture; widespread; general; of frequent occurrence; usual; familiar". It cannot be accurately claimed that something found in a small minority of the totality of psychiatric diagnoses pertains to the entire community (of diagnoses); is widespread; is a frequent occurrence; is usual, or familiar. I would point out to you what the definition of a Hasty Generalisation logical fallacy is: "This fallacy occurs when one attempts to form a general rule from particular cases when there is not enough evidence to do so". [73]

Returning to the author's statement in his/her response to my first letter: "The evidence is less clear for other conditions but still suggestive—more research is needed—but is enough to justify our general statement". There are several real problems with this assertion. You will recall that the statement in question in *Davidson* 21st edition is made as a clearly unequivocal statement of fact: "The function of the brain is commonly altered, however, with for example, changes in neurotransmitters such as dopamine, noradrenaline (norepinephrine) and 5-hydroxytryptamine (5-HT, serotonin)".

The unequivocal message of this passage is that reliable scientific evidence has established beyond all doubt that the function of the brain is commonly altered in relation to dopamine, noradrenaline and serotonin. Yet, in the author's response, there is no validation of the supposedly factual nature of altered brain function for all other diagnoses other than schizophrenia claimed in the passage published in Davidson's textbook. Regarding all other diagnoses, the author's comments— "the evidence is less clear but still suggestive"—fall far short of verifying the claim of altered brain function as an established fact. The author's admission that "more research is needed" is an implicit acknowledgement that research to date has *not* established altered brain functioning in these other conditions as a fact but that future research will do so, which is itself a major assumption that may or may not come to fruition in the future. The author's subsequent statement that this is "enough to justify our general statement" is therefore logically unsound. How can "evidence that is less clear", that is merely "suggestive", regarding which "more research is required" be logically concluded as "enough to justify our original statement", which was a statement of fact regarding commonly altered brain function?

The definition of a Begging the Question/Circular Reasoning logical fallacy is: "An argument is circular if its conclusion is among its premises, if it assumes (either explicitly or not) what it is trying to prove. Such arguments are said to beg the question. A circular argument fails as a proof because it will only be judged as sound by those who already accept its conclusion". [74]

The authors seemed to be suggesting that the "more research" that "is needed" will definitely confirm the premise that "the function of the brain is commonly altered". If so, then the authors are clearly jumping the gun here, concluding that an unproven premise regarding future research is a foregone conclusion.

In support of their sweeping statement regarding altered brain function in psychiatric disorders, the chapter authors provided no supportive evidence regarding depression or any other psychiatric diagnosis other than schizophrenia. I will include more details on this in my future book on the medical approach to schizophrenia, but a few comments are relevant here. The one research paper alluded to by the authors as evidence in relation to schizophrenia was published in 2012, two years *after* the 21st edition of *Davidson's Principles and Practice of Medicine*. The authors could not therefore have been using this research paper as grounds for what they wrote in a book published in 2010, two years previously. As I wrote in my second letter to the commissioning letter:

> I would have thought it patently obvious that quoting a paper published two years later cannot be used as supportive evidence of a supposed statement of fact published in a very important and prestigious medical textbook published two years earlier. This simply does not add up.

There were several other problems associated with this research paper on schizophrenia, all of which I described in my second letter to the book's commissioning editor. These questions made the reliance on this paper as solid "evidence" of altered brain function very tenuous indeed. The final paragraph of my second letter read as follows:

> In conclusion, I do not believe that my concerns have been satisfactorily addressed to any significant degree in the author's response. I formally request that my concerns, both in my previous letter and also in this letter, be addressed fully.

I am sure that the editors of *Davidson's* 21st edition share my conviction that it is imperative that the information contained within the pages of this widely-used and much-trusted textbook be scientifically accurate, with all possible effort to minimize the risk of misinforming medical students and post-graduates who rely on the accuracy and the veracity of their textbooks. I again request that you give this matter your serious consideration. I look forward to your response.

I did not receive much of a response to my second letter. The commissioning editor replied:

Many thanks for your letter. All I can do is pass this on to the chapter authors and if they wish to take this further with you I will ask them to be in touch directly. As far as my role in this is concerned I am reassured by the authors that no change is required to the printed text. [75]

The commissioning editor had apparently asked the authors for their response to my first letter. They advised him that no further action was necessary. The commissioning editor apparently took their advice on face value and decided that nothing more was required of him. Not satisfied with this response, I emailed the commissioning editor:

Thank you for your response. I note your comment that you are accepting the authors' reassurance that no change is necessary to the wording because the wording is correct as it is. Are you aware of the Appeal to Authority logical fallacy? It occurs when an argument is accepted because of the apparent authority of the arguer rather than on the merits of the argument. I presented you with about ten pages of reasons as to why this wording is factually incorrect, misinformation, and misleading. The authors provided you with just one piece of so-called supportive evidence. In my last letter to you, I set out very clearly and in detail why the authors' response to my questions was very inadequate. Yet it appears you are accepting the authors' reassurance without question, rather than taking seriously my comprehensive setting out of the reality as to why this wording is fallacious and should therefore not be in print in such an august publication as *Davidson's* 21st edition. As you are the commissioning editor, I find this disappointing.

The commissioning editor's reply was brief:

I acknowledge receipt of your email. Yours sincerely . . . [76]

Three weeks later, I received a further and apparently final brief email from the commissioning editor:

I am writing to let you know that we have taken advice from an external third party in connection with the matter raised in your correspondence. As a result of this we are completely satisfied that no change is required to the printed text of *Davidson*. We regard the matter as now closed. [77]

Since I had yet to receive anything resembling an adequate response to the important issues I raised, I did not regard the matter as closed. I again wrote to the commissioning editor:

> In regard to previous correspondence regarding a factual error I brought to your attention in the psychiatry chapter of *Davidson's* 21st edition; in your last email to me dated 30 January 2014, you wrote "I am writing to let you know that we have taken advice from an external third party in connection with the matter raised in your correspondence. As a result of this we are completely satisfied that no change is required to the printed text of *Davidson*. We regard this matter as now closed."
> I am aware that while you did forward the original reply from the authors to me, you did not forward to me the advice you referred to in your email of 30 January 2014. I am therefore at a disadvantage in this, since I have not been given access to the advice upon which you are acting. I therefore would be grateful for your attention to the following questions. They will not take up much of your time. If the advice was in writing, I would be grateful if you would please forward a copy to me. If the advice was verbal, I would be grateful if you would inform me as to the precise nature of this advice. Please also inform me regarding who provided this advice, and the position and professional status of the person from whom you received this advice.

Two weeks later I received the following reply:

> As I mentioned previously we have taken advice from an external third party in connection with the matter raised in your correspondence. As a result of this I am satisfied that no change is required to the printed text of *Davidson*. Your reservations about this aspect of the textbook are noted but I feel we have investigated them thoroughly. The text has been carefully reviewed again by the textbook's Editors as well as the authors of the chapter, and an independent third party has fully supported what is written in the book. We appreciate you raising this with us—we always check any points raised with us to ensure the book is accurate. Having undertaken an investigation I regard this matter as now closed and no further correspondence is I think necessary. [78]

I replied:

> Thank you for your email of March 17th. I note that my request to see the third party advice you received has not been granted to me. It would appear that this error of fact will continue in *Davidson's* textbook into the foreseeable future. What a pity. I will do what I can to ensure that the public are made aware of this misinformation and of how this matter was dealt with by your company.
> You say that this matter has been investigated thoroughly and is now closed. I beg to differ. The author's only reply to me, the only reply that I have seen in this regard, was grossly inadequate, and I find it remarkable that you and your publishing company are willing to accept this as adequate. To remind you, the

author's only defence of their assertions was a single research paper, published two years AFTER *Davidson's* 21st Edition, and therefore could not possibly have been a source of "evidence" for their assertions. I presented you with a host of reasons as to why that research paper was not a credible source upon which to base such assertions in any case, including several such reservations raised by the study authors themselves. I have received no response that addressed these matters. Your chapter authors were apparently unable to provide even a single item of evidence in regard to depression to back up their unequivocally-asserted statements in the book.

You say that you "appreciate" my "raising this" with you. I can't say that was the feeling I sensed at my end. I felt, based on the responses—or at times the lack of adequate responses—that I received, that I was seen as somewhat of a nuisance. You, your company and your authors might bear that in mind for future reference. In conclusion; your conviction regarding the correctness of the text is erroneous. The facts remain the facts. There is no reliable scientific basis for the assertions in question, and your conversations with the authors or third parties do not alter this fact. This whole exercise has been interesting and illuminating for me. In my opinion, when faced with a rather difficult issue, collegiality rather than truth has won the day. Therefore for me, this matter is not closed.

The last time I challenged wording in similar fashion was in 2002-3. Then, I questioned the Irish Medicines Board about two aspects of the wording on the Seroxat patient information leaflet that I knew to be false, yet had been on the patient information leaflet for many years. Within six months, the Irish Medicines Board advised the drug company to change both of these wordings; one concerned incorrect claims re correcting chemical levels, and the other was an emphatic yet scientifically unsubstantiated statement relating to the medication being non-addictive. I knew I was right then, and I know I am right now. I only embark on such questioning when I know the truth of the situation. [79]

I believe this is an example of the prioritising of collegiality above truth. There is no reliable scientific evidence that confirms any degree of altered function of any neurotransmitters including the three specifically mentioned by the authors of that chapter. It appears that the commissioning editor primarily satisfied himself by asking the authors to adjudicate on my letter. Other than eventually seeking other advice which I was not permitted to see, in my opinion the textbook's publishing company could and should have done much more to get to the truth of the matter. I am not familiar with the duties of a commissioning editor, but surely someone within a major publishing company is responsible for ensuring the veracity of the content of such a prominent medical textbook.

The consequence of all this is that an important error of fact continues in print in this medical textbook. Thousands of medical students will upon reading this be misinformed regarding neurotransmitter functioning. It could be argued that such misinformation is in the interest of mainstream psychiatry, since it credits psychiatry with a degree of scientific prowess and reliability that is not consistent with the actual evidence.

I believe that the publishing company chose to run with the status quo. Medicine is a very hierarchical profession. It is rare that specialists such as the authors of this chapter would be asked to account for themselves, and certainly not by a "mere" GP. Acknowledging the error might be quite embarrassing for both the authors and the publishing company; better perhaps to play the hierarchy card and conclude that because the supposed expert said the wording was correct they could run with it. None of this changes the reality of the factual error in the book however.

A FLAWED DISEASE MODEL

Throughout this book I have given examples of the flawed logic and distorted thinking that is characteristic of the chemical imbalance notion of depression. Claims that brain chemical imbalances occur in depression when there is no reliable scientific evidence to confirm this conclusion are typical examples of a Wishful Thinking logical fallacy. [80]

For over thirty years, the brain chemical imbalance delusion has been the bedrock of the medical and drug company promotion of depression as a disease like any other. Those who promote a supposedly disease-centred understanding of depression might do well to consider psychiatrist Daniel Carlat's honest admission in his 2010 book *Unhinged: The Trouble with Psychiatry—A Doctor's Revelations about a Profession in Crisis*:

> In virtually all of the psychiatric disorders—including depression, schizophrenia, bipolar disorder and anxiety disorders—the shadow of our ignorance overwhelms the few dim lights of our knowledge. [81]

Behaviour is sometimes related to disease. For example, low blood glucose—known as hypoglycaemia—is associated with alterations in behaviours such as agitation and aggression. Hypoglycemia arises most commonly in people diagnosed with diabetes who have taken too much insulin, causing their blood sugar level to reduce to suboptimal levels. Hypoglycemia is very rare in non-diabetic situations, usually being caused by a pancreatic tumour causing overproduction of insulin. The behaviours associated with hypoglycaemia are quite different to those of depression, and clearly point to a biological problem. They generally occur suddenly, often quite dramatically. Blood glucose testing confirms the low blood level. If left untreated, coma within minutes is likely, leading to irreversible brain damage and possibly death pretty quickly if untreated. Hypoglycemia responds within minutes to treatment with glucose. Provided the low blood glucose is reversed quickly enough, no damage ensues and full consciousness is restored within minutes, though the person may need to sleep for a while afterwards. The biological mechanisms involved in hypoglycemia are fully understood within medicine. The brain needs glucose to function. Without a constant supply of glucose, brain cells quickly run into serious trouble. A deficiency of glucose lasting even a few minutes will seriously compromise brain function, leading to the clinical situation described above that is so typical of hypoglycemia.

There is no scientific basis for the disease model for depression that is espoused and promoted by psychiatrists and GPs. In this book I set out how fundamentally flawed the brain chemical imbalance aspect of the medical disease-oriented approach

264 Depression Delusion: The Myth of the Brain Chemical Imbalance

to depression is. In my next book I address other major flaws in the disease-model approach to depression, including whether depression meets the medical criteria for a disease, and claims of genetic abnormalities in depression.

CONFUSION ABOUT CAUSE AND EFFECT

Prozac Nation: Young and Depressed in America is a personal memoir written by Elizabeth Wurtzel. Published in 1994, *Prozac Nation* quickly became a best-seller, one of the best-known books of the Prozac era. The author described a meeting with a psychiatrist in hospital who was impressively honest regarding depression and medication. Having listened to Wurtzel's story, the psychiatrist said:

> Elizabeth, there is no pill in the world that's going to make you feel better. We have no way of measuring whether you have any sort of deficiency or not. The way we diagnose people for mental illness is purely anecdotal, and then we prescribe medications that we believe will suit the patient best by trial and error. Since there's not a blood test to detect depression or schizophrenia, we just have to figure out what works as best we can . . . I assure you, from what you've told me, and what I'm reading here, that your problem is not chemical. [82]

Wurtzel described meeting a psychiatrist some time later at the Affective Disorders Clinic at McLean, a centre where psychiatrists were "gung ho about a new pill . . . brand name Prozac". [83] Informed by her consultation with this psychiatrist, Wurtzel describes antidepressants as "drugs" that:

> Mainly act on the production of norepinephrine and serotonin, two chemicals . . . that the brains of depressives are either lacking or not using efficiently. Essentially, these drugs prevent secreting cells from reabsorbing these neurotransmitters, thus allowing them to circulate and stimulate the next nerve cell into production. [84]

Toward the end of her book, the author reflected:

> In the case of my own depression, I have gone from a thorough certainty that its origins are in bad biology to a more flexible belief that after an accumulation of life events made my head such an ugly thing to be stuck in, my chemicals started to agree . . . regardless of how I got started on my path of misery, by the time I got treatment the problem was certainly chemical. What many people don't realize is that the cause-and-effect relationship in mental disorders is a two-way shuttle: It's not just that an a priori imbalance can make you depressed. It's that years and years of exogenous depression (a malaise caused by external events) can actually fuck up your internal chemistry so much that you need a drug to get it working properly again. [85]

As described in these passages, Elizabeth Wurtzel erroneously came to believe the rhetoric that brain chemical imbalances occur in depression. Like many others, including several mentioned earlier in this book, her questioning of the prevailing view of depression concerned whether the often-claimed chemical imbalances cause depression or are caused by it. It would certainly be correct to state that years of malaise and unhappiness can cause the experiences and behaviours that become diagnosed as depression. It is unnecessary to conclude that this happens because brain chemistry becomes abnormal.

American physician Andrew Weil is highly regarded internationally for his holistic approach to health and disease. In his 1997 book *Natural Health, Natural Medicine*, Weil is critical of psychiatry's preoccupation with brain chemical deficiencies. Yet it is the cause-and-effect issue he questions rather than the more fundamental issue, the fact that no such abnormalities have even been identified:

> Of all the branches of medicine today, psychiatry is most mired in materialistic thinking. It believes that all mental problems result from disordered brain biochemistry, hence its total commitment to the use of drugs. It makes equal sense to me that disordered moods and thinking *cause* disordered chemistry, and I am inclined to look for other ways to treat depression. [86]

Since misinformation about depression and brain chemical imbalances is widespread, it is to be expected that people will express these beliefs as facts in various situations. Following treatment for depression, Diane Patrick, wife of Massachusetts Governor Deval Patrick gave a press briefing:

> I've done a little reading in the time I've had. And what I know is that depression is really a chemical imbalance which is triggered by systemic stress. [87]

Diane Patrick is an intelligent and successful woman. A lawyer and teacher, it is likely that when she decided to learn about depression, she did so methodically. It is a testament to the widespread nature of the depression brain chemical imbalance delusion that she would come to such an erroneous conclusion. She certainly *believed* that depression is a chemical imbalance but she cannot *know* this, since one cannot know something that has not been demonstrated to exist. One might reasonably think her comments an advance on the prevailing view, which dictates that the chemical imbalance is the cause of depression. Diane Patrick stated that the brain chemical imbalance in depression is the result of systemic stress.

Well known Irish broadcaster Gareth O'Callaghan came to similar conclusions in his 2003 book *A Day Called Hope: A Personal Journey Beyond Depression*:

> I believe depression is related to moods and emotions. Scientists might claim that chemical imbalances in the brain are the root of different emotions and moods, and that chemical imbalances cause depressed behaviour. I would turn this back to front. My own experience makes me believe that tangled emotions and low moods, over a prolonged period of time, actually cause these chemical imbalances. [88]

This argument is an advance on the prevailing medical view, since it honours the distinct possibility that our bodies may react to our experiences in various ways. There is however a fundamental flaw in this position. Both Diane Patrick and Gareth O'Callaghan could certainly be forgiven for not knowing this, given the piecemeal and misleading approach with which depression is discussed in society and the degree to which respected professionals and drug companies regularly mention brain chemical abnormalities as if these were established facts. Both positions—that depression is caused by or causes chemical imbalances—presuppose the existence of known and reliably identified chemical imbalances. Such assumptions are unjustified given the absence of scientific evidence to support them. These assumptions are therefore Begging the Question logical fallacies. [89]

The billions of dollars invested in the serotonin and other theories has conveniently bypassed some obvious questions. When a substance has a certain effect and the substance has been found to interefere with brain chemistry, it does not follow that the underlying problem was a defect relating to the action of the substance without establishing this deficiency in the first instance.

NOTES TO CHAPTER ELEVEN

1.   Edward Shorter, *How Everyone Became Depressed,* Oxford: Oxford University Press, 2013, p. 160.
2.   Edward Valenstein, *Blaming the Brain: The Truth About Drugs and Mental Health,* New York: The Free Press, 1998, pps. 96, 235.
3.   Author Marian Keyes, interviewed on the Marian Finucane Show, RTE Radio One, 08 November 2014, http://www.rte.ie/radio1/podcast/podcast_marianfinucane.xml, Marian Keyes, 08 November 2014, accessed 08 November 2014.
4.   Charles Medawar & Anita Hardon, *Medicines out of Control?: Antidepressants and the Conspiracy of Goodwill,* The Netherlands: Aksant Academic Publishers, 2004.
5.   Daniel Carlat, *Unhinged: The Trouble with Psychiatry—a Doctor's Revelations about a Profession in Crisis,* London: Free Press, 2010, p. 13.
6.   Andrew Scull biography, Department of Sociology, University, of California, San Diego, http://sociology.ucsd.edu/faculty/bio/scull.shtml, accessed 27 February 14.
7.   Andrew Scull Ph.D., Professor of History of Psychiatry, Princeton University, in *the Lancet,* Volume 375, Issue 9722, 10 April 2010, pps. 1246-1247.
8.   Eliott S. Valenstein, *Blaming the Brain: The Truth About Drugs and Mental Health,* New York: The Free Press, 1998.
9.   Marcia Angell, "The Truth about the Drug Companies", *New York Review of Books,* 15 July 2004, http://www.nybooks.com/articles/archives/2004/jul/15/the-truth-about-the-drug-companies/, accessed 18 August 2014.
10. Marcia Angell, "Drug Companies and Doctors: A Story of Corruption", *New York Review of Books,* 15 January 2009, http://www.nybooks.com/articles/archives/2009/jan/15/drug-companies-doctorsa-story-of-corruption/, accessed 18 August 2014.
11. Michael Corry & Aine Tubridy, *Depression: An Emotion not a Disease,* Cork: Mercier Press,2005,p.11.
12. J. Moncrieff & D. Cohen, "Do Antidepressants Cure or Create Abnormal Brain States? *PLoS Med* 3(7), 06 June 2006: e240. doi:10.1371/journal.pmed.0030240, http://www.plosmedicine.org/article/info%3Adoi%2F10.1371%2Fjournal.pmed.0030240, accessed 30 December 2013.
13. David Burns, *When Panic Attacks: The New Drug-Free Anxiety Therapy That Can Change Your Life,* Harmony, 2006.

14. Catherine DeAngelis, "Impugning the Integrity of Medical Science: The Adverse Effects of Industry", *Journal of the American Medical Association*, 16 April 2008, Vol 299, No. 15, http://jama.jama network.com/article.aspx?articleid=181748, accessed 27 February 2014.

15. Ben Goldacre, "Bad Science: Depression—the facts and the fables", *The Guardian,* 26 January 2008, http://www.theguardian. com/commentisfree/2008/jan/26/badscience, accessed 29 December 2013.

16. Richard Bentall, *Doctoring the Mind: Why Psychiatric Treatments Fail,* London: Penguin Books Ltd, 2009, p. 77.

17. Kirsch, Irving, *The Emperor's New Drugs Exploding the Antidepressant Myth,* 2009, London: Random House.

18. Fresh Air Interview, "A Psychiatrist's Prescription for his Profession", 13 July 2010, http://www.npr.org/templates/transcript/transcript.php?storyId=128107547, accessed 13 May 2014.

19. Vivek Datta, "Chemical Imbalances and Other Black Unicorns", Mad in America website, 25 June 2012, http://www.madinamerica.com/2012/06/chemical-imbalances-and-other-black-unicorns/, accessed 27 February 2014.

20. Vivek Datta, "Chemical Imbalances and Other Black Unicorns", Mad in America website, 25 June 2012, http://www.madinamerica.com/2012/06/chemical-imbalances-and-other-black-unicorns/, accessed 27 February 2014.

21. www.anxiety.com website, "The 'chemical imbalance' theory as a cause for anxiety and depressive disorders officially put to rest!", p. 3, http://www.anxietycentre.com/downloads/Chemical-Imbalance-Theory-is-False.pdf, accessed 27 February 2014.

22. David Healy, "The Antidepressant Era: The Movie", 23 January 2013, www.davidhealy.org, accessed 20 November 2013.

23. Edward Shorter, *How Everyone Became Depressed,* Oxford:Oxford University Press, 2013,pps.156-157.

24. Psychiatrist Stuart Shipko, Choose Help website, in an answer to the question, "Can long term tramolol permanently deplete my serotonin?", 10 February 2014, http://www.choosehelp.com/experts/addictions/addictions-stuart-shipko/can-long-term-tramadol-permanently-deplete-my-serotonin, accessed 11 May 2014.

25. John Sommers-Flanagan, http://www.anxietycentre.com/downloads/Chemical-Imbalance-Theory-is-False.pdf, accessed 27 February 2014.

26. Shane Ellison, http://www.anxietycentre.com/downloads/Chemical-Imbalance-Theory-is-False.pdf, accessed 27 February 2014.

27. A. Coppen, "The Biochemistry of Affective Disorders", *British Journal of Psychiatry,* 113 (504): 1237-64, 1967.

28. Regarding the exaggerated effectiveness of antidepressants see note 53 in the Notes to Chap. Five.

29. Stephen Reidbord, "Chemical imbalance—Sloppy thinking in psychiatry 1", "Reidbord's Reflections", 29 April 2012, http://blog.stevenreidbordmd.com/?p=561, accessed 25 May 2014.

30. Steven Sharfstein, interviewed on NDC's *Today,* 27 June 2005, in Jan Eastgate, "Introduction: They Lied", http://www.cchr.co.za/they_lied.html, accessed 26 February 2014.

31. Steven Sharfstein, in *People* magazine, 11 July 2005, in Jan Eastgate, "Introduction: They Lied", http://www.cchr.co.za/they_lied.html, accessed 26 February 2014; also, "American Psychiatric Association Admits There Is No Test For 'Chemical Imbalance'", http://rockrivertimes.com/wpapp/archives/1993/07/01/american-psychiatric-association-admits-there-is-no-test-for-39 chemical-imbalance39/, accessed 18 August 2014.

32. Joanna Moncrieff, *The Myth of the Chemical Cure,* Basingstoke: Palgrave Macmillan, 2009.

33. "Television adverts of antidepressants cause anxiety", *New Scientist,* 12 November 2005, Issue no. 2525.

34. For information on Begging the Question logical fallacies see note 22 in the Notes to the Introduction.

35. The definition of a metaphor, as defined in the online Merriam Webster dictionary, http://www.merriam-webster.com/dictionary/metaphor, accessed 30 December 2013.

36. The definition of a mixed metaphor on the online Merriam Webster Dictionary, http://www.merriam-webster.com/dictionary/mixedmetaphor, accessed 30 December 2013.

37. Fresh Air Interview, "A Psychiatrist's Prescription For His Profession", 13 July 2010, http://www.npr.org/templates/transcript/transcript.php?storyId=128107547, accessed 13 May 2014.

38. Fresh Air Interview, "A Psychiatrist's Prescription For His Profession", 13 July 2010, http://www.npr.org/templates/transcript/transcript.php?storyId=128107547, accessed 13 May 2014.

39. Fresh Air Interview, "A Psychiatrist's Prescription For His Profession", 13 July 2010, http://www.npr.org/templates/transcript/transcript.php?storyId=128107547, accessed 13 May 2014.

40. Fresh Air Interview, "A Psychiatrist's Prescription For His Profession", 13 July 2010, http://www.npr.org/templates/transcript/transcript.php?storyId=128107547, accessed 13 May 2014.

41. J. Leo & J. Lacasse, "Psychiatry's Grand Confession", Mad in America website, 23 January 2012, http://www.madinamerica.com/2012/01/psychiatrys-grand-confession/, accessed 20 July 2014.

42. Alix Speigal, "When It Comes To Antidepressants, Serotonin Isn't The Whole Story", NPR website, 23 January 2012, http://www.npr.org/blogs/health/2012/01/23/145525853/when-it-comes-to-depression-serotonin-isnt-the-whole-story, accessed 04 January 2014.

43. Alix Speigal, "When It Comes To Antidepressants, Serotonin Isn't The Whole Story", NPR website, 23 January 2012, http://www.npr.org/blogs/health/2012/01/23/145525853/when-it-comes-to-depression-serotonin-isnt-the-whole-story, accessed 04 January 2014.

44. See note 12 in the Notes to Chapter Ten.

45. Alix Speigal, "When It Comes To Antidepressants, Serotonin Isn't The Whole Story", NPR website, 23 January 2012, http://www.npr.org/blogs/health/2012/01/23/145525853/when-it-comes-to-depression-serotonin-isnt-the-whole-story, accessed 04 January 2014.

46. Kay Tasman, Jerald Kay & Jeffrey A. Lieberman, eds, *Psychiatry,* 2003, Volume 1, p. 290.

47. Ronald Fieve, *Moodswing: Dr. Fieve on Depression,* Bantam, 1989.

48. Ronald Pies, "Doctor, Is My Mood Disorder Due To A Chemical Imbalance?", Psych Central website, 04 August 2011, http://psychcentral.com/blog/archives/2011/08/04/doctor-is-my-mood-disorder-due-to-a-chemical-imbalance/ accessed 27 February 2014.

49. Ronald Pies, "Doctor, Is My Mood Disorder Due To A Chemical Imbalance?", Psych Central website, 04 August 2011, http://psychcentral.com/blog/archives/2011/08/04/doctor-is-my-mood-disorder-due-to-a-chemical-imbalance/ accessed 27.02.14.

50. Ronald Pies, "Doctor, Is My Mood Disorder Due To A Chemical Imbalance?", Psych Central website, 04 August 2011, http://psychcentral.com/blog/archives/2011/08/04/doctor-is-my-mood-disorder-due-to-a-chemical-imbalance/ accessed 27.02.14.

51. Ronald Pies, "Doctor, Is My Mood Disorder Due To A Chemical Imbalance?", Psych Central website, 04 August 2011, http://psychcentral.com/blog/archives/2011/08/04/doctor-is-my-mood-disorder-due-to-a-chemical-imbalance/ accessed 27.02.14.

52. John Murtagh, *Murtagh's General Practice,* 5th edition,McGraw-Hill Medical Publications,2011,p. 37.

53. I discuss this in Chapter Twelve under the heading "Do GPs generally treat brain disorders?"

54. Mark Graff, interview, CBS Studio Two, July 2005, in Jan Eastgate, "Introduction: They Lied", http://www.cchr.co.za/they_lied.html, accessed 26 February 2014, and in "The Pharmaceutical Industry And Pharmaceutical Endeavour", p. 286, http://www.ghwatch.org/sites/wwwghwatch.org/files/ D4_ 0.pdf, p. 286, accessed 26 February 2014.

55. Ronald Pies, "Psychiatry's New Brain-Mind and the Legend of the 'Chemical Imbalance'", *Psychiatric Times,* 11 July 2011, http://www.psychiatrictimes.com/blogs/couch-crisis/psychiatrys-new-brain-mind-and-legend-chemical-imbalance, accessed 24 February 2014.

56. Ronald Pies, "Psychiatry's New Brain-Mind and the Legend of the 'Chemical Imbalance'", *Psychiatric Times,* 11 July 2011, http://www.psychiatrictimes.com/blogs/couch-crisis/psychiatrys-new-brain-mind-and-legend-chemical-imbalance, accessed 24 February 2014.

57. Phil Hickey, "Psychiatry DID Promote The Chemical Imbalance Theory", 06 June 2014, Mad in America website, http://www.madinamerica.com/2014/06/psychiatry-promote-chemical-imbalance-theory/, accessed 13 June 2014.

58. Phil Hickey, "Psychiatry DID Promote The Chemical Imbalance Theory", 06 June 2014, Mad in America website, http://www.madinamerica.com/2014/06/psychiatry-promote-chemical-imbalance-theory/, accessed 13 June 2014.

59. Michael Kimmelman, "The Creative Mind Reader", *The New York Times* magazine, 31 December 2006, http://www.nytimes.com/2006/12/31/magazine/31wwln_schildkraut.t.html?_r=0, o 29 December 2013.

60. Michael Kimmelman biography, on the American Program Bureau Speakers International website, http://www.apbspeakers.com/speaker/michael-kimmelman, accessed 29 December 2013.

61. Jonathan Leo & Jeffrey R. Lacasse, "The Media and the Chemical Imbalance Theory of Depression", 28 November 2007, *Society*, 2008, 45: 35-45, DOI 10.1007/s12115-007-9047-3, http://link. springer.com/article/10.1007%2Fs12115-007-9047-3#page-1/, accessed 24 May 2014.
62. Harry Barry, *Flagging the Problem: A New Approach to Mental Health*, Dublin: Liberties Press, 2007.
63. Psychiatrist P. Mohl, in a statement made at the 1986 American Psychiatric Association, as quoted in "Data accumulating to support concept that psychotherapy is biologic treatment", *Clin. Psychiatric News*, 1986, 14, 1, 28.
64. Daniel Carlat, *Unhinged: The Trouble with Psychiatry—a Doctor's Revelations about a Profession in Crisis*, London: Free Press, 2010, pps. 75 and 81.
65. For information on selfhood see note 2 in the Notes to Chapter Four.
66. Abraham H. Maslow quoted in Abraham Kaplan, *The Conduct of Inquiry: Methodology for Behavioural Science*, San Francisco: Chandler Publishing Co., 1964, p. 28.
67. A. H. Maslow, *The Psychology of Science: A Reconnaissance*, New York, NY: Harper & Row, 1966, p.15.
68. Daniel Carlat, *Unhinged: The Trouble with Psychiatry—a Doctor's Revelations about a Profession in Crisis*, London: Free Press, 2010, p. 16.
69. Nicki R. Colledge, Brian R. Walker and Stuart H. Ralston, eds, *Davidson's Principles and Practice of Medicine*, 21st edition, Churchill Livingstone Elsevier, 2010.
70. Michael C. Sharpe, Professor of Psychological Medicine, Psychological Medicine Research, University of Edinburgh, UK and Stephen M. Lawrie, Professor of Psychiatry and Neuro-imaging, University of Edinburgh, UK, in *Davidson's Principles and Practice of Medicine* 21st edition, eds Nicki R. Colledge, Brian R. Walker and Stuart H. Ralston, 2010, Churchill Livingstone Elsevier, p. 231.
71. For information on False Cause logical fallacies see note 42 in the Notes to Chapter Five.
72. In an email to me from Laurence Hunter, Commissioning Editor, dated 08 January 2014.
73. Definition of a Hasty Generalization logical fallacy, Pegasus, University of Central Florida, http://pegasus.cc.ucf.edu/~stanlick/fallacylist.html, accessed 08 January 2014.
74. http://www.logicalfallacies.info/presumption/begging-the-question/, accessed 08 January 2014.
75. In an email to me from Laurence Hunter, Commissioning Editor, 09 January 2014.
76. In an email to me from Laurence Hunter, Commissioning Editor, 10 January 2014.
77. In an email to me from Laurence Hunter, Commissioning Editor, 30 January 2014.
78. In an email to me from Laurence Hunter, Commissioning Editor, 17 March 2014.
79. In an email from me to Laurence Hunter, Commissioning Editor, 21 March 2014.
80. For information on Wishful Thinking logical fallacies, see note 115 in the Notes to Chapter Two.
81. Daniel Carlat, *Unhinged: The Trouble with Psychiatry – a Doctor's Revelations about a Profession in Crisis*, London: Free Press, 2010, pps. 79-80.
82. Elizabeth Wurtzel, *Prozac Nation: Young and Depressed in America*, New York: Riverhead Books, 1994, p. 147.
83. Elizabeth Wurtzel, *Prozac Nation: Young and Depressed in America*, New York: Riverhead Books, 1994, p. 296.
84. Elizabeth Wurtzel, *Prozac Nation: Young and Depressed in America*, New York: Riverhead Books, 1994, Ibid, p. 297.
85. Elizabeth Wurtzel, *Prozac Nation: Young and Depressed in America*, New York: Riverhead Books, 1994, Ibid, pps. 345-6.
86. Andrew Weil, *Natural Health, Natural Medicine*, London: Warner Books, 1997, p. 280.
87. Diane Patrick, in J. Leo & J.R. Lacasse, "The Media and the Chemical Imbalance Theory of Depression", *Society*, 45:35-45, 2008, DOI 10.1007/s12115-007-9047-3, http://download.springer.com/static/pdf/285/art%253A10.1007%252Fs12115-007-9047-3.pdf?auth66=1419804289_14472b2ea29966924c320d60dfb0115f&ext=.pdf, accessed 29 December 2014.
88. Gareth O'Callaghan, *A Day Called Hope: A Personal Journey Beyond Depression*, London: Hodder & Stoughton, 2003.
89. For information on Begging the Question logical fallacies see note 22 in the Notes to the Introduction.

12. THE MEDICAL PROFESSION AND THE BRAIN

A picture regularly painted by psychiatrists is that the bulk of their work involves treating mental illnesses with known biological abnormalities in the brain. In the media and in consultations with patients, many psychiatrists portray themselves as experts on the brain.

This is a charade. Psychiatrists do not treat any known organic disorders of the brain for which a definite treatable biological abnormality has been established. No conditions characterised by known brain malfunctions that are amenable to treatment are treated by psychiatry. All such illnesses are treated by other medical specialties, principally neurology and neurosurgery. Brain diseases or disorders likely to require surgical treatment are dealt with by neurosurgeons. Brain diseases or disorders not requiring surgery come under the mantle of neurology. Patients with no demonstrable organic pathology come under the domain of psychiatry.

On the rare occasions where an organic cause is identified for psychiatric-like experiences and behaviours, the patient is quickly transferred under the care of the appropriate specialty. Patients found to have an organic brain illness such as a brain tumour, brain injury or encephalitis are immediately transferred to a neurologist, intracranial hemorrhage to a neurosurgeon, pernicious anemia to a haematologist, thyroid and adrenal problems to an endocrinologist, Lupus (SLE) to an immunologist or rheumatologist. This is how the medical system has always worked and will continue to work. The medical profession is conservative by nature. Sudden, radical change in its modus operandi is not how the medical profession operates. Psychiatrists treating known biological illnesses from which people can recover would represent a seismic shift within medicine. Such seismic shifts within the traditionally conservative medical profession are extremely rare occurrences.

WHAT DO PSYCHIATRISTS DO? ARE THEY BRAIN EXPERTS?

Psychiatry is seen and portrayed as a modern scientific medical specialty, standing proud and tall alongside neurology, cardiology and all other medical specialties. This position gives psychiatry an aura of respectability and status that puts its principles and practice almost above questioning. Psychiatry has thus firmly established itself as *the* field of expertise in mental health matters.

Most people presume that psychiatrists have singular expertise in the brain. This view has been repeatedly fuelled by psychiatrists themselves. As illustrated in a claim from an 1858 *Editorial in the Journal of Mental Science,* this position has been actively promoted for over 150 years:

Insanity is purely a disease of the brain. The physician is now the responsible guardian of the lunatic and must ever remain so. [1]

Psychiatrists and GPs regularly inform the public that psychiatry and the treatment of what are called psychiatric illnesses are grounded upon the specialist understanding of the brain possessed by psychiatrists and to a lesser extent, GPs. This stated position is not consistent with the realities of medical practice.

Every medical specialty has an organ or system within the body regarding which they have gained special expertise. Psychiatrists regularly claim to have special expertise regarding the brain, asserting that the illnesses they treat are brain disorders. In their utterances and writings, many psychiatrists and GPs express considerable enthusiasm for brain biology, repeatedly emphasising its relevance and application to current mental health practice.

As discussed in the previous section, it is clear from everyday medical practice that the medical experts in brain function, investigation and brain disease treatment are neurologists and neurosurgeons, not psychiatrists. This fact raises a question; if the brain and the nervous system is not the organ or system in which psychiatry has recognized specialist expertise that is routinely employed and practiced in psychiatric wards and clinics, what is the organ or anatomical system in which psychiatry has specialized knowledge and daily application in clinical practice? The answer is—none. This reality is confirmed by the complete absence of any meaningful investigation of brain function or of the function of any other system in everyday psychiatric practice, other than to exclude organic brain disease requiring treatment by neurology or neurosurgery.

It is often said that actions speak louder than words, that what people do is generally more revealing that what they say. Danny Santagato expressed this truth well:

To know a person, watch what they do, not what they say. How a person describes themselves is one thing. How a person conducts themselves is the real thing. A person's actions speak the truth about themselves, who they really are, more than their own verbal or written description of themselves. [2]

This truth also applies to groups and organizations. As science writer John Horgan wrote in his 2000 book *The Undiscovered Mind: How the Brain defies Replication, Medication and Explanation:*

Like politicians, scientific theories, especially those with medical pretensions, should perhaps by judged not for what they say but for what they do. [3]

If assessment of the brain really was a core characteristic of psychiatry, this would be obvious in everyday psychiatric practice. Regularly evaluating the brain would be central to their diagnostic and therapeutic approach, in accordance with the methods and practices of all other medical specialties. Walk through any medical, surgical, paediatric or gynaecology ward and you will see groups of doctors regularly reviewing the wide array of investigations they carry out on their patients. One might therefore expect that in psychiatric wards there would similarly be groups of doctors deep in discussion about the brain investigations they regularly carry out such as CT and MRI scans and brain angiograms that are pivotal to their diagnostic and treatment processes. One might expect that laboratory tests evaluating various brain chemical levels such as serotonin and other brain neurotransmitters would be routinely carried out on admission to a psychiatric ward and at regular intervals during admission, as always happens with diabetic patients in hospital.

None of this happens on a psychiatric ward. The lack of any investigative tests relating to the diagnosis and management of psychiatric disorders is striking. Not even the worst cases of depression in the psychiatric ward have their diagnosis confirmed by any brain tests, by any chemical, radiological or laboratory investigations. When such tests are carried out, they are done in order to rule out actual organic illnesses. Psychiatric disorders such as depression are only diagnosed when such tests are found to be normal. The authors of the 2013 psychiatry textbook *The Oxford Handbook of Psychiatry* admitted:

> In the main, psychiatrists base diagnosis and treatment on symptom clusters, not brain imaging or other investigations. [4]

The authors also conceded that investigations such as brain scans "are generally investigations of exclusion". [5] Under the heading "Why don't psychiatrists look at the brain?" the authors also acknowledged:

> Psychiatrists are the only medical specialists who rarely directly examine the organ they treat. The chances that a patient with even a serious psychiatric disorder for example schizophrenia, bipolar disorder, severe depression has even had a brain scan are fairly slim. [6]

This textbook attempts to square the circle created by this glaring inconsistency in relation to all other medical specialties:

> Psychiatrists may not yet examine the brain directly, but they are certainly concerned with the functioning of the brain in health and disease. [7]

Psychiatrists may indeed be "concerned with the functioning of the brain", but this concern rarely stretches to checking or engaging with brain functioning in their everyday work in any real hands-on way. They do not engage directly in the functioning of the brain relating to the human experiences and behaviour that ends up being treated by psychiatry. The following passage from investigative reporter Kelly Patricia O'Meara's book *Psyched Out: How Psychiatry Sells Mental Illness and Pushes Pills that Kill* is accurate:

> Neither under-grad nor post-grad training in psychiatry involves hands-on practical study and work with the human brain. Every other specialty involves this, i.e. practical applied study and learning of the biological nuts and bolts of the

organs specific to that specialty. Not psychiatry. This does not happen, not to a meaningful extent in any case. [8]

According to the authors of the 2013 psychiatric textbook *The Oxford Handbook of Psychiatry*:

Psychiatrists prescribe their various treatments including antidepressants, ECT and mood stabilizers, all of which have a major impact on brain function, but do not know beforehand which areas of the brain are working well and which are not functioning properly. [9]

The authors do not seem to notice that assuming that some parts of the brain do not function properly when there is no evidence to confirm this is a major assumption, a leap of faith, a Begging the Question logical fallacy. [10] They do acknowledge that:

It is certainly true that the level of knowledge about causation and treatment of mental disorders is less advanced that for other branches of medicine. [11]

"Less advanced than for other branches of medicine" is quite an understatement of the truth. At best, such major discrepancies between what psychiatrists and GPs say regarding biology and depression and what they do might be put down to lack of awareness or perhaps a fixed delusion. At worst, one might consider it wilful deception. One thing you will find on psychiatric wards that you won't find on other hospital wards is a lot of people in various stages of tranquillization. This is because sedation is one of the most prominent actions of substances used in psychiatric treatment.

Psychiatrists do not examine or investigate their patients' brains because they cannot do so. They have identified no reliable biological abnormalities for any of the diagnoses they apply and treat. There is therefore no point in carrying out blood tests, scans, or any other tests, except to exclude the presence of true organic illnesses. And that is why psychiatrists do not investigate the brains of their patients.

In practice, psychiatry does not have an organ or system of expertise, not in any currently applicable sense. If not the brain, what do psychiatrists specialize in? In a candid 2010 radio interview, psychiatrist Daniel Carlat did not mention assessing the brain when asked what psychiatrists actually did:

We are in the business of making diagnoses using the *DSM*, which is the official diagnostic manual for the psychiatric disorders of the American Medical Association. We make our diagnoses, and then we usually prescribe medications . . . And then once I have a diagnosis, essentially I match these symptoms up with the medication. So modern psychiatry is really a conversation, a series of symptoms, and then a matching process of medication to these symptoms. [12]

Diagnosing and prescribing, that's about the extent of psychiatry's focus, according to psychiatrist Daniel Carlat. It can be rather embarrassing for mainstream psychiatrists to acknowledge how little they really knew about the brain and brain function. They often dress their comments up in confusing and contradictory language designed to make themselves look more expert than they actually are. I include several such examples in this book. This practice is referred to by neuroanatomist Jonathan Leo in his 2004 article titled "The Biology of Mental Illness":

> For students interested in learning how to become critical readers, there is nothing quite like the psychiatry literature. A recent brochure about clinical depression from the National Institute of Mental Health (NIMH) states: "Substantial evidence from neuroscience, genetics and clinical investigation shows that depressive illnesses are disorders of the brain. However, the precise causes of these illnesses continue to be a matter of intense research". Statements like this, where the theory is affirmed while simultaneously acknowledging that there is no specific evidence to support it, are common in the psychiatric literature. Rather than a straightforward statement that the chemical theory of mental illness is a theory in search of evidence, instead, these authors try to put on a good face, or a good spin, on a theory whose usefulness as a marketing tool has far exceeded its scientific validity. [13]

An ironic truth is that psychiatrists generally have little or no experience in treating confirmed biological brain diseases such as Parkinson's disease and multiple sclerosis.

BETWEEN A ROCK AND A HARD PLACE

As just described, contrary to claims of doing so continually, psychiatrists do not treat known organic illness. Known organic illnesses come under the appropriate medical specialty. Emotional and psychological distress comes generally under the realm of psychology and the counselling professions. So where exactly does psychiatry fit in?

Psychiatrists have invented the term "mental illness", the diagnosis and treatment of which is their bread and butter, their supposed area of expertise. They have fed the public with unsubstantiated ideas about neurotransmitters and chemical imbalances. People generally trust doctors. Most people are happy to let doctors get on with it, presuming that they have the public interest primarily at heart. Few people realize that psychiatry is a house of cards without a solid scientific foundation that could easily crumble if properly and independently examined, and psychiatry's position with it. One can therefore understand why psychiatrists might resist the questioning of their profession; there is a great deal at stake for them.

Psychiatry finds itself between a rock and a hard place, somewhere between the medical specialties that treat known brain diseases—neurology and neurosurgery—and the various forms of talk therapies including psychology and psychotherapy. The challenge for psychiatry has been to carve out its own distinct identity. Claims that depression and other psychiatric diagnoses are biological illnesses are crucial to psychiatry's identity and its unmerited position at the top of the mental health tree. These assertions separate psychiatry from the talk therapies and ensure that psychiatry has first claim to these "diseases" and the people they diagnose as having them. It is in psychiatry's interest to be more closely aligned to neurology than to talk therapies, given neurology's respected standing as a scientific branch of medicine dealing with biological brain disorders. But to maintain its own identity, psychiatry needs to be perceived as distinct from neurology. Specializing in "mental illnesses" provides the needed distinction, since neurologists do not treat "mental illnesses". Most psychiatrists have convinced themselves and the public that what they refer to as psychiatric disorders are biological illnesses. They get around the fact that there is no reliable corroborative scientific evidence for this by employing a number of strategies. These include misleading the public and perhaps themselves regarding the current state of medical knowledge through exaggeration and distortion of the facts, misrepresenting theories as facts, and confidently claiming that the assumed biological basis of depression will definitely be established at some time in the near future.

For over a century, psychiatry has reassured the public that both the necessary understanding and more effective solutions lie just around the corner. "Bear with us, we are almost there", psychiatry's catchphrase for the past 100 years and more, buys them more time, every time. As sociology professor Andrew Scull wrote in 1990:

> Biological psychiatry, as always, promises that a medical solution is almost within our grasp. It would be nice if one could believe it. I fear one might as well be waiting for Godot. [14]

Positioned precariously between a rock and a hard place, psychiatry has so far managed to straddle this position very effectively. Actually, the current situation suits mainstream psychiatry's priorities perfectly. Psychiatry has succeeded in persuading the public that it is different from psychology and psychotherapy, so that's one side of the equation sorted. Maintaining their position in regard to neurology and other medical specialties is more delicate. Psychiatrists claim that the "diseases" they treat are fundamentally biological and that biological evidence is just around the corner. But psychiatrists know that it is neurologists and not psychiatrists who treat brain diseases with known abnormalities of brain structure and function. If brain abnormalities were actually identified in depression and other psychiatric diagnoses, psychiatry would be presented with a potential nightmare scenario. Precedent within the medical profession would dictate that the responsibility for these patients would immediately shift to neurology or whatever the relevant specialty might be. In the case of depression, this would mean that psychiatry would lose the majority of the patients who currently attend them. This would represent a catastrophe for psychiatry. Earlier in this book I mentioned psychiatrist Steven Reidbord's 2012 blog on brain chemical imbalances. In this blog Dr. Reidbord wrote (italics his):

> Historically, whenever chemical or structural abnormalities *were* found to account for abnormal mental functioning, those conditions were no longer considered psychiatric and were adopted by another branch of medicine. If this trend continues, psychiatry will never include pathophysiology in the usual medical sense. It certainly does not at present. [15]

Pathophysiology is defined as the study of functional changes in the body that occur in response to disease or injury. Steven Reidbord is correctly stating that if structural or functional brain abnormalities were ever found in psychiatric disorders including depression, care of these people would immediately transfer away from psychiatry to a specialty that deals with known brain abnormalities, that is, to neurology or neurosurgery.

The most beneficial position for psychiatry is therefore the one that currently pertains. By nailing its colours to the biological mast, psychiatry has successfully set itself apart from talk therapies. As long as no biological abnormalities are reliably identified, there is no threat that their bread and butter will be removed from them to other medical specialties. Maintaining the myth that biological solutions are just around the corner satisfies the public and maintains psychiatry's position quite satisfactorily from psychiatry's perspective, albeit between a rock and a hard place. This position has no solid scientific foundation, but as long as the public do not realize this and psychiatry does not attempt to encroach on the territory of other medical specialties such as neurology, psychiatry's position is secure.

Psychiatry's survival in its present form requires the delusion that is the disease-focused model of mental illness to remain supreme. Only then can psychiatry remain at the top of the mental health pyramid. The current biologically-dominated psychiatric model can only dominate if biology is accepted as the core issue without this actually being established. Having such a vested interest in and being so tied to biology as the core issue in mental health, the widely assumed scientific objectivity of mainstream psychiatry is highly questionable.

I believe that the bias in favour of biology that pertains within psychiatry is linked to psychiatry's desire to stand out as *the* experts on mental health. After all, if biology isn't central to the experiences that have become known as mental illnesses, what special expertise do psychiatrists really possess?

When doctors defend their pronouncements on depression, they are not just defending a diagnosis; they are defending themselves, their ideology, their modus operandi and ultimately, their status and role in society as the prime experts in mental health. For doctors who have vehemently promoted the notion that depression is caused by a chemical imbalance or another brain problem as a fact or near-fact, belatedly acknowledging that this is not the case risks losing credibility. The same goes for the other untrue pieces of the jigsaw that constitute the medical construction of depression which I will address in my next book.

GPs also find themselves in a difficult situation, but it too is of their own making. The medical jacks-of-all-trades and masters-of-no-specialty other than general practice itself, within the medical hierarchical system GPs are subservient to the supposedly superior expertise of psychiatry. GPs are often accused from many directions including some psychiatrists of overprescribing antidepressants and prescribing them for the wrong people. Conversely, some psychiatrists assert publicly that depression is a significantly underdiagnosed and undertreated condition, sometimes criticizing GPs for underdiagnosing depression. Such contrasting positions do not occur with known biological diseases like diabetes where objective clinical tests are a prerequisite to diagnosis, making the diagnosis of diabetes watertight scientifically. GPs are further criticized from several quarters for being a main driver of the explosion of antidepressant prescribing. Such mixed messages put GPs in an invidious position. One can understand how some GPs might feel they cannot win, being damned if they do and damned if they do not diagnose and treat depression. This uncomfortable juxtaposition is a case of the chickens coming home to roost, a direct consequence of assigning disease status to depression by deviating from longstanding medical standards regarding the definition of disease. Doctors created this problem by insisting that depression is a medical illness like any other, for which only doctors have the expertise to lead the way.

I sensed some of this frustration in British GP Margaret McCartney's 2013 *Guardian* article titled "Depression is more than simple unhappiness". She wrote:

> Ruby Wax told the Radio 4 Today programme on Monday that GPs, like me, overprescribe medication "like M&Ms . . . probably to get them off their backs.[16]

In response to Ruby Wax' comments that "teachers could recognize a pupil's depression", because in their eyes was "a deadness not a sadness", Dr. McCartney retorted: "This is not a validated test for depression I've ever come across". The idea that a teacher might be able to identify depression did not seem to sit well with this doctor. Having come across such comments on many occasions, I feel that they are often a coded way of saying, "We doctors are the experts, don't tell us how to do our job and don't encroach on our territory". Perhaps it did not strike Dr. McCartney that doctors themselves do not have any scientifically validated tests for depression. In what is in my opinion a common and possibly unconscious distortion of reality made by doctors in an effort to justify their lack of hard scientific mental health data such as laboratory tests, Dr. McCartney wrote:

> As with other conditions, such as migraine, there is no blood test or scan to confirm it; the diagnosis rests on talking to the person and understanding the symptoms in the context of their life. [17]

Using migraine as justification for no tests being available for depression is flawed logic, a Weak Analogy logical fallacy. [18] While there certainly can be a psychological or emotional aspect to migraine, it is very clear that the trademark characteristic of migraine—extremely severe headache—is primarily an intense physical pain that lasts for many hours, usually with other physical characteristics largely specific to migraine such as photophobia (light hurting the eyes), sudden onset of quite severe dizziness, tinnitus, various optical phenomena such as seeing zigzag lines, and nausea and vomiting. Often there are tell-tale specific warning signs before the migraine such as seeing an aura or flashing lights. This is not the case for the experiences that are commonly deemed to be evidence of depression, which are generally predominantly emotional and psychological. Regarding depression, "the diagnosis rests" not on "understanding the symptoms" but on a particular way of interpreting people's experiences. Dr. McCartney continued:

Unhappiness is normal; depression . . . is not . . . If people in exquisite mental agony hear a message—no matter how well-intentioned—saying that they may just be merely unhappy, we have failed them . . . We must be careful not to stigmatize people who are mentally ill with the idea that they are simply unhappy.[19]

These comments provide insights into medical thinking and its limitations. Only two possible explanations for people's "exquisite mental agony" are considered; depression and unhappiness. This is a False Dilemma logical fallacy. [20] There is a third possibility, one that offers far more accuracy, that this and many other doctors apparently do not see, possibly because they have been "educated" into not seeing it. I discussed this possibility in chapter four. Such comments by doctors that portray the limited medical understanding of emotional and mental health are a major reason for my concern regarding the suitability of doctors to be society's appointed leaders in these fields. This doctor's own reference to "exquisite mental agony" portrays the emotional and mental nature of the majority of the experiences that become diagnosed as depression. This leads into another medical inconsistency surrounding depression and general medical practice; do GPs generally treat brain disorders?

DO GPS GENERALLY TREAT TREATABLE BRAIN DISEASES AND DISORDERS?

GPs treat 90% of the mental health workload that presents to the medical profession. GPs diagnose most cases of depression and prescribe the majority of antidepressant medication. The following comment made in a 1973 psychiatry textbook by two British professors of psychiatry articulates the medical position regarding the accepted appropriateness of GPs treating depression:

Depression is a disorder that can be reliably diagnosed by non-specialists as part of primary health care. [21]

The World Health Organization website contains a similar statement:

Depression is a disorder that can be reliably diagnosed and treated by non-specialists as part of primary care. [22]

As Canadian psychiatrist Kwame McKenzie says in his 2009 book *Understanding Depression*, "Eighty per cent of people with depression are treated by their GP alone".[23] If they were true, claims by both the medical profession and the pharmaceutical industry that depression is a brain disorder create a scenario that is inconsistent with medical practice generally. As a general rule within the medical profession, GPs do not diagnose and treat diseases of the central nervous system without the direct involvement and oversight of a neurologist or neurosurgeon. That GPs would diagnose and treat eighty per cent of cases of any established brain disorder that is amenable to treatment without referral to specialist services is therefore contrary to accepted medical practice. The vast majority of such patients are quickly referred to specialist services by GPs. Even when a GP is pretty certain that a patient has a brain or central nervous system disorder and is confident about the diagnosis and treatment, the patient will generally be referred on to specialist neurological services where thorough examinations and investigations will be carried out to either confirm or refute a diagnosis. In such cases GPs will not initiate treatment prior to referral to hospital except in serious or life-threatening situations. Yet with depression, GPs treat the majority without reference to any specialist or any investigations to confirm the supposed brain disorder. Some GPs might argue that they are happy to treat migraine without referral to a specialist. However, migraine is not a potentially life-threatening disorder of brain tissue characterized by subtle delicate brain abnormalities, as depression is promoted to be. Migraine is a medically benign vascular disorder, relating to excessive dilation and constriction of blood vessels.

Given their pivotal position in the diagnosis and treatment of depression, it is vital that GPs have the necessary understanding and skills required to execute their responsibilities effectively, in the best interests of their patients. To ascertain the level of GPs' understanding of depression as a brain disorder, I researched several current textbooks of general practice in the University of Limerick library. The University of Limerick is home to a recognized and approved four-year GP training scheme. Course participants are qualified doctors who wish to learn the craft of being a general practitioner. In addition to textbooks specifically oriented toward general practice, trainee GPs will refer to psychiatry books during their training.

Prominent among the textbooks in the Limerick University library's general practice section, *Murtagh's General Practice* is an impressive 2011 tome of some 1,508 pages. A great deal of care obviously went into the creation of this book. Fifty-three "content consultants" are listed as having reviewed content and 151 are listed as "survey respondents" who also contributed to reviewing the book prior to publication. It can therefore be taken as a fair and considered reflection of current thinking and practice in the field of general practice. The principal author, general practitioner GP John Murtagh, is clearly well respected within his profession. He holds professorial-level ranking at four universities, three in Australia and one in Beijing. [24] In the "Depression" chapter under the heading "Cause" the authors stated:

> The cause is somewhat mysterious but it has been found that an important chemical is present in smaller amounts than usual in the nervous system. It is rather like a person low in iron becoming anaemic. [25]

Every reader of this medical textbook is being exposed here to blatant misinformation. These three lines contain one important falsehood and a logical fallacy. The authors are utterly incorrect in their assertion that "it has been found that an important chemical is present in smaller amounts that usual in the nervous system". In comparing depression to anaemia, the author provides a classic Weak Analogy logical fallacy, since the similarities between the two are exaggerated and the differences ignored. A diagnosis of anaemia requires confirmatory blood tests and identification of the cause of anaemia so it can be treated appropriately, a very different scenario to depression, for which there is no chemical abnormality and no diagnostic laboratory tests. Under the heading "Treatment", the authors inform their readers that:

> The basis of treatment is to replace the missing chemicals with antidepressant medication. [26]

Under an "Important points" heading the authors assert:

> Depression is an illness; it just happens; it can be lethal if untreated; the missing chemicals need to be replaced; it responds well to treatment. [27]

On two occasions here, the author referred unequivocally to "the missing chemicals". The clear message is that "missing chemicals" are a known scientific fact, which of course they are not. Trainee GPs who read this misinformation are likely to believe it, become misinformed, and bring this misinformation into their future everyday work with their patients.

These authors are intelligent people, yet it not does appear to strike them as odd that they made definitive statements about missing brain chemicals without any laboratory or other investigations even being carried out to confirm the stated deficiencies. The contrast between this approach and the approach of GPs to known chemical imbalance conditions such as diabetes could hardly be more striking.

I also reviewed the general practice textbook *Practical General Practice: Guidelines for Effective Clinical Management*. In the eight pages on depression in this 770-page book, no mention is made of possible causes, biology, abnormalities or tests, which is the typical way an understanding of a disease is set out in medical textbooks. In contrast, the authors provide considerable detail regarding the biology of and tests for diabetes on nine of the eleven pages on diabetes. While blood glucose monitoring, urine glucose testing and glucose tolerance test all appear in the book's comprehensive index, there is no mention of serotonin or of biological tests for depression in the index. [28]

This is the extent of knowledge regarding depression in general practice textbooks for a group of doctors who diagnose and treat eighty per cent of diagnoses of depression, which we are told is a brain disorder. I genuinely believe that these well-intentioned authors, along with the vast majority of their GP colleagues, have quite a limited understanding of depression. The lack of precision and joined-up thinking in these textbooks do little to undermine this view. The level of knowledge and understanding of mental health demonstrated by GPs does not inspire much confidence in this regard. Many GPs privately admit that their understanding of mental health is quite limited. In a 2014 interview, former Irish professor of general practice Bill Shannon acknowledged:

> Unfortunately many GPs don't have the necessary skills or resources in terms of time to deal properly with complex mental health issues. [29]

RED HERRINGS AND THE BRAIN

Many books on depression written by psychiatrists and GPs contain impressive-looking descriptions and illustrations of the brain and brain cells, without clarifying how little is truly understood about the brain and that no abnormality of any neuron or neurotransmitter has ever been found in depression. In an effort to convince the readers of how much they know, many doctors write in considerable detail about normal brain and neurotransmitter function. Many websites that promote the biochemical imbalance notion of depression engage in the same practice. Many readers are thus seduced into an exaggerated sense of how much doctors understand the brain and depression. The public are dazzled into a state of receptivity regarding the erroneous belief that the biochemical imbalance notion is scientifically well established. Since no brain abnormality relating to neurotransmitter function has been identified in depression, this practice is a Red Herring logical fallacy. [30] Detailed presentations regarding normal brain function deflect the reader's attention from noticing the elephant in the room—the fact that no brain chemical abnormalities have been found in depression.

Nancy Andreasen has been one of the world's most influential psychiatrists of the past thirty years. Andreasen devoted four pages of her 1984 book *The Broken Brain: The Biological Revolution in Psychiatry* to "neurochemical factors" under the heading "What causes affective disorders". [31] The bulk of this text referred to the neurotransmitter hypotheses and the effects of drugs on neurotransmitters. Not one sentence of this referred to any confirmed neurochemical brain abnormality that might have any practical application for patients. Andreasen included a chapter titled "The Revolution in Neuroscience: What is the Brain?" There are 56 pages in this chapter, the vast majority of which contain information regarding the known structure and function of the brain. [32] She did not contextualise this by stating that in everyday medical practice, the brain falls within the remit of neurology and neurosurgery rather than psychiatry. She failed to acknowledge that little of this is of any real practical value or application in psychiatry, as evidenced by the fact that psychiatrists do not generally examine the brain. But it was good public relations for psychiatrists, since it conveyed quite an appealing albeit misleading impression of psychiatry as a specialty with a solid grasp of the biology of the diagnoses it treats.

Psychiatrist Jesse Wright and psychologist Monica Ramirez Basco provided another example of this common practice in their 2002 book *Getting Your Life Back: The Complete Guide to Recovery from Depression*:

> In order to understand the biology of depression, you will need to know some of the basics of how brain cells function and what changes occur when people are depressed. We'll begin with a few definitions. [33]

The authors then provided detailed definitions of a neuron (brain cell), a neurotransmitter, a synapse and other impressive sounding stuff, none of which have been   identified as abnormal in depression. Such impressive irrelevancies soften up the reader to believe what is coming, which appeared on the next page (italics mine):

In depression, there *can* be abnormalities in the activities of neurons that are controlled by any one of three different types of neurotransmitters—serotonin, norepinephrine, and dopamine. Doctors often describe depression to their patients as being caused by a chemical imbalance. What they mean by this is that there is a lowering of the activity of the serotonin, norepinephrine, or dopamine in the brain, or a disturbance in the function of these neurotransmitters. [34]

Later in their book, this "can" has become "may", a very different picture of conjecture where previously the authors claimed certainty (italics mine):

When a person becomes depressed, there *may* be a decrease of the amount of the neurotransmitter available in the brain, or the chemical messages *may* have a harder time getting through. [35]

In his 2009 book *Understanding Depression*—a book endorsed by the British Medical Association—psychiatrist and author Kwame McKenzie begins a paragraph with the statement:

The symptoms of depression may be caused by low levels of certain chemicals in the brain. [36]

Then comes the persuasive red herring:

To understand why this might be, we need to look at how the brain works. [37]

Five pages of text regarding normal brain function follow—what little is currently known about it—including an impressive-looking diagram of a brain cell. The author does not inform the reader that this discussion about *normal* brain function offers no confirmation of the assumed *abnormal* brain function that he and many of his colleagues assume to be a foregone conclusion in depression.

A similar classic Red Herring logical fallacy is present in the *New York Times* depression "In-depth Report" webpage. [38] At the centre of the "causes" webpage of this Report is a representation of a human being. Highlighted in this illustration are organs that produce hormones including the pituitary, thyroid and adrenal glands, the pancreas, testes and ovaries. The caption beneath the picture concerns the production of hormones in these organs, their release into the bloodstream and their subsequent actions elsewhere in the body. Insulin and its role in regulating blood sugar is specifically mentioned, as is thyroid hormone and its action in regulating metabolism within the body. There is no reference in the caption to the content of the article and there is no direct reference in the article to the diagram. Neither the picture nor the caption beneath it mention serotonin or any other neurotransmitter. The diagram is a complete red herring as far as the article content is concerned, but its presence adds a persuasive scientific feel to the story. Many readers might erroneously conclude that the presence of the diagram in this article means that the claimed chemical "abnormalities" in depression are as reliably understood as the organs and chemicals referred to in the diagram. [39] In her 2005 and 2010 book *Dealing with Depression: Understanding and Overcoming the Symptoms of Depression,* British GP Caroline Shreeve similarly included an impressive illustration and discussion of how brain nerve cells communicate with one another. [40]

The eMedTV webpage contains a video titled "The brain and its chemicals", which lasts 3 minutes 48 seconds. This video consists of a sophisticated presentation of how neurotransmitters operate in the gaps between cells, otherwise known as synapses. [41] This is a Red Herring logical fallacy, since no abnormality relevant to the content of this video has been established as a known feature of depression.

Under the heading "Biology Review: The Neuron" and adjacent to two sophisticated illustrations of the neuron and of neurotransmission, the Brain-physics.com website states:

> To understand how Prozac works, it may be helpful to review some basic brain biology. [42]

"Prozac" is the next heading, under which the following content appears:

> When serotonin is released from the "sending" nerve cell, the leftover serotonin is normally reabsorbed by the uptake pump. By blocking the uptake pump, Prozac increases the amount of active serotonin that can be delivered to the "receiving" nerve cell. This means that the neurons steep for a longer period of time in the serotonin you already produce . . . There are other mechanisms as well. The drug blocks the sensor on the axon that tells the cell when enough serotonin has been produced. This causes the axon to release even more serotonin. Finally, over a period of 2-3 weeks, the receiving cell becomes more sensitive to serotonin, and this is the point at which the anti-depressant effect becomes experienced by the patient. It will take several more weeks, however, for the anti-obsessional effects to become completely realized. [43]

Placing the two sophisticated diagrams of brain function in this passage was a clever move, but it is a Red Herring logical fallacy. The reader is encouraged to believe that normal brain function—primitive though our understanding of brain function is—is relevant to and explains the action of Prozac. Since there is no reliable evidence that brain function is compromised in depression, these diagrams and the impressive-sounding discussion on so-called normal brain function have no relevance here. The reader is unlikely to realize this, being far more likely to mistakenly conclude that brain function in depression is indeed compromised and that Prozac and other antidepressants fix the supposed chemical problem.

NOTES TO CHAPTER TWELVE

1. Editorial in the *Journal of Mental Science*, 1858, cited in Rogers & Pilgrim 2001, *Mental Health Policy in Europe*, Basingstoke, Hampshire: Palgrave MacMillan, p. 46.

2. Danny Santagato, http://www.searchquotes.com/search/A_Persons_Actions/, accessed 13 April 2014.

3. John Horgan, *The Undiscovered Mind: How the Brain defies Replication, Medication and Explanation*, Weidenfeld, London, 2000, p. 77.

4. David Semple & Roger Smyth, *The Oxford Handbook of Psychiatry*, 3rd edition, Oxford: Oxford University Press, 2013, p. 10.

5. David Semple & Roger Smyth, *The Oxford Handbook of Psychiatry*, 3rd edition, Oxford: Oxford University Press, 2013, p. 10.

6. David Semple & Roger Smyth, *The Oxford Handbook of Psychiatry*, 3rd edition, Oxford: Oxford University Press, 2013, p. 10.

7. David Semple & Roger Smyth, *The Oxford Handbook of Psychiatry*, 3rd edition, Oxford: Oxford University Press, 2013, p. 11.

8. Kelly Patricia O'Meara, *Psyched Out: How Psychiatry Sells Mental Illness and Pushes Pills that Kill*, Authorhouse, 2006.

9. David Semple & Roger Smyth, *The Oxford Handbook of Psychiatry*, 3rd edition, Oxford: Oxford University Press, 2013, p.10.

10. For information on Begging the Question logical fallacies see note 22 in the Notes to the Introduction.

11. David Semple & Roger Smyth, *The Oxford Handbook of Psychiatry*, 3rd edition, Oxford: Oxford University Press, 2013, p. 2.

12. Daniel Carlat in a 2010 NPR radio interview, http://www.npr.org/templates/transcript/transcript.php?storyId=128107547, accessed 30 December 2013.

13. Jonathan Leo, "The Biology of Mental Illness" *Society*, July/August 2004, Volume 41, Issue 5, pp. 45-53, http://link.springer.com/article/10.1007%2FBF02688217#page-1, accessed 19 August 2014.

14. Andrew Scull, "Cycles of Despair", *Journal of Mind and Behavior*, 1990, 11, 301-12.

15. Steven Reidbord, "Chemical imbalance—Sloppy thinking in psychiatry 1", in " Reidbord's Reflections", 29 April 2012, http://blog.stevenreidbordmd.com/?p=561, accessed 25 May 2014.

16. Margaret McCartney, "Depression Is More Than Simple Unhappiness", *The Guardian*, 12 August 2013, http://www.theguardian.com/commentisfree/2013/aug/12/depression-unhappiness-antidepressants-overprescribed, accessed 30 December 2013.

17. Margaret McCartney, "Depression Is More Than Simple Unhappiness", *The Guardian*, 12 August 2013, http://www.theguardian.com/commentisfree/2013/aug/12/depression-unhappiness-antidepressants-overprescribed, accessed 30 December 2013.

18. For information on Weak Analogy logical fallacies see note 69 in the Notes to Chapter Five.

19. Margaret McCartney, "Depression Is More Than Simple Unhappiness", *The Guardian*, 12 August 2013, http://www.theguardian.com/commentisfree/2013/aug/12/depression-unhappiness-antidepressants-overprescribed, accessed 30 December 2013.

20. For information on False Dilemma logical fallacies see note 38 in the Notes to Chapter Five.

21. E. Anderson & W, Trethowan, *Psychiatry*, London: Bailliere Tindall, 1973.

22. World Health Organization website, "Depression", http://www.who.int/topics/depression /en/, accessed 05 October 2014.

23. Kwame McKenzie, *Understanding Depression*, Poole: Family Doctor Publications in association with the British Medical Association, 2009, pps. 2, 14.

24. John Murtagh, *Murtagh's General Practice*, Fifth Edition, McGraw-Hill Medical Publications, 2011, p. v.

25. John Murtagh, *Murtagh's General Practice*, Fifth Edition, McGraw-Hill Medical Publications, 2011, p. 181.

26. John Murtagh, *Murtagh's General Practice*, Fifth Edition, McGraw-Hill Medical Publications, 2011, p. 181.
27. John Murtagh, *Murtagh's General Practice*, Fifth Edition, McGraw-Hill Medical Publications, 2011, p. 181.
28. Alex Khot & Andrew Polmear, *Practical General Practice: Guidelines for Effective Clinical Management*, Sixth Edition, Elsevier, 2011.
29. Tivoli Institute News, "An Interview with Bill Shannon by Edward Boyne", http://www.tivoliinstitute.com/news-details.php?ID=4, accessed 21 March 2014.
30. For more information on Red Herring logical fallacies see note 23 in the Notes to the Introduction.
31. Nancy Andreasen, *The Broken Brain: The Biological Revolution in Psychiatry*, New York: Harper & Row, 1984, p. 231.
32. Nancy Andreasen, *The Broken Brain: The Biological Revolution in Psychiatry*, New York: Harper & Row, 1984.
33. Jesse Wright & Monica Ramirez Basco, *Getting Your Life Back: The Complete Guide to Recovery from Depression*, Free Press, 2002.
34. Jesse Wright & Monica Ramirez Basco, *Getting Your Life Back: The Complete Guide to Recovery from Depression*, Free Press, 2002, p. 158.
35. Jesse Wright & Monica Ramirez Basco, *Getting Your Life Back: The Complete Guide to Recovery from Depression*, Free Press, 2002, p. 183.
36. Kwame McKenzie, *Understanding Depression*, Poole: Family Doctor Publications in association with the British Medical Association, 2009, p. 17.
37. Kwame McKenzie, *Understanding Depression*, Poole: Family Doctor Publications in association with the British Medical Association, 2009, p. 17.
38. *New York Times* "Major Depression In-depth Report", http://www.nytimes.com/health/ guides/disease/major-depression/causes.html accessed 24 January 2014.
39. *New York Times* "Major Depression In-depth Report", http://www.nytimes.com/health /guides/disease/major-depression/causes.html accessed 24 January 2014.
40. Caroline Shreeve, *Dealing with Depression: Understanding and Overcoming the Symptoms of Depression*, London: Piatkus, 2010, p. 39.
41. eMedTV webpage, video titled "The brain and its chemicals", http://depression.emedtv.com/depression-video/depression-introduction-video.html, accessed 11 May 2014.
42. The Brainphysics.com website, "Biology Review: The Neuron", http://www.brainphysics.com/howprozacworks.php, accessed 11 May 2014.
43. The Brainphysics.com website, "Biology Review: The Neuron", http://www.brainphysics.com/howprozacworks.php, accessed 11 May 2014.

13. THE DEPRESSION DELUSION: WHAT IS REAL AND WHAT IS NOT REAL

THE EXPERIENCES AND BEHAVIOURS OF DEPRESSION ARE VERY REAL

The experiences and behaviours that become diagnosed as depression are no delusion. Not for one second would I question the realness of these often excruciating experiences and behaviours. However, I am not alone in questioning the medical interpretation of human distress. Professor Richard Smith CBE, former editor and chief executive officer of the *British Medical Journal* delivered a lecture at University College, Cork in November 2003. During his lecture Professor Smith spoke of the danger of over-medicalization in society:

> I am not saying that people are not suffering; of course there is a lot of distress and suffering. What I am sceptical about is whether some things are best thought of as medical problems and approached in a medical way. [1]

In the opening line of his foreword to the 2001 edition of my book *Beyond Prozac*, psychologist and author Tony Humphreys wrote:

> It was an unfortunate event in history that individuals who were psycho-socially distressed ever came under the umbrella of the medical profession. [2]

The reality that some people feel better on medication is not a delusion either. Many people report considerable benefit from these drugs. However, the effectiveness of antidepressants has consistently been exaggerated, their adverse effects insufficiently recognised, and alternate approaches have received insufficient attention. I discuss these issues in detail in my books *Beyond Prozac: Healing Mental Distress* [3], *Selfhood* [4] and in future books.

DELUSION DEFINED

The dictionary.com website defines a delusion as "a false belief or opinion", and a delusion as understood within psychiatry as "a fixed false belief that is resistant to reason or confrontation with actual fact". [5] Known as psychiatry's bible, the 2013 *Diagnostic and Statistical Manual of Mental Disorders-5* defines delusions as:

> Fixed beliefs that are not amenable to change in light of conflicting evidence. Their content may include a variety of themes. Delusions are deemed bizarre if they are

clearly implausible and not understandable to same-culture peers and do not derive from ordinary life experiences. The distinction between a delusion and a strongly-held idea is sometimes difficult to make and depends in part on the degree of conviction with which the belief is held despite clear or reasonable contradictory evidence regarding its veracity. [6]

According to psychiatrist Kwame McKenzie in his 2009 book *Understanding Depression*, "A delusion is a false belief that is held unshakably by the person who has it". [7] The *Shorter Oxford Textbook of Psychiatry* defines a delusion as:

A belief that is firmly held on inadequate grounds, is not affected by rational argument or evidence to the contrary, and is not a conventional belief that the person might be expected to hold given their educational, cultural and religious background . . . Delusions are not beliefs shared by others in the same culture. [8]

In 1949 psychiatrist A.M. Meerloo wrote:

A delusion is a substitute belief. It is the enforcement of certainty instead of the acceptance of uncertainty. Delusion is the fear of uncertainty, of hesitation and skepticism . . . an incorrigible error . . . an impenetrable mental armour . . . Delusion is a disturbance in reality confrontation . . . There is no longer any growth, reciprocity or dialectic development . . . Because the delusion is incapable of integral and agile thinking, it gives rise to a subjective feeling of certainty. The delusion is not subject to discussion. The delusion has lost the attempt at self-correction . . . Every delusion starts as a form of expansion. When the delusion becomes fixed, however, it is a pathological process. [9]

According to the *Stanford Encyclopedia of Philosophy:*

All types of delusions are rigid to some extent, that is, they are not easily given up because they tend to resist counterevidence. All delusions are reported sincerely and with conviction, although the behaviour of people with delusions is not always perfectly consistent with the content of their delusions. [10]

In chapter twelve under the heading "What do psychiatrists do?" I described how the behaviour of doctors who claim that brain chemical imbalances occur in depression is not matched by their behaviour. While we have been cultured into linking delusions with mental illness, the assertion on the *Stanford Encyclopedia of Philosophy* website that "there is an abundance of evidence that delusional phenomena are widespread in the normal population" is correct. [11] The title of an article on the Science Brainwaves website concurs with this view: "How delusions occur, and why they may be widespread". [12]

Psychiatry tends to attribute no meaning or purpose to delusions, quickly concluding them to be simply evidence of psychosis, of immersion in unreality and therefore unworthy of any further consideration other than as evidence of severe mental illness. This is an erroneous interpretation. Delusions serve a purpose. Allen Frances, psychiatrist and lead author of *DSM-4*—the predecessor of the 2013 psychiatric *Diagnostic and Statistical Manual of Mental Disorders-5*—has correctly stated that:

A lot of false beliefs help people cope with life. [13]

According to the *Encyclopaedia Britannica*:

Delusions may represent pathological exaggeration of normal tendencies to rationalization, wishful thinking and the like. [14]

In 1949, psychiatrist A.M. Meerloo wrote:

The delusion defends us against the great leap into the obscure and the unknown. Delusion is a fear of realistic, critical thinking, the kind of thinking which is subject to criticism from without and the criticism from within that illuminate's one's own subjective notions. [15]

Meerloo provided further insights:

People are hard to convince of the incorrectness of their thinking. The majority are fixated to their own thoughts to such a degree that they are unable to listen to those of others. They fear doubt and close their ears . . . A philosophical system can be justification and delusion. There is a tendency to escape into ivory tower philosophy and empty theorizing out of impotence. [16]

To summarize; delusions are quite common. They serve a purpose for the holder of the delusion, either as a means of avoiding reality and uncertainty or to maintain power and position. Each characteristic just described applies to the depression delusion.

THE DEPRESSION DELUSION

The depression delusion I refer to concerns how the experiences and behaviours that become diagnosed as depression are commonly interpreted and understood. In this book I examine the best known aspect of the depression delusion; the widely accepted view that brain chemical imbalances are a known feature of depression.

Let us look again at the characteristics of a delusion as described in the psychiatrist's bible, the *Diagnostic and Statistical Manual of Mental Disorders-5*, in more detail and apply them to brain chemical imbalances and depression. The *DSM-5* defines delusions as:

Fixed beliefs that are not amenable to change in light of conflicting evidence. Their content may include a variety of themes. Delusions are deemed bizarre if they are clearly implausible and not understandable to same-culture peers and do not derive from ordinary life experiences. The distinction between a delusion and a strongly-held idea is sometimes difficult to make and depends in part on the degree of conviction with which the belief is held despite clear or reasonable contradictory evidence regarding its veracity. [17]

The dominant fixed belief about depression for the past fifty years has been the notion that brain chemical abnormalities are known to occur in depression. I have described in this book how claims of brain chemical imbalances in depression are fixed beliefs held steadfastly without any direct supporting evidence and in spite of much conflicting evidence. This belief is so fixed that its maintenance regularly defies logic, given the absence of supporting scientific evidence. This unproven hypothesis has been repeatedly presented as a fact, despite there being no evidence to confirm it and considerable evidence to discredit it. The notion that depression is caused by a deficiency of serotonin has long taken hold within society, despite the fact that the link remains utterly unproven.

The content of this delusion includes a variety of themes. Several brain chemicals have been implicated as the supposed culprits. These fixed beliefs do not arise from ordinary life experiences. Indeed they run contrary to life experiences, ignoring and minimising the relevance of life experiences in favour of these fixed beliefs. The medical profession has held rigidly to these beliefs with steadfast conviction. This despite over fifty years of failure to find hard evidence to support these fixed beliefs, considerable unclear and contradictory evidence regarding their veracity and the presence of other more plausible ways of understanding depression. Immovable conviction of the rightness of one's position is a core characteristic of delusions, held regardless of the lack of evidence for or the weight of evidence contradicting it. There has been much conviction within psychiatry and general practice regarding the idea that brain chemical imbalances are a known characteristic of depression. Thousands of research projects have been designed in an attempt to prove this, with no success.

This just leaves one aspect of the *DSM-5* definition of a delusion: "Delusions are deemed bizarre if they are clearly implausible and not understandable to same-culture peers". [18] The *Shorter Oxford Textbook of Psychiatry* definition of a delusion contains a similar statement: "Delusions are not beliefs shared by others in the same culture". [19]

The majority of psychiatrists and GPs have promoted the chemical imbalance notion as a perfectly acceptable explanation for depression for almost fifty years. Taking their lead from the medical profession, this position is widely accepted as truth within society. The prevailing understanding has become wholly acceptable to psychiatrists, GPs and the general public, not at all "bizarre, implausible and not understandable". At first glance, this may seem to eliminate any possibility that the medical approach to depression might be delusionary. Yet, when compared to the principles and practices of other medical specialties, the ways of psychiatry are quite bizarre, implausible and not understandable. The repeated practice for over forty years of proclaiming the existence of brain chemical abnormalities in depression and basing the medical approach to depression on such claims without a shred of direct supporting evidence would not be considered acceptable or plausible in any other specialty of medicine. Any doctor who diagnosed diabetes or any other medical condition characterized by a chemical imbalance without first confirming the chemical imbalance with blood tests and without regularly carrying out laboratory tests to assess the ongoing status of the chemical imbalance would likely find themselves in a very difficult situation, including a seriously ill patient, a major complaint to the Medical Council, and a law suit for medical negligence. I recall as a medical student being on a ward round with a leading physician at the Mid-West Regional Hospital in Limerick, Ireland. He confided to me and a fellow student that he did not understand psychiatry, but that he sometimes needed psychiatrists to tranquillize disruptive patients on the wards so he didn't ask too many questions. In chapter twelve I described the reality that while psychiatrists regularly talk about the brain with authority and apparent expertise, they never carry out brain investigations to make psychiatric diagnoses. This reality clearly raises major questions about the plausibility of their claims of having expertise in the brain and that psychiatric diagnoses are illnesses caused by brain abnormalities.

Because of the collegiality that exists within the medical profession, the majority of doctors who have reservations about psychiatry remain silent. A significant minority of doctors and other mental health professionals see through the delusion and do publicly express their concerns about psychiatric beliefs and practices. While the number of psychiatrists who do not accept the picture of depression painted by psychiatry as grounded in reality is small, in medical terms the numbers are significant. Psychiatry is the only specialty of medicine within which such significant degrees of dissent about core matters of ideology and practice exist. The views of these doctors are not welcomed by the majority within psychiatry. Those who hold them generally become ostracized within the medical brotherhood. Members of other medical specialties who publicly dissent significantly from their psychiatry colleagues are therefore a rare commodity. The level of dissent that exists outside of the profession is also unique to psychiatry. Ex-patients of cardiology, neurology and other specialties might consider themselves as survivors of their illness or treatment. Psychiatry is the only medical specialty where considerable numbers of recipients of psychiatric treatment consider themselves to be survivors of the actual system itself.

When one considers the prevailing view of depression in the context of two related phenomena, the view of depression shared by most psychiatrists and GPs falls very much within the definition of a delusion. These phenomena are groupthink and mass delusion.

GROUPTHINK, MASS DELUSION AND DEPRESSION

Groupthink is a psychological phenomenon that can occur within groups in which the desire for conformity and harmony dominates, often resulting in incorrect or deviant decision-making outcomes. The term was first coined by social psychologist Irving Janis. In his 1972 book *Victims of Groupthink: A Psychological Study of Foreign-Policy Decisions and Fiascoes*, Janis wrote that groupthink happens when a group makes faulty decisions because group pressures can lead to a deterioration in "mental efficiency, reality testing and moral judgement". [20] He defined groupthink as:

The psychological drive for consensus at any cost, that suppresses disagreement and prevents the appraisal of alternatives in cohesive decision-making groups. [21]

Groupthink happens when group members seek to minimize conflict within the group by prioritizing consensus decision-making, without sufficient consideration or critical evaluation of other ideas or viewpoints. Loyalty to the group is imperative. Actions considered disloyal to the group are often met with considerable reprisals and if considered serious enough, expulsion. This threat diminishes independent thinking and individual creativity. Groupthink takes precedence over realistic appraisals of other possible understandings and courses of action that might go against the mindset of the group. Within the groupthink mindset, devil's advocates are not welcome. A regular feature of groupthink is the consistency of the story that is presented in public.

The characteristics of groupthink are firmly present within psychiatry. Doctors who subscribe to the prevailing psychiatric view present a united front. Occasions where psychiatrists contradict each other in public in ways that might damage the perception of the group in the eyes of the public are rare indeed. They tend to occur around differences on issues that are not core values of the group. Psychiatrists may differ considerably on issues that are important but that do not threaten or question the core values of psychiatry. On such occasions, chinks in the armour of the groupthink may be unintentionally revealed.

For example, in 2013 on Irish national radio two Irish professors of psychiatry disagreed profoundly regarding whether or not the availability of abortion in a jurisdiction reduced the risk of suicide. [22] The discussion became quite heated. One professor referred to research mentioned by the other in support of her argument as "not a valid survey", "not science", "an absolute farce", "incomprehensible", "garbled", "analysed by a group of people with stated bias and that is anti-scientific" and "didn't make any sense". The other professor said on air that she would have to leave the studio, which as it turned out she did not. While I imagine both psychiatrists may have felt somewhat upset by this public conflict, they both left the studio with their shared fundamental beliefs about psychiatry intact and unquestioned. In my opinion, it is extremely unlikely that these two psychiatrists would disagree on fundamental fixed psychiatric beliefs such as the assumed biological basis of depression. In my thirty years as a medical doctor, I have never seen any such public disagreement, not amongst doctors who share the same fundamental beliefs about the biological basis of psychiatric diagnoses including depression. In 1999 psychologist Mary Boyle, author of *Schizophrenia: A Scientific Delusion?* wrote that while mainstream psychiatrists may sometimes differ regarding what diagnostic category a person "belongs" to, there is never any debate or questioning of the validity of the fundamental beliefs of psychiatry. [23]

The mental health system is built not on scientifically verifiable methods but on interpretation of people's experiences and behaviours. Interpretation is by its nature a subjective practice, including group interpretation, where a group of like-minded individuals makes similar interpretations as occurs within psychiatry. Doctors working in mental health have generally convinced themselves that they are real doctors like any other medical specialty treating real physical illnesses. The general public has accepted this too. When the delusion is a collective one, shared by the vast majority of group members, it becomes collectively accepted as truth, becoming increasingly familiar, comfortable and invisible over time.

As Abacus news correspondent Charles Wilson wrote in an article titled "Serotonin Depression Myth":

> The facts bandied about with such frivolous confidence by well-meaning doctors are actually hypotheses and speculation. These hypotheses are taught in medical schools as facts, for lack of any substantial theories. Before Copernicus everyone in Europe thought the sun revolved around the earth every 24 hours. If everyone looks at a problem from the same perspective, they will see the same thing and draw the same conclusions. [24]

In 1919, American schoolbook author Emma Miler Bolenius wrote that Christopher Columbus had to navigate his way around a mass delusion in the fifteenth century:

> When Columbus lived, people thought that the world was flat. They believed the Atlantic Ocean to be filled with monsters large enough to devour their ships, and with fearful waterfalls over which their frail vessels would plunge to destruction. Columbus had to fight these foolish beliefs in order to get men to sail with him.[25]

While some historians question the modern-day belief that most people in past centuries were convinced that the world was flat, at times in the past many people did believe that the world was indeed flat.

The word "mass" is derived from the Latin word "massa" which means "that which can be moulded or kneaded". When repeated often and convincingly enough by people who are highly trusted in society, a theory may become accepted as fact, a delusion accepted as reality, and public opinion moulded and kneaded into believing what suits the persuaders. As Marxist revolutionary Vladimir Lenin once said, "A lie told often enough becomes the truth". [26] Adolf Hitler's propaganda officer Joseph Goebbels said in 1939, "Tell a lie a hundred times and it becomes the truth". [27] Psychiatrist A.M. Meerloo wrote in 1949 that:

> A lie repeated ten times becomes believable, and one repeated a hundred times exerts a hypnotic effect. [28]

This is precisely what has happened regarding the depression brain chemical imbalance delusion. Because they have repeatedly heard and read claims that brain chemical abnormalities are a characteristic of depression, the general public are so familiar with the notion that they accept it without reservation or critique. Following the direction of the medical profession, the majority of the general public have understandably come to accept that what doctors say about depression must be true.

Theory is not necessarily as benign as it might appear. Dutch psychiatrist Joost Meerloo once wrote that "Theory aims at subjecting reality to its own dictatorship".[29] This is what psychiatry has been doing for the past one hundred years. Through the imposition of its theories that are regularly misrepresented as facts, psychiatry and the pharmaceutical industry have dictated mass thinking regarding mental health including depression. Consequently a mass collective delusion about the nature and causation of what is called "depression" has become rooted within society.

In 1959, psychiatrist A.M. Meerloo cautioned against the dangers of mass thinking:

> All propaganda utilizes this psychological experience to imbue the masses with subjective truths or lies . . . Mass thinking is a living reality within us . . . The mass leaves no room for particularity and individuality. The individual must learn to howl with the wolves. Mass thinking intimidates the individual. Only a very few are able to withdraw in critical isolation . . . There are . . . suggestive weapons, fascinating catchwords and penetrating formulas, which inoculate the masses so effectively that hardly anyone can escape mass-infection. Some thoughts can be hammered in with great suggestiveness . . . Democracy is easily tired and lazy and there are few who offer mental resistance. We are not trained to be individualists . . . Who has the courage to be the one-man opposition in a large meeting? . . . Mass psychology has the potentiality for becoming a dangerous science . . . Even illogicality is a form of power. The aphorism need not be proven, provided the formula is repeated often and brilliantly enough . . . Among huge masses, especially, reason can easily turn into delusion . . . In mass delusion all coming to terms with reality is lost . . . The masses are rather easy to hypnotize because of the action of suggestive words, the cooperation of common unconscious longings and the increased suggestibility of a group . . . there is also an increased tendency to follow uncritically . . . It is difficult to immunize people against mass-seduction.[30]

As is generally the case with delusions, the core aspects of the depression delusion have remained largely unchanged for over fifty years. These core aspects could be paraphrased as follows:

> Depression is a known to be a medical illness like any other illness. Depression is a disease like any other, a disorder of the brain, a psychiatric disorder that has reached pandemic levels worldwide. It is imperative that all those who suffer from this disease receive appropriate medically-based treatment as advised by their doctors, *the* experts on medical illnesses. Biological abnormalities are a characteristic of all mental illnesses including depression. Brain chemical imbalances and depression go hand in hand. Antidepressants work by correcting a brain problem such as correcting chemical imbalances in the brain.

In her foreword to my 2004 book *Beyond Prozac: Healing Mental Distress*, author and psychologist Dorothy Rowe referred to this collective delusion regarding depression within the medical profession in the following passage:

> The only way to maintain the belief that mental disorder has a physical cause is steadfastly to refuse to be aware of what is going on and what has gone on in the lives of individual people. Terry Lynch was incapable of doing this. He listened to

his patients, and so he came to see that there were direct connections between the form of the patient's distress and the life of the patient. [31]

The only thing I would add to Dorothy Rowe's comments is that it wasn't really that I was incapable of refusing to be aware of what was going on. Rather, I was not willing to turn a blind eye and carry on working within a delusionary system. In her 2009 book *The Myth of the Chemical Cure: A Critique of Psychiatric Drug Treatment*, psychiatrist Joanna Moncrieff referred to this bizarre situation:

> The institution of psychiatry, aided and abetted by the pharmaceutical industry and ultimately backed by the state, has constructed a system of false knowledge about the nature of psychiatric drugs. [32]

To this I would add that psychiatry and general practice, aided and abetted by the pharmaceutical industry, has also created a system of false knowledge regarding the nature of what become known as psychiatric diagnoses, depression included.

Ben Goldacre is a British physician, academic and science writer. He became a member of the Royal College of Psychiatrists in 2005 and a research fellow at the Institute of Psychiatry in London in 2008. In his 2012 book *Bad Pharma*, Goldacre described how consolidated the brain chemical imbalance delusion has become within society:

> The idea that depression is caused by low serotonin is now deeply embedded in popular folklore, and people with no neuroscience background at all will routinely incorporate phrases about it into everyday discussion of their mood, just to keep their serotonin levels up. Many people also "know" that this is how antidepressant drugs work: depression is caused by low serotonin, so you need drugs which raise serotonin levels in your brain, like SSRI antidepressants, which are "selective serotonin reuptake inhibitors". But this theory is very wrong. The "serotonin hypothesis" for depression, as it is known, was always shaky, and the evidence now is hugely contradictory . . . But in popular culture the depression-serotonin link is proven and absolute, because it has been marketed so effectively . . . This is not a belief that arose spontaneously out of nowhere: it has been carefully fostered and maintained. [33]

A major concern regarding any mass delusion is the reluctance to examine the validity of the fundamental beliefs and tenets of the delusion. Jonathan Rottenberg is an associate professor of psychology at the University of South Florida. In a 2014 article he wrote about the failure to challenge the most fundamental beliefs about depression and the consequences of not doing so (brackets mine):

> Perhaps the most troubling and ironic thing about the toll of depression is that it has risen while more research and treatment resources have been poured into combating it. In fact, depression represents an $83-billion annual burden to the United States economy in lost productivity and increased medical expenses.

Why aren't we winning this fight? I have come to believe that we are failing in part because our most fundamental idea about depression—the intuitively tidy notion that it stems from some kind of defect—is misconceived. There are different versions of the defect model . . . Pre-eminent among the defect models is the notion of the correctible chemical imbalance. We live in a biological age and this comforting idea is popular, embraced by media, patient groups and mental health professionals alike. It is a mind-set borne out in prescriptions filled: 27 million Americans take antidepressants. Yet for all the searching, in none of the defect models has the deficiency been found. There are no biological tests for depression, despite the hundreds of physical assays (tests) available. [34]

Why is it that the problem of depression has continued to escalate despite vast resources being aimed toward the problem and supposedly highly effective treatments available at the stroke of the doctor's pen? If antidepressants are as effective as the public have been led to believe, why is it that 27 million Americans taking antidepressants has not resulted in more people back at work, lower instead of higher disability rates, and fewer rather than ever-increasing costs to the US and other Westernized economies? It is because, as Rottenberg asserts, the very basis upon which the prevailing understanding of depression is built is fundamentally wrong. A thorough independent examination of the fundamental tenets of psychiatry would reveal that they have no basis in fact, which is why mainstream psychiatry is so reluctant to have its core beliefs subjected to independent rigorous examination.

The brain chemical imbalance depression delusion is alive and well. It has been promoted by those with power and authority in mental health for over half a century and has become accepted as fact by the majority of the public. Only a set of circumstances combining great public trust and financial backing could facilitate such a global delusion. The medical-pharmaceutical alliance, the main drivers of the depression delusion, has both. The drug industry has supplied much the money to establish and maintain this delusion. The public generally trust what doctors say, including doctors' pronouncements regarding brain chemical imbalances and depression. The psychiatric disease model of depression has been consistently promoted as though such abnormalities have been demonstrated to exist. Their existence is assumed as definite, it being only a matter of time before the abnormalities and imbalances are discovered. As psychologist and author Mary Boyle wrote in her 1990 book *Schizophrenia: A Scientific Delusion?*

The crucial difference between medicine and psychiatry can perhaps best be summarized by saying that whereas medical scientists study bodily functioning and describe patterns in it, psychiatrists behave *as if* they were studying bodily functioning and *as if* they had described patterns there, when in fact they are studying behaviour and have assumed—but not proved—that certain types of pattern *will be* found there. [35]

Many psychiatrists and GPs go to considerable lengths to convince the public that psychiatry is a specialist field of medical knowledge based on a solid scientific foundation like all medical specialties. The public might understandably assume that like other medical specialties, psychiatry is an objective branch of medicine with a solid scientific grounding. People might naturally expect psychiatrists to be open to promising new ideas. Neither of these presumptions is correct. Psychiatry's quest for truth is conditional and compromised. Psychiatry is willing to seriously consider only ideas that are consistent with the beliefs and ideology of mainstream psychiatry, ideas that are unlikely to diminish psychiatrists' standing as *the* experts in mental health.

With few exceptions, the overall impression conveyed by those who express the prevailing view of depression is generally one of assuredness in their knowledge and in their sound scientific grounding in which the public can trust. When one digs deeper, beneath the apparently convincing and reassuring words of those who espouse the prevailing view of what depression is, one enters quite a different world. Inconsistencies and contradictions are commonplace within psychiatry, though these recurring features may not be visible to the untrained eye. This is inevitable, since the profession is attempting to dress depression up as something it is has not been demonstrated to be, a biological illness like diabetes or multiple sclerosis. It is therefore inevitable that cracks appear when the arguments of psychiatry are subjected to rigorous examination. As we have seen, many such examples of double-speak and slight-of-hand occur when we get to the core questions.

An admission by psychiatrist Daniel Carlat points to a mass delusion within the groupthink system that is mainstream psychiatry (brackets mine):

> We (psychiatrists) have convinced ourselves that we have developed cures for mental illnesses, when in fact we know so little about the underlying neurobiology of their causes that our treatments are often a series of trials and errors. [36]

In his 1974 book *Not Made of Wood*, Dutch psychiatrist Jan Foudraine described how he gradually moved from the idea that people experiencing psychosis were suffering from a disease. In the process he became acutely aware of psychiatry's fixed beliefs:

> I discovered that this idea—that psychotic people were suffering from a "disease"—was a delusion entertained by a lot of psychiatrists and very much harder to tackle than the "fantasies" of people I met in the psychiatric institutions. [37]

In her 2010 book *Why we Lie*, psychologist and author Dorothy Rowe outlined a major reason for the persistence of untruths within psychiatry such as the depression delusion:

> Abandoning a theory on which you have built your career and reputation with your peers will threaten your sense of being a person, and so you are likely to deny the evidence that shows your theory to be wrong. [38]

Anthropologist E. E. Evans-Prichard similarly spoke of a common desire to maintain our belief systems at all costs, even in the face of convincing evidence to the contrary:

He cannot think that his thought is wrong. [39]

I experienced this phenomenon myself when a young doctor wryly joked at the end of a two-hour talk I gave to trainee general practitioners fifteen years ago in which I invited them to maintain a healthy questioning attitude to the fundamental beliefs of their training:

Great! Now we don't know who we are!

Those who have subscribed to the depression brain chemical imbalance delusion and have a major vested interest in the delusion being maintained will generally not contemplate that they might be looking for a needle in the wrong haystack. The delusion works for them. Their need to hold on to their fixed belief is to them more important than their willingness to see reality as it is. Maintaining the delusion enables them to maintain their worldview, their dominant position in mental health, their way of working and living. Maintaining the delusion enables them to avoid facing up to reality and to avoid taking full responsibility for their actions. They can continue living the way they want to live and keep reaping the many benefits proffered upon them as a consequence of the mass public belief in brain chemical imbalances in depression that have never been shown to exist.

NOTES TO CHAPTER THIRTEEN

1. Richard Smith, *The Guardian*, 14 January 2004.
2. Tony Humphreys, in the foreword to *Beyond Prozac: Healing Mental Suffering without Drugs*, by Terry Lynch, Dublin: Mercier Press, 2001, p. 11.
3. Terry Lynch, *Beyond Prozac: Healing Mental Distress*, Ross-on-Wye: PCCS Books, 2004.
4. For information about Selfhood see note 2 in the Notes to Chapter Four.
5. The definition of a delusion, dictionary.com website, http://dictionary.reference.com/browse/delusion, accessed 02 April 2014.
6. American Psychiatric Association, *The Diagnostic and Statistical Manual of Mental Disorders, (DSM-5)*, American Psychiatric Publishing, May 2013.
7. Kwame McKenzie, *Understanding Depression*, Poole: Family Doctor Publications in association with the British Medical Association, 2009, pps. 12-14.
8. Philip Cowen, Paul Harrison & Tom Burns, *The Shorter Oxford Textbook of Psychiatry*, Oxford: Oxford University Press, 2012, p. 8.

9. A, M. Meerloo, "Delusion and Mass Delusion", 1949, http://www.lermanet.com/exit/ mass-delusion-meerloo.htm, accessed 02 April 2014.
10. *Stanford Encyclopedia of Philosophy*, http://plato.stanford.edu/entries/delusion/, accessed 22 November 2013.
11. *Stanford Encyclopedia of Philosophy*, http://plato.stanford.edu/entries/delusion/, accessed 22 November 2013.
12. Science Brainwaves website, "How delusions occur, and why they may be widespread", http://www. sciencebrainwaves.com/uncategorized/how-delusions-occur-and-why-they-may-be-widespread/, accessed 22 November 2013.
13. Allen Frances, in Gary Greenberg, *The Book of Woe: The DSM and the Unmaking of Psychiatry,* London: Scribe Publications, 2013, p. 281.
14. *Encyclopaedia Britannica*, http://www.britannica.com/EBchecked/topic/156888/delusion, accessed 22 November 2013.
15. A.M. Meerloo, "Delusion and Mass Delusion", 1949, http://www.lermanet.com/exit/ mass-delusion-meerloo.htm, accessed 23 November 2013.
16. A.M. Meerloo, "Delusion and Mass Delusion", 1949, http://www.lermanet.com/exit/ mass-delusion-meerloo.htm, accessed 23 November 2013.
17. American Psychiatric Association, *The Diagnostic and Statistical Manual of Mental Disorders, (DSM-5),* American Psychiatric Publishing, May 2013.
18. American Psychiatric Association, *The Diagnostic and Statistical Manual of Mental Disorders, (DSM-5),* American Psychiatric Publishing, May 2013.
19. Philip Cowen, Paul Harrison & Tom Burns, *The Shorter Oxford Textbook of Psychiatry*, Oxford: Oxford University Press, 2012.
20. Irving Lester Janis, *Victims of Groupthink: A Psychological Study of Foreign-Policy Decisions and Fiascoes,* Houghton Mifflin, 1972.
21. Irving Lester Janis, *Victims of Groupthink: A Psychological Study of Foreign-Policy Decisions and Fiascoes,* Houghton Mifflin, 1972.
22. "Today with Pat Kenny" radio programme, Radio One, 03 May 2013, with Professor Veronica O'Kane and Professor Patricia Casey.
23. Mary Boyle, "Diagnosis", in C. Newnes, C. Holmes and C. Dunn (Eds.), *This is Madness*, Ross-on-Wye: PCCS Books, 1999, pps 75-90.
24. Charles Wilson, "Serotonin depression myth", .http://www.abacus-news.co.uk/depression /08/serotonin-depression-myth.php, accessed 15 April 2014.
25. Emma Miler Bolenius, American Schoolbook Author, 1919, http://scienceblogs.com/ startswithabang/2011/09/21/who-discovered-the-earth-is-round/, accessed 15 April 2014.
26. Vladimir Lenin, http://www.brainyquote.com/quotes/quotes/v/vladimirle132031.html, accessed 02 April 2014.
27. Joseph Goebbels, 1939, http://www.ius.bg.ac.yu/apel/materijali/info-warfare.html, accessed 02 April 2014.
28. A.M. Meerloo, "Delusion and Mass Delusion", 1949, http://www.lermanet.com/exit/ mass-delusion-meerloo.htm, accessed 02 April 2014.
29. A.M. Meerloo, "Delusion and Mass Delusion", 1949, http://www.lermanet.com/exit/ mass-delusion-meerloo.htm, accessed 24 April 2014.
30. A.M. Meerloo, "Delusion and Mass Delusion", 1949, http://www.lermanet.com/exit/ mass-delusion-meerloo.htm, accessed 02 April 2014.
31. Dorothy Rowe, foreword to *Beyond Prozac: Healing Mental Distress,* by Terry Lynch, Ross-on-Wye: PCCS Books, 2004.
32. Joanna Moncrieff, *The Myth of the Chemical Cure: A Critique of Psychiatric Drug Treatment*, Basingstoke: Palgrave Macmillan, 2009, p. 237.
33. Ben Goldacre, *Bad Pharma*, London: Fourth estate, 2012, p. 258.
34. Jonathan Rottenberg, "An Evolved View of Depression", 27 January 2014, *The Chronicle Review*, http://chronicle.com/article/An-Evolved-View-of-Depression/144199/, accessed 26 February 14.
35. Mary Boyle, *Schizophrenia: A Scientific Delusion?* London and New York: Routledge, 1990, p. 179.
36. Daniel Carlat, *Unhinged: The Trouble with Psychiatry—a Doctor's Revelations about a Profession in Crisis,* London: Free Press, 2010.
37. Jan Foudraine, *Not Made of Wood*, Quartet Books, 1974.

38. Dorothy Rowe, *Why We Lie*, Fourth Estate, London, 2010, p. 64.
39. Anthropologist E.E. Evans-Prichard, quoted in Ingleby, D., "Understanding 'Mental Illness'", in D. Ingleby, ed, *Critical Psychiatry: The Politics of Mental Health,* Harmondsworth, Middx: Penguin, 1981, p. 37.

14. QUESTIONABLE PRACTICES AND STANDARDS IN HIGH PLACES

Psychiatry is fundamentally an ideology, a belief system. The brain chemical imbalance story has for fifty years been at the heart of this belief system. The ideology that has shaped both psychiatric practice and public perception is built not on evidence but on faith. American psychotherapist Dr. Dan Edmunds Ph.D. described this phenomenon as follows:

> The religion of psychiatry: Bio-psychiatry has its creed, the creed that all problems of life are the result of so-called chemical imbalances. Any professional or individual challenging such conception is branded a heretic and subject to sanction. [1]

As one who has been treated like a heretic within the medical profession for the past fourteen years, I know exactly what Dan Edmunds means.

DEPRESSION IS A FLAW IN CHEMISTRY NOT CHARACTER, RIGHT?

The catchy claim that "depression is a flaw in chemistry not character" is one of the most commonly used ways of expressing the popular view that depression is caused by abnormalities in people's brain chemistry and not due to any character flaw or personal weakness. I include several such examples in this book. It is not difficult to see the attraction of this interpretation of depression. It implies that if you are depressed, you do not have a flawed character and it is not your fault. The fault lies with your brain chemistry.

Two major problems arise regarding this phrase. Since no abnormal brain chemistry has ever been found in depression, claims that "depression is a flaw in chemistry" have no basis in fact. Secondly, only two possible explanations for depression are considered—flawed chemistry or flawed character. Faced with just these two choices, flawed chemistry is obviously a more attractive option. This is a False Dilemma logical fallacy. [2] As I discuss in chapter four, there is another way of understanding depression, which is a far more accurate in regard to the experiences and behaviours of depression without resorting to either the fiction of chemical abnormalities or the judgement of a flawed or weak character.

FLAWED PERCEPTION

We human beings are multidimensional. We are sentient beings with many aspects to our being. We have a physical aspect; our physical body. We have an emotional aspect; we feel. We have a psychological aspect; we think. We have a social and relational aspect; we relate to others at many levels. There is a sexual aspect to our being and for many, their spiritual aspect is important to them. Common sense would suggest that the more aspects of the human being that are taken into consideration, the better we will understand and respond to human experiences and behaviour. Yet the medical profession's approach to what is called depression remains primarily one-dimensional, with little real importance placed on the contexts within which the person finds themselves in life.

In its ideology and practice, psychiatry focuses primarily on possible biological questions and answers. This approach is consistent with medical training, which derives fundamentally from the Cartesian split, in which body and mind are portrayed as two separate and unrelated entities. Psychiatry pays scant attention to the other aspects of the human being and when is does, it generally does so from a biological perspective. Being primarily one-dimensional in its assessment of human suffering creates a major risk that important aspects of human experience will be missed, which is precisely what happens. This narrow biological perspective is itself distorted and seriously flawed, being further compromised due to the illogical and unscientific approach that is often taken, of which the depression brain chemical imbalance delusion is a prime example. Discounting the other aspects in this manner should only be done based on strong evidence in support of doing so, but no such evidence exists. Convinced that the fundamental basis of depression is biological, the medical profession assumes that the physical biological aspect is by far the primary aspect worthy of their attention and research.

Sometimes the innocence of youth enables young people to see truths that many older and supposedly wiser adults do not or will not see. In Hans Christian Andersen's tale *The Emperor's New Clothes*, it took a young child to see and to name the fact that the emperor was wearing no clothes. On 29 September 2013, the Irish *Sunday Independent* newspaper published a letter from a sixteen-year-old girl. She questioned the widespread interpretation of distress in young people as depression. "Are we making too big a deal of 'depression' among teens?" she asked. Regarding the stresses experienced by teenagers, she asked whether this is:

A form of mental illness or just a rite of passage during teen years? Are we right to brand one in three teenagers as mentally ill? Telling girls they are depressed because they worry about looks and weight isn't good for their mental state, nor will it benefit them in later years. Learning to accept who you are is more important that being diagnosed with depression.

How striking that a sixteen-year-old girl can see more clearly than many adults including supposed professional experts.

FLAWED SCIENCE

The 2013 *Oxford Handbook of Psychiatry* discussed myths in mental health and how to deal with them:

> Myths matter. Throughout history myths have served the central function of explaining the inexplicable: creating the illusion of understanding . . . in our professional lives we (psychiatrists) are afforded the benefit of authority based on our expertise. This is why there are professional examinations and qualifications. We must guard against misinformation and protect ourselves and our patients from treatments and explanatory models for which evidence is decidedly lacking.[3]

The authors of this psychiatry textbook seem satisfied that they and their profession guard effectively against myth-making in psychiatry. They are mistaken. The true expertise of psychiatry is far less than is commonly assumed in society and within psychiatry itself. The fact that there are examinations and qualifications in psychiatry is no guarantee of accurate and true understanding. Examinations and qualifications that contain mistaken premises may reinforce rather than diminish any myths upon which they might be constructed. While claiming to "guard against misinformation and protect ourselves and our patients from treatments and explanatory models for which evidence is decidedly lacking", these authors are blind to the reality that many psychiatrists and GPs are spreading misinformation about depression and brain chemicals every day on a vast scale and have been doing so for thirty years or more. Telling people that their depression is definitely or probably caused by brain chemical imbalances is a daily practice in most GP surgeries and psychiatric clinics, claims for which "evidence is decidedly lacking". Has psychiatry protected patients and the public from the falsehoods and half-truths that have persistently promoted by drug companies for almost thirty years? These authors continue (brackets mine):

> Fortunately we have the Scientific Method to help us sift the evidence and the testable biopsychosocial model of the aetiology (causation) of psychiatric illness. [4]

The degree to which psychiatric principles and practice adhere to the Scientific Method is questionable. It is clear that regarding the brain chemical imbalance notion, psychiatry does not adhere to the Scientific Method to help "sift through the evidence", since there is no confirming evidence for this notion. The fundamental belief that biology is at the root of all psychiatric diagnoses including depression is rarely questioned within mainstream psychiatry, never mind tested. Core fundamental tenets of the "biopsychosocial model of the aetiology of mental illness" such as the deeply-held but unevidenced conviction that depression is fundamentally a biological disorder are rarely if ever put to rigorous testing within psychiatry. Elsewhere in this book these same authors admitted that psychiatrists do not even examine or test the brain. [5]

The Scientific Method has long been at the heart of the scientific approach to life. This method involves the stages of observation, research, hypothesis, experimentation and conclusion. Applying these to psychiatry's approach to brain chemical imbalances and depression, the observation was that some people have experiences and engage in behaviours that doctors interpret as depression. The hypothesis was then created that depression is an illness caused by biological abnormalities in the brain. Doctors then tested this hypothesis by setting up experiments and research projects. The conclusion involves summarizing the results of the research and reviewing how they match up with their hypothesis.

Mainstream psychiatry has not followed the sequence described in the Scientific Method to its logical conclusion. Thousands of research projects designed to identify brain chemical abnormalities over more than half a century have repeatedly drawn a blank. Yet mainstream psychiatry has continued relentlessly with the same basic approach, seeking primarily to identify only biological answers. If it were a truly objective profession, psychiatry should long ago have approached other equally valid hypotheses with equal vigour. This has not happened. One obvious and valid hypothesis is that depression consists primarily of an emotional and psychological set of experiences and behaviours that naturally also involve the body, since the body is an important aspect of our existence and experiences. This hypothesis has largely been shelved by psychiatry for many decades in favour of biological hypotheses which they have wrongly adopted and promoted as if they are established facts.

This behaviour falls far short of the standards required in true scientific endeavour. It is entirely reasonable as a scientific endeavour to create a hypothesis and test the hypothesis to ascertain whether it is a fact that can be incorporated into the existing body of knowledge. It is not acceptable to stick primarily to one fundamental hypothesis for more than five decades, to build much of their research projects around this hypothesis, and to draw unfounded conclusions while largely ignoring other potentially promising hypotheses because they are not consistent with their beliefs and ideology.

The LiveScience website states that science is based on fact, not opinion or preferences. [6] In science, something is only accepted as a fact when it can be accurately and reliably verified. By prematurely concluding that brain chemical imbalances are a key feature of depression and promoting this as fact to the general population, drug companies, mainstream psychiatry and GPs have repeatedly contravened this fundamental rule of science. Regarding depression, no solid evidence confirming brain biological abnormalities exists. Brain abnormalities have not been accurately and reliably verified. Psychiatry has jumped light years ahead of itself and has drawn conclusions that are utterly inconsistent with the level of actual scientific evidence. For decades, psychiatry has put this hypothesis into the public domain as if it were an established fact. The public has been misinformed for decades and continues to be misinformed. Misinforming the public regarding such an important aspect of life as emotional and mental health is a very serious matter.

Many psychiatrists describe themselves as scientists and therefore as objective and trustworthy, and they are seen as such by most people. As Dr. Rupert Sheldrake described in his 2012 book *The Science Delusion: Freeing the Spirit of Enquiry*, the issue of objectivity in science is rather more complicated than it might seem at first glance:

> The assumption that the sciences are uniquely objective not only distorts the public perception of scientists, but affects scientists' perception of themselves. The illusion of objectivity makes scientists prone to deception and self-deception. It works against the noble idea of seeking truth. [7]

In my opinion, a hallmark of a true scientist is the willingness and honesty to see the validity and value of evidence that runs contrary to their hypotheses. True scientists are happy to have their theories questioned and tested by others. This is not how psychiatry and the pharmaceutical industry have generally operated in relation to the depression brain chemical imbalance delusion. In my experience, the majority of psychiatrists are rarely prepared to engage in open debate about the validity of their biological hypotheses and of other ways of understanding and responding to human distress. Many of those who do engage in open debate often react with irritation or anger at the very idea of being asked to account for themselves and their beliefs. Psychiatry has adopted the biological hypothesis of depression for so long and to such a degree that objectivity in psychiatry has long been replaced by fixed ideas. Mainstream psychiatry has nailed its colours to the biological mast to such a degree and for so long that it is difficult to see a way back for psychiatry in its current form. If the biological hypothesis crumbles, then the collapse of psychiatry in its present form may not be far away. There is therefore a great deal at stake for psychiatry and psychiatrists. Defending the biological view is critically important for psychiatry's survival and position in society. At this stage, virtually the entire profession of psychiatry is built upon the biological idea. This major vested interest makes it extremely difficult for psychiatrists to properly question their fundamental beliefs. Rupert Sheldrake described this phenomenon in his 2012 book *The Science Delusion: Freeing the Spirit of Enquiry*:

> Most scientists are unconscious of the myths, allegories and assumptions that shape their social roles and political power. These beliefs are implicit rather than explicit. If they are unconscious, they cannot be questioned; and in so far as they are collective, shared by the scientific community, there is no incentive to question them. [8]

PROPAGANDA, HEGEMONY AND SOPHISTRY

These three related phenomena have been features of the medical and pharmaceutical approach to depression and mental health for many decades. They have been used by vested interests to maintain power and control of mental health. The persuasion and deception of the majority of the public into believing that brain chemical imbalances occur in depression illustrates the success of the process of persuasion in which propaganda, hegemony and sophistry have been employed by those with power in mental health.

The *Oxford dictionary* defines propaganda as:

> Information, especially of a biased and misleading nature, used to promote a political cause or a point of view. [9]

In 1996, professor in mass communications Richard Alan Nelson defined propaganda as:

A systematic form of purposeful persuasion that attempts to influence the emotions, attitudes, opinions and actions of specified target audiences for ideological, political or commercial purposes through the controlled transmission of one-sided messages which may or may not be factual via mass and direct media channels. [10]

In their 2011 book *Propaganda and Persuasion*, Garth S. Jowett and Victoria J. O'Donnell defined propaganda as:

The deliberate, systematic attempt to shape perceptions, manipulate cognitions and direct behaviour to achieve a response that furthers the desired intent of the propagandist. [11]

The promotion of depression as a brain chemical imbalance by the medical profession, drug companies and other interested parties falls within all three of these definitions of propaganda. The origins of this propaganda go back a long way. In 1845 leading German psychiatrist Wilhelm Griesinger claimed:

Mental diseases are brain diseases . . . It is only from the neuropathological standpoint that one can try to make sense of the symptomatology of the insane. [12]

This continues to be the position of mainstream psychiatry, a position that reflects the limited vision of its proponents rather than any established scientific reality. Over 150 years later, this claim remains in the realm of conjecture. In his 1998 book *Blaming the Brain: The Truth about Drugs and Mental Health*, Professor Emeritus of Neuroscience Elliot Valenstein summarized the scientific data in regard to the SSRI antidepressants:

What physicians and the public are reading about mental illness is by no means a neutral reflection of all the information that is available. [13]

Throughout this book I have presented many pronouncements from drug companies and medical doctors that meet the definitions of propaganda described in the previous page. In a 2006 editorial in the *British Journal of Psychiatry*, psychiatrist Joanna Moncrieff wrote about the phenomenal expansion of the brain chemical imbalance notion:

The activities of the pharmaceutical industry in recent years have greatly expanded its application. Disease awareness campaigns for depression . . . have been wholly or partly funded by drug companies . . . The effect of these activities has been to increase the number of people who define themselves as psychiatrically ill and to create the impression that the biochemical basis of psychiatric disorders is well established. For example, the well-informed public (e.g. specialist journalists) has been shocked to hear that research has not established that serotonin abnormality is the cause of depression. [14]

In their 2007 book *Your Drug May Be Your Problem: How and Why to Stop Taking Psychiatric Medications*, psychiatrist Peter Breggin and professor of social work David Cohen wrote:

> The notion that Prozac corrects biochemical imbalances is sheer speculation—propaganda from the biological psychiatric industry . . . Our emotional and spiritual problems are not only seen as psychiatric disorders, they are declared to be biological and genetic in origin. The propaganda for this remarkable perspective is financed by drug companies and spread by the media, by organized psychiatry and individual doctors, by "consumer" lobbies, and even by government agencies such as the National Institute of Mental health (NIMH). As a result, many educated Americans take for granted that "science" and "research" have shown that emotional upsets or "behavior problems" have biological and genetic causes and require psychiatric drugs. Indeed, they believe they are "informed" about scientific research. Few if any people realize that they are being subjected to one of the most successful public relations campaigns in history . . . Claims that "mental illness" is caused by "biochemical imbalances" is the major public relations thrust of current drug promotion. In magazine advertisements, and during consultations with doctors in their offices, potential patients are repeatedly told that psychiatric drugs "work" by correcting known "biochemical imbalances" in their brains. Media reports treat these claims as gospel truth, and the American Psychiatric Association reports that 75 percent of Americans believe in them . . . we have no techniques for measuring the actual levels of neurotransmitters in the synapses between the cells. Thus all the talk about biochemical imbalances is pure guess work. [15]

In her 2009 book *The Myth of the Chemical Cure*, psychiatrist Joanna Moncrieff wrote:

> Intense publicity from the combined forces of the pharmaceutical industry and the psychiatric profession has started to mould public attitudes to reflect professional and commercial ones. [16]

In his 2013 book *How Everyone Became Depressed* Canadian psychiatrist Professor Edward Shorter described the major process of persuasion that has occurred regarding the brain chemical imbalance notion in depression:

> What is happening here is the turning of a massive crank, to make the concept of depression scientifically acceptable to physicians, and thus indirectly appealing to their patients. Yet another crank was simultaneously grinding as well: the media crank that sold the neurotransmitter doctrine of depression directly to a mass audience. From the 1970s onwards, the public was increasingly exposed to the concept of neurotransmitters as the scientific basis for confidence in the antidepressants and the whole doctrine of depression, on the logic that if it responds to Prozac, it must exist. [17]

The Wisegeek website contains a detailed description of hegemony:

> The term "hegemony" refers to the leadership, dominance or great influence that one entity or group of people has over others . . . Modern uses of "hegemony" often refer to a group in a society having power over others within that society. Hegemony more often refers to the power of a single group in a society to essentially lead and dominate other groups in a society . . . Besides money, other forms of influence can be used by one group to dominate others. [18]

In an article titled "Hegemony", Professor Michael Lewis Goldberg of the University of Washington described Italian Marxist Gramsci's concept of cultural hegemony as:

> The success of the dominant classes in presenting their definition of reality, their view of the world, in such a way that it is accepted by other classes as "common sense". The general "consensus" is that it is the *only* sensible way of seeing the world. Any groups who present an alternative view are therefore marginalized . . . Domination is not simply imposed from above, but has to be won through the subordinated group's spontaneous consent to the cultural domination which they believe will serve their interests because it is "common sense". [19]

A 2008 *New York Times* article discussed the nature and importance of hegemony:

> Hegemony describes the dominance of one social group or class in a society. This control can be exercised subtly rather than forcefully through cultural means and economic power, and rest on a mixture of consent and coercion . . . The modern concept of hegemony—often attributed to the 1920s Italian social theorist Antonio Gramsci—was used to explain how a powerful economic or social group came to dominate a society without maintaining a state of constant fear. Rather than using force or explicit coercion, hegemonic power rested on the successful manipulation of cultural and social institutions—such as the media—to set the limits of economic and political opportunities for citizens. This gave the dominant group in society a position to influence the preferences of others in favour of the existing order; and to ensure that representatives of these dominant interests served in key monetary, regulatory, judicial and bureaucratic posts. [20]

You might be surprised to read that the prevailing societal understanding of depression is a form of hegemony. It might appear impossible that psychiatry and general practice could ever be a hegemonic force in society. Surely psychiatry and general practice puts the health and wellbeing of the public above all else? The words and actions of doctors within these two medical disciplines can surely be fully trusted and taken as truth? Regrettably in the field of mental health, this is often not the case.

In 2005, Mark Cresswell of the Department of Sociology at the University of Manchester defined psychiatric hegemony as:

The political process by which dominant forms of medical knowledge work to produce subjects within a broader normative order. [21]

Earlier in this book I mentioned science writer and physician Ben Goldacre's 2008 *Guardian* article in which he referred to the hegemony of the widespread acceptance of the depression brain chemical imbalance delusion as absolute truth:

> In popular culture the depression/serotonin story is proven and absolute, because it was never about research, or theory, it was about marketing, and journalists who pride themselves on never pushing pills or the hegemony will still blindly push the model until the cows come home. [22]

As a hegemony is created and maintained by those with power and authority, a consensus culture develops in which those subject to the dominant forces come to see the dominion as for their own good, as "common sense". The masses are therefore willing to maintain the status quo and there is little or no revolt. Journalist Robert Whitaker identified powerful key players in the creation of the consensus culture that has wrongly re-framed human experience and behaviour as brain diseases:

> A powerful quartet of voices came together during the 1980s eager to inform the public that mental disorders were brain diseases. Pharmaceutical companies provided the financial muscle. The American Psychiatric Association and psychiatrists at top medical schools conferred intellectual legitimacy upon the enterprise. The National Institute of Mental Health put the government's stamp of approval on the story. The National Alliance on Mental Illness provided the moral authority. [23]

I have no issue with the dominance of medical knowledge and practice as long as it is grounded upon sound logic and solid scientific evidence and it is open to public scrutiny. I was fully willing to entrust my life to Professor Calvin Coffey, an excellent surgeon in Limerick, Ireland, when I developed a bowel problem in 2011 that required surgery. Without that surgery I would not be here today. I will always be grateful to that doctor, his team and the care I received while I was ill. I accept the validity of the medical approach to known diseases such as diabetes and cancer and to all conditions where the medical thinking and practice is logical and scientifically verified. In contrast, claims of biochemical imbalances in depression are devoid of scientific verification and contain major gaps, leaps of faith and contradictions in logic.

The prevailing societal understanding of and approach to depression has all the hallmarks of a hegemony. This understanding has been promoted as "common sense" and propagated by powerful, wealthy and trusted groups, primarily the pharmaceutical industry, the medical profession and other groups for whom this delusion is beneficial. The groups who have actively sought to persuade the general public that the depression brain chemical imbalance delusion is real have much to gain from the societal and cultural dominance the widespread acceptance of the brain chemical imbalance depression delusion provides for them.

In 1996 psychiatrist David Kaiser expressed grave concern about what he termed "the hegemony known as biological psychiatry". Kaiser wrote:

> As a practicing psychiatrist, I have watched with growing dismay and outrage the rise and triumph of the hegemony known as biologic psychiatry. Within the general field of modern psychiatry, biologism now completely dominates the discourse on the causes and treatment of mental illness, and in my view this is a catastrophe with far-reaching effects in individual patients and the cultural psyche at large. It has occurred to me with forcible irony that psychiatry has quite literally lost its mind, and along with it the minds of the patients they are presumably supposed to care for . . . the field has gone far down the road into a kind of delusion, whose main tenets consist of a particularly pernicious biologic determinism and pseudo-scientific understanding of human nature and mental illness . . . Biologic psychiatrists as a whole are unapologetic in their view that they have found the road to the truth . . . Although they admit a role for environmental and social factors, these are usually relegated to a secondary status. Their unquestioning confidence in their biologic paradigms of mental illness is truly staggering". [24]

Hegemonic behaviour involves the often subtle imposition of views upon others. The depression delusion, including the brain chemical imbalance notion, has been imposed on the public for almost fifty years by psychiatry, general practice, drug companies and other groups with a vested interest in this delusion. Psychologist and author Lucy Johnstone has expressed concern regarding this imposition:

> Upholders of the (psychiatric) orthodoxy have every right to their own view. What they do not have the right to do, and cannot do without undermining their claim to be part of a legitimate scientific enterprise, is impose their views on others, and attack and suppress those who put forward critiques and alternatives. Nevertheless, this frequently happens. [25]

In a 2005 *Wall Street Journal* article, journalist Sharon Begley articulated her concern regarding the dominance of the brain chemical imbalance notion in depression:

> The hegemony of the serotonin hypothesis may be keeping patients from a therapy that will help them more in the long term. The relapse rate for patients on pills is higher than for those getting cognitive-behavioural therapy. [26]

Some hegemonies are pretty obvious, such as the dominance of one country over another within empires of various kinds. Others, like this one, are far more subtle. The collective depression brain chemical imbalance delusion has helped to ensure that people do not notice psychiatry's hegemonic domination of emotional and mental health globally. A superstructure now exists in mental health, whose ideas have become dominant and pervasive throughout society. The interests of the groups that control mental health thinking and practice are presented not as the interests of the dominant group but as national interests that are widely shared, a strategy common to most hegemonies.

Also in 2005, psychiatrist Grace Jackson wrote in her book *Rethinking Psychiatric Drugs: A Guide for Informed Consent* that:

> One unfortunate consequence of the monoamine theory of depression has been the recent hegemony of the opinion that low serotonin causes depression, anxiety, impulsivity, compulsions and violence. [27]

According to neuroscientist Elliot Valenstein in his 1998 book *Blaming the Brain: The Truth about Drugs and Mental Health,* since the 1930s, when psychiatry became a board-certified medical specialty, psychiatry began to:

> Mobilize itself against any and all competition in treating mental disorders. Those not trained in psychiatry were perceived as intruders. [28]

There remains to this day a general assumption that mental health issues must be seen as biological with doctors at the helm. As far as mainstream psychiatry is concerned, this position is wrongly taken as firmly established and therefore beyond questioning.

The Free Online Dictionary defines sophistry as:

> A method of argument that is seemingly plausible but is actually invalid and misleading . . . A plausible but misleading or fallacious argument. [29]

The term is applied to reasoning that appears sound but is actually misleading or fallacious. The handing of the brain chemical imbalance notion by psychiatry, drug companies and other interested parties fits this definition. It appears plausible and is presented as such, but a detailed examination of the brain chemical imbalance and depression notion reveals it to be invalid, misleading and without substance.

A PERVERSE IMPLANTATION

In his 1978 book *The History of Sexuality*, French philosopher and social theorist Michael Foucault observed a recurring phenomenon of social construction he called the "perverse implantation", whereby categories of behaviour become named and widely accepted. They are subsequently internalized by members of societies where those named categories are used. Once internalized, these categories become formative aspects of people's perception of existence and interpretation of experience.

Robert Krause of the Yale School of Nursing is the author of a 2005 article titled "Depression, antidepressants and an examination of epidemiological changes". In this article, Krause contended that the characteristics of a perverse implantation apply to depression:

A concerted effort has been made by government, corporate and public health groups to market the category of depression broadly. This raises the concern that depression may be the sort of category members of society have internalized, leading to specifically designed behavioural changes and changes to one's relationship to oneself. [30]

The implantation of the idea of depression in the consciousness of the public has been highly successful. The belief that depression is a medical illness caused by chemical brain imbalances is solidly embedded within modern societies. The notion that psychiatrists are *the* experts on mental health and mental illness has also taken a firm hold, having penetrated the hallowed halls of the law courts. Psychiatrists are seen within most legal systems as the foremost experts on mental health matters. The evidence of a psychiatrist expert witness will generally trump all other mental professionals including psychologists except in exceptional cases and situations that are not considered to fall primarily within the remit of psychiatry.

NOTES TO CHAPTER FOURTEEN

1. Dan Edmunds, "The Religion of Bio-Psychiatry", Mad in America website, 26 March 2012, http://www.madinamerica.com/2012/03/the-religion-of-bio-psychiatry/, accessed 11 May 2014.
2. For information on false Dilemma logical fallacies see note 38 in the Notes to Chapter Five.
3. David Semple & Roger Smyth, *The Oxford Handbook of Psychiatry*, 2013, 3rd edition, Oxford: Oxford University Press, p. 20.
4. David Semple & Roger Smyth, *The Oxford Handbook of Psychiatry*, 2013, 3rd edition, Oxford: Oxford University Press, p. 20.
5. I refer to the admission in the *Oxford Handbook of Psychiatry* that psychiatrists do not generally examine the brain in note 6 in the Notes to Chapter Twelve. See also the associated text in Chapter Twelve.
6. Livescience website, "What is Science and the Scientific Method?" http://www.livescience.com/20896-science-scientific-method.html, accessed 24 July 2014.
7. Rupert Sheldrake, *The Science Delusion: Freeing the Spirit of Enquiry*, London: Hodder and Stoughton, 2012, p. 292.
8. Rupert Sheldrake, *The Science Delusion: Freeing the Spirit of Enquiry*, London: Hodder and Stoughton, 2012, p. 293.
9. Definition of propaganda, Oxford Dictionaries, http://www.oxforddictionaries.com/definition/english/propaganda, accessed 23 July 2014.
10. Richard Alan Nelson, A Chronology and Glossary of Propaganda in the United States, Greenwood, 1996, pps. 232-233.
11. Gareth S. Jowett & Victoria J. O'Donnell, *Propaganda and Persuasion*, Sage Publications, 2011.
12. K. Arens, "Wilhelm Griesinger: Psychiatry between Philosophy and Praxis", *Philosophy, Psychiatry & Psychology*, 1996; 3(3):147-163.
13. Elliot Valenstein, *Blaming the Brain: The Truth about Drugs and Mental Health*. New York: Free Press, 1998, p. 220.

14. Joanna Moncrieff, "Psychiatric drug promotion and the politics of neoliberalism, *The British Journal of Psychiatry* (2006) 188: 301-302 doi: 10.1192/bjp.188.4.301, http://bjp.rcpsych.org/content/188/4/301.full, accessed 11 May 2014.

15. Peter Breggin & David Cohen, *Your Drug May Be Your Problem: How and Why to Stop Taking Psychiatric Medications,* Da Capo Press, 2007.

16. Joanna Moncrieff, *The Myth of the Chemical Cure: A Critique of Psychiatric Drug Treatment,* Basingstoke: Palgrave Macmillan, 2009, p. 62.

17. Edward Shorter, *How Everyone Became Depressed*, Oxford: Oxford University Press, 2013, p. 160.

18. Wisegeek website, "What is Hegemony?", http://www.wisegeek.org/what-is-hegemony. htm, accessed 01 May 2014.

19. Michael Goldberg, "Hegemony", https://faculty.washington.edu/mlg/courses/definitions /hegemony.html, accessed 04 May 2014.

20. *New York Times*, "Hegemony", 01 May 2008, http://www.nytimes.com/2008/05/01/ news/01iht - 30oxan.12491269.html, accessed 04 May 2014.

21. M. Creswell, "Psychiatric 'survivors' and testimonies of self-harm", *Soc Sci Med.* 2005 Oct; 61(8): 1668-77. Epub 2005 April 22.

22. Ben Goldacre, "Bad Science: Depression—the facts and the fables", *The Guardian*, 26 January 2008, http://www.theguardian. com/commentisfree/2008/jan/26/badscience, accessed 29 December 2013.

23. Robert Whitaker, *Anatomy of an Epidemic: Magic Bullets, Psychiatric Drugs and the Astonishing Rise of Mental Illness in America,* New York: Random House, 2010.

24. David Kaiser, "Against Biologic Psychiatry", *Psychiatric Times*, December 1996, Vol. XIII, Issue 12.

25. Lucy Johnstone, *Users and Abusers of Psychiatry: A Critical Look at Psychiatric Practice,* Second Edition, London: Routledge, 2000, p. 212.

26. Sharon Begley, "Some Drugs Work To Treat Depression, But It Isn't Clear How", *Wall Street Journal*, 18 November 2005, http://www.mindfreedom.org/kb/psych-drug-corp/ fraud/more-media-articles-about-fraud-in-psychiatric-drug-ads, accessed 07 May 2014.

27. Grace Jackson, *Rethinking Psychiatric Drugs: A Guide for Informed Consent,* Bloomington: Authorhouse, 2005, p. 84.

28. Elliot Valenstein, *Blaming the Brain: The Truth about Drugs and Mental Health,* New York: Free Press, 1998, p. 148.

29. The Free Dictionary definition of sophistry, http://www.thefreedictionary.com/sophistry, accessed 23 July 2014.

30. Robert Krause, "Depression, antidepressants and an examination of epidemiological changes", Spring 2005, radicalpsychiatry.org website, http://www.radicalpsychology.org /vol4-1/krause. html, accessed 24 May 2014.

15. FUTURE DELUSIONS

While the majority of the public remain convinced that brain chemical imbalances are a known characteristic of depression, it has become increasingly clear to many psychiatrists and drug companies that the days of being able to keep the public persuaded on this issue are numbered. While in their offices and in public many doctors continue to misinform people that depression is characterised by a chemical brain deficiency, there has been a decrease in the promotion of this idea in recent years. This has happened because no evidence has been found to verify the theory, and the weight of evidence against it has become so strong. In recent years, the leaders of psychiatry have been searching for new bright ideas to replace the old ones.

Having been so wrong about the biochemical imbalance notion, one might expect that in the public interest the medical profession would inform the public of this error with a level of emphasis similar to that given to the promotion of this misinformation over a fifty-year period. This has not happened. Instead, the leaders of psychiatric thinking have been quietly shifting their focus from brain chemical abnormalities to other biological notions. They change the detail while maintaining the fundamental aspects of the depression delusion; that depression is a genetically inherited brain disease characterised by brain abnormalities. Indeed many have attempted to present this shift in emphasis as evidence of progress, a clever trick indeed. By doing so, mainstream psychiatry seeks to quietly move on from the biochemical imbalance debacle without people noticing, minimising the awkward questions that might follow if the public really knew what was going on. Mainstream psychiatrists also buy themselves more time, by convincing governments and the public that they are indeed progressing, whereas in fact they are just looking for a different needle within the same biological haystack.

In a 2006 editorial in the *British Journal of Psychiatry*, psychiatrist Joanna Moncrieff correctly described the brain biochemical imbalance idea as an example of the long-standing psychiatric belief that psychiatric diagnoses are fundamentally biological abnormalities:

> This idea is a popular version of the longstanding psychiatric model of mental disorder as arising from potentially identifiable deviations from "normal" biological functioning. [1]

As with all previous biological notions, the brain chemical imbalance idea will be replaced by other new notions when the current concept becomes more of a liability than an advantage, provided there is an exciting new idea or two waiting in the wings to take its place. The primary idea—that depression is a fundamentally biological illness—does not change, nor will it as long as mainstream psychiatry is in charge, since psychiatry's dominant position in mental health is dependent upon it.

A great new idea is needed to sustain belief in the massive industry that depression as a biological illness has become, to replace the brain chemical imbalance idea that has become jaded and torpedoed by truth.

THE DELUSION IS DYING, LONG LIVE THE NEXT DELUSIONS

Vested interests groups, principally the pharmaceutical industry, mainstream psychiatry and to a lesser extent general practitioners have used their position, power and money to resist those who have questioned the chemical imbalance delusion for the past fifty years. It has become increasingly difficult in recent years to defend the indefensible, due largely to the courage and persistence of those who have spoken out and the equalizing effect the internet has provided by making information more readily available.

Many doctors and drug companies realize that the chemical imbalance notion in depression is living on borrowed time. These powerful players have a major vested interest in the public continuing to believe that depression is a biological disease. As Dorothy Rowe observed in relation to the Royal College of Psychiatrists, [2] many doctors have stopped talking and writing about chemical imbalances in depression, without alerting the public of this shift in their position.

This change does not represent a full and open consideration of all possible causes and characteristics of depression. It is a move away from a delusion that has become increasingly porous to new ones that allow those in power to start the delusional cycle all over again. This shift will steer well clear of the type of approach I discussed in chapter four. If successful, it will buy the medical profession and pharmaceutical industry another ten to twenty years. A key priority of the medical profession and drug companies is to keep the sleeping giant that is public opinion on side, that is, to keep the public believing that (a) depression is fundamentally a biological issue, and (b) the public is best served by continuing to entrust doctors and drug companies with ultimate responsibility for its resolution. If this situation were to continue, it would be a very serious mistake as far as the public interest—and the welfare of the considerable number of vulnerable people who experience great distress—is concerned.

In recent years, the emphasis has moved somewhat from the brain chemical imbalance notion to genetic causation and other ideas. I address genetics and depression in my next book, which should be available within a year of this publication. The change in emphasis is already under way, being heralded and flagged in various media publications. According to one such article which appeared in the *Boston Globe* in 2008, titled "Head fake: How Prozac sent the science of depression in the wrong direction":

> In recent years scientists have developed a novel theory of what falters in the depressed brain. Instead of seeing the disease as the result of a chemical imbalance these researchers argue that the brain's cells are shrinking and dying. This theory has gained momentum in the past few months, with the publication of several high profile scientific papers. The effectiveness of Prozac, these scientists say, has

little to do with the amount of serotonin in the brain. Rather, the drug works because it helps heal our neurons, allowing them to grow and thrive again . . . In this sense, Prozac is simply a bottled version of other activities that have a similar effect, such as physical exercise. They are not happy pills, but healing pills. These discoveries are causing scientists to fundamentally reimagine depression. [3]

The article referred to the words of psychiatrist Ronald Duman:

"The best way to think about depression is as a mild degenerative disorder", says Ronald Duman, a professor of psychiatry and pharmacology at Yale. "Your brain cells atrophy, just like in other diseases—such as Alzheimer's and Parkinson's. The only difference with depression is that it's reversible. The brain can recover".

The author of the article continued:

Given the prevalence of depression, a more accurate scientific understanding of the disease is of immense value. In fact, research is already being used to develop more effective treatments for the mental illness, some of which are currently in clinical trials.

Many concerns arise from this article. The title itself is misleading. Prozac did not send "the science of depression in the wrong direction"; enthusiastic and zealous medical researchers, psychiatrists and drug companies did. The use of the term "the science of depression" conveys an impression of scientific practice and endeavour in relation to depression that is not supported by the evidence. The article's statement that "scientists have developed a novel theory of what falters in the depressed brain" contains a subtle but enormous assumption. Since it has not been scientifically established that anything "falters in the depressed brain", any claim that is based on this inappropriate assumption is a Begging the Question logical fallacy. [4]

The fact that the idea that brain cells are "shrinking and dying" in depression "has gained momentum" and that "several high profile scientific papers" have been published proves nothing other than a growing interest in the theory. The chemical imbalance theory has had immense momentum for over thirty years. Thousands of high profile scientific papers have been written about it. Yet the chemical imbalance theory remains utterly unproven and discredited scientifically.

According to this article, scientists now maintain that "the effectiveness of Prozac has little to do with the amount of serotonin in the brain. Rather, the drug works because it helps heal our neurons, allowing them to grow and thrive again". The shift away from serotonin is presented as though it is a major advance, whereas it is merely a move from one theory to another. Stating that the drug works to "heal our neurons, allowing them to grow and thrive again" is a remarkable claim filled with wishful thinking. There is no evidence that people's neurons are damaged in depression to begin with. The claim that "Prozac is simply a bottled version of other activities that have a similar effect, such as physical exercise" is clearly questionable, a Weak Analogy logical fallacy. [5] To compare taking a chemical that interferes with brain function to such a natural activity as exercise is not appropriate, but it will likely appear convincing to many readers.

Claims made in the article that antidepressants "aren't happy pills, but healing pills. These discoveries are causing scientists to reimagine depression" merit scrutiny. There is no evidence that antidepressants are "healing pills". This shift in emphasis is not a "discovery". It is not "these discoveries" that are "causing scientists to reimagine depression", but the fact that the chemical imbalance theory is reaching the end of the line. If another convincing theory is not found to take its place, psychiatry and drug companies will find themselves in an awkward position, having millions of people taking substances for which no convincing though bogus rationale of action exists. The author's use of the phrase "to reimagine depression" is interesting, and very accurate. That is precisely what these scientists are doing. They are reimagining and reframing their theories of depression, but only within an overall biological framework of depression. All the reimagining in the world has no true scientific validity unless it is backed up by hard evidence, which does not exist for any biological theory of depression, old or new.

The quotes in this article attributed to Ronald Duman, a professor of psychiatry and pharmacology at Yale University, are very problematic: "The best way to think about depression is as a mild degenerative disorder. Your brain cells atrophy, just like in other diseases—such as Alzheimer's and Parkinson's. The only difference with depression is that it's reversible. The brain can recover". Readers are likely to believe these words since they originate from a perceived expert. Any person who does believe these comments has been seriously misinformed. No scientific evidence verifies the notion that "depression is a mild degenerative disorder". Not one of the many medical textbooks I refer to in this book provide any evidence that verifies this claim. In my next book, I look in detail at claims that depression is a disease and a genetic disorder. I have already carried out detailed research for that book. The evidence does not support claims that in depression "your brain cells atrophy, just like in other diseases such as Alzheimer's and Parkinson's diseases". I believe it is very wrong for any perceived expert to make such claims as thought they were facts when in truth they are unsubstantiated theories. These claims are classic Weak Analogy logical fallacies. [6] Duman's assertion that "The best way to think about depression is as a mild degenerative disorder" requires some adjustment. This is not *the* best way to think about depression; it is *his* best way, his preferred way. It is a way of thinking about depression that is attractive to many, including primarily biologically-focused psychiatrists, which the majority of psychiatrists are in practice. But there is no reliable scientific evidence that verifies this claim.

According to this article, "Given the prevalence of depression, a more accurate scientific understanding of the disease is of immense value." It does not seem to have occurred to the author that the substitution of one unevidenced theory for another does not constitute "a more accurate understanding". Such commentaries inadvertently become part of a broader attempt to generate a new marketing strategy when the credibility of the old one is no longer sustainable.

THE NATIONAL INSTITUTE OF MENTAL HEALTH FORGES AHEAD

The American National Institute of Mental Health is perhaps the world's most powerful and influential mental health organization. In recent years the leadership of the National Institute of Mental Health has been attempting to spearhead a shift in thinking about depression, from the biochemical brain imbalance notion toward other ways of imagining depression. The underlying assumption that depression is fundamentally a biological condition remains sacrosanct and unquestioned.

Psychiatrist Thomas Insel has been Director of the U.S. National Institute of Mental Health since 2002. Insel is therefore one of the most influential figures in mental health in the world. During his tenure as head of this agency, Insel has championed a biological perspective on mental illness. According to Insel in a presentation to psychiatrists in 2011:

> We can think of mental disorders not just as brain disorders but as disorders of neural circuits. [7]

We can think anything we like about anything. Our thinking does not make the content of our thought any more real, although we may delude ourselves that it does. There is no solid scientific evidence that so-called mental disorders are "disorders of neural circuits". The following is an extract from an American Psychiatric Association report on Thomas Insel's 2011 presentation: [8]

> Insel told psychiatrists at the meeting that psychiatric diagnosis today is made by observation of symptoms, detection of illness is late, prediction of illness is poor, etiology (cause) is unknown, and treatment is trial and error. There are no cures and no vaccines.

This is an accurate reflection of the state of psychiatry and psychiatric practice. Out of the ashes of this dismal picture, Insel promised all manner of wondrous developments within psychiatry:

> But that will change. Psychiatric research today promises to produce a true science of the brain based on three core principles:
> Mental disorders are brain disorders.
> Mental disorders are developmental disorders.
> Mental disorders result from complex genetic risk plus experiential factors. [9]

These claims are very problematic. Arguably the world's most influential psychiatrist is prepared to "promise" that research will deliver a host of wonderful discoveries. One cannot and should not "promise" that the outcome of research will yield results favoured by the researchers. Psychiatric research is not something that is just beginning. For over a century, psychiatrists have been relentlessly seeking to identify the very discoveries that Insel promises will happen as a result of psychiatric research, with little success.

Though not uncommon within psychiatry, Insel's logic and reasoning is questionable. He is willing to claim that "mental disorders are brain disorders" is a "core principle" of "psychiatric research today". But what he terms "mental disorders" have *not* been identified to be brain disorders. Like many of his colleagues, this director of the National Institute of Mental Health has apparently convinced himself that something which is in truth a major assumption is instead a fact, a "core principle". I have provided many examples of Begging the Question logical fallacies in this book. This one, by such a senior and influential figure in world mental health, is a most serious Begging the Question logical fallacy. [10]

In a 2005 article, Thomas Insel and fellow psychiatrist Remi Quirion set out their vision for psychiatry. It is a vision infused with wishful and limited thinking. The hope of the authors is that, as a consequence of some future wonderful discoveries, psychiatry will "emerge once again as the most compelling and intellectually challenging medical specialties" and be "integrated into the mainstream of medicine".[11] These comments reveal a major investment of hope by the authors. Truly objective scientists have no such investment in the outcome. They are dispassionate regarding the outcome of the Scientific Method as it is applied to their hypothesis. Clearly, these very important authors are not impartial, since they see their preferred outcomes as delivering the redemption of psychiatry. The authors' opening line read:

> One of the fundamental insights emerging from contemporary neuroscience is that mental illnesses are brain disorders. [12]

One might expect that these leading psychiatrists would understand the meaning of the word "insight". The Merriam-Webster Dictionary defines insight as:

> An understanding of the true nature of something . . . the ability to understand people and situations in a very clear way. [13]

These psychiatrists claimed that "mental illnesses are definitely brain disorders" is now a "fundamental insight"; a *fact*. Believing in something for which there is no credible solid evidence cannot be legitimately referred to as an insight. Since there is no credible scientific evidence that confirms mental illnesses to be brain disorders, concluding that they are indeed brain disorders is an *assumption*, and certainly not an *insight*. Such basic distortions of truth, whether intentional or unintentional, are rife within psychiatry. This is yet another major Begging the Question logical fallacy. [14] All of these falsehoods and distortions of truth have one thing in common; they all paint a positive picture of psychiatry, making psychiatry appear more scientific than it actually is.

What if mental disorders are not brain disorders? This very real possibility has been totally discounted by Insel and the others, though not because it is not a legitimate possibility. It is discounted because it does not fit into the medical wish list, and because many doctors have such limited vision that they cannot conceive mental disorders as anything but biological brain disorders. Indeed, serious societal consideration of the very real possibility that depression is not a biological "mental illness", but rather an understandable and largely psychic set of experiences and behaviours—that is, primarily emotional and psychological but with physical aspects also—could be disastrous for mainstream psychiatry and the pharmaceutical industry. This is because these powerful groups have invested their identity and modus operandi in a predominantly biological understanding and approach. Little wonder then that mainstream psychiatry does not exactly encourage debate, apart from that which takes the assumed biological basis of depression as a given.

According to a 2012 article on the American Psychological Association website, Thomas Insel believes that the diagnosis and treatment of mental illness today is where other specialties such as cardiology were 100 years ago: "Like cardiology of yesteryear, the field is poised for dramatic transformation, he says." Interviewed for this article, Insel enthused:

> We are really at the cusp of a revolution in the way we think about the brain and behaviour, partly because of technological breakthroughs. We're finally able to answer some of the fundamental questions. [15]

One might not expect the words from a world leader in mental health to contain flaws and misinformation. Insel's belief that "We are really at the cusp of a revolution in the way we think about the brain and behaviour, partly because of technological breakthroughs" bears little resemblance to reality. No more than the rest of us, Thomas Insel is not able to predict the future. His claim that "we are on a cusp of a revolution" is utter conjecture, but it keeps people happy and on side. Such grandiose claims from within psychiatry are not uncommon and not new. The truth is that we are no nearer than we were thirty years ago when another major international figure in mental health—Insel's fellow psychiatrist Nancy Andreasen—unequivocally claimed in her 1984 book *The Broken Brain: The Biological Revolution in Psychiatry* that:

> The biological revolution has already occurred. [16]

Such claims of biological revolutions in psychiatry create a veneer of real science and progress, buying time, public trust and funding for mainstream psychiatry. They are just some of the many examples of superlatives that are regularly used by supporters of a biological understanding of depression. They are also examples of William Shakespeare's famous "she doth protest too much" quote from his play *Hamlet*. In other medical specialties, where a solid body of evidence of organic disease is well established, specialists do not have to attempt to convince the public of the authenticity of their work and their approach to it. The absence of evidence of any biological abnormalities in depression and other psychiatric diagnoses repeatedly tempts psychiatrists and general practitioners to overstate and exaggerate in order to compensate for their actual lack of true tangible scientific progress during the past fifty years.

Insel's statement that "We're finally able to answer some of the fundamental questions" is both revealing and incorrect. It is revealing because it is an admission of psychiatry's failure to answer any "fundamental questions" up to now. It is incorrect and misleading because psychiatry is still unable to answer any fundamental questions regarding the biology of depression. As Insel's fellow psychiatrist Edward Shorter has acknowledged:

> Psychiatric illness has tended to be classified on the basis of symptoms rather than causes, which was where the rest of medicine was in the nineteenth century. [17]

Psychiatrist Helen Mayberg M.D. is somewhat less optimistic about the state of psychiatry that her influential colleague Thomas Insel. Interviewed for the same article in which Insel made the above claims, Mayberg acknowledged:

> Syndromes are so nonspecific by our current criteria that the best we can do is flip a coin. We don't do that for any other branch of medicine. [18]

The following assertion by James Hunter and the National Institute of Mental Health from an article currently on the Psych Central website is another example of the National Institute of Mental Health's extravagant claims of new discoveries in depression:

> Recent advances in research technology are bringing National Institute of Mental Health scientists closer than ever before to characterizing the biology and physiology of depression in its different forms and to identifying effective treatments for individuals based on symptom presentation. [19]

This passage conveys some very misleading impressions. The author is greatly exaggerating the impact of research technology. By writing "closer than ever", the public are being misled into thinking that research has been close to the answers for quite some time and is even closer to those answers now. This is simply not true. The "biology and physiology of depression" remains as much of a mystery now as it was half a century ago, perhaps even more so now as the extraordinary complexity of the human brain has become increasingly apparent. Medical research is nowhere near characterising the biology and physiology of depression or understanding its significance. The last few words of this passage are revealing. According to the author, the hope is that effective treatments will be found "based on symptom presentation". Since for fifty years the search for effective treatments has largely revolved around symptom presentation, this statement contains no new information. One of the many weaknesses of the depression disease notion is that it is based almost entirely on symptoms, which is not how any other medical speciality operates.

In a 2013 article posted in the National Institute of Mental Health website, the article's author—Thomas Insel again—enthused about the latest new great hope, Research Domain Criteria. The importance of this notion to Thomas Insel is illustrated by the article title; "Director's Blog: Transforming Diagnosis". It is an example of the pattern in psychiatry to substitute a new idea in place of an older idea that is no longer tenable as a persuasive argument. This fledgling new idea, which few readers will have heard of, is the National Institute of Mental Health's next new big thing:

Research Domain Criteria is, for now, a research framework, not a clinical tool. This is a decade-long project that is just beginning. [20]

In this passage, I believe that Insel sought to buy more time and more funding for the National Institute of Mental Health, since this is a "decade-long project that is just beginning". As is often the case with psychiatrists, Insel makes remarkable claims regarding the outcome of this project:

Patients and families should welcome this as a first step toward "precision medicine", the movement that has transformed cancer diagnosis and treatment. Research Domain Criteria is nothing less than a plan to transform clinical practice to bring a new generation of research to inform how we diagnose and treat mental disorders. [21]

By inferring that this new and unproven initiative will lead to "precision medicine" within psychiatry, the National Institute of Mental Health's Thomas Insel has made a giant leap of faith. If Insel and his colleagues are sufficiently persuasive, this new initiative will buy the National Institute of Mental Health and the medical profession at least another ten years of acceptance and credibility within the general public. These are remarkable claims indeed, but they are probably seductive enough to secure funding for ten years. These claims also ensure that the illusion that psychiatry will definitely provide the answers is maintained for at least another decade; yet another ten years within which properly considering other possible understandings apart from the prevailing biological one does not happen.

The Research Domain Criteria concept has currently no solid scientific evidence to support it. According to Insel and the National Institute of Mental Health:

It became immediately clear that we cannot design a system based on biomarkers or cognitive performance because we lack the data. We need to begin collecting the genetic, imaging, physiologic and cognitive data to see how all the data cluster and how these clusters relate to treatment response. [22]

This is being presented as if collecting the necessary data is a wonderful new idea that they have suddenly discovered. Every third year medical student knows that collecting such data is fundamental to the operation of every area of medicine. There are no substantive genetic, imaging, physiologic or cognitive data specific to any so-called mental illness. If such data existed, those who formulated the 2013 *The Diagnostic and Statistical Manual of Mental Disorders-5* (the *DSM-5*) would undoubtedly have included it, since any such data would have strengthened the highly questioned credibility of the *DSM-5*.

Thomas Insel has made some interesting pronouncements in his time. At the American Psychiatric Association's annual conference in 2004, Insel told his audience that the psychiatrist's bible, the *Diagnostic and Statistical Manual of Mental Disorders* had zero percent validity. He told the conference:

Brain imaging in clinical practice is the next major advance in psychiatry. Trial-and-error diagnosis will move to an era where we understand the underlying biology of mental disorders. We need to identify biomarkers, including brain imaging, to develop the validity of these disorders. We need to develop treatments that go after the core pathology, understood by imaging. The end game is get to an era of individualized care. [23]

The certainty with which Insel and others put forward their convictions is striking. We *will* move to this era. We *will* find these biomarkers. We *know* there an "underlying biology", we just have not found it yet. We *know* the outcome, or at least we have convinced ourselves regarding what the outcome will be. We just haven't managed to join up the dots regarding how to get there. But what if there are no biological markers? What if there are no dots, or if the dots are very different from those assumed by Insel and others? The radar of mainstream psychiatry is only designed to identify biology. What if the dots are largely emotional and psychological rather than biological?

In commentaries about the future of psychiatry and mental health, both Insel and his predecessor as director of the U.S. National Institute of Mental Health are united in their primary focus on biology. In a 2013 interview, Thomas Insel said that his goal was to reshape the direction of psychiatric research to focus on biology, genetics and neuroscience. [24] Insel neglected to mention that psychiatric research has primarily focused on biology, genetics and neuroscience for over 50 years, and that this focus has to date yielded no reliable evidence regarding biology or biomarkers in relation to psychiatric diagnoses. Also in a 2013 interview, Insel's predecessor as Director of the National Institute of Mental Health, neuroscientist Steven Hyman said:

Our best hope is that the genetics will unfold over the next several years, due to the efforts of large international consortia that have formed to recruit and to study patients. [25]

If genetics really is "our best hope", then perhaps we should not get our hopes up, since genetics in mental health have been studied intensely for half a century without any breakthroughs. It is more accurate to describe genetics as Steven Hyman's and mainstream psychiatry's best hope. It certainly isn't mine.

Meanwhile, scant attention is given to what is right there in front of these doctors and researchers but regularly missed. The person, and the context of their life and life story, their emotional and psychological pain and distress, their woundedness, loss of self and the defence mechanisms they utilise to get by in life, all contain valuable indicators of what is wrong and how the situation might be remedied. These key issues are regularly missed by the medical radar system that is designed primarily to pick up anything that might point to physical or biological answers.

Notes to Chapter Fifteen

1. Joanna Moncrieff, "Psychiatric drug promotion and the politics of neoliberalism", *British Journal of Psychiatry*, 2006, 188: 301-302 doi: 10.1192/bjp.188.4.301, http://bjp.rcpsych.org/ content/188 /4/301.full, accessed 11 May 2014.
2. See note 54 in the notes to chapter two and the associated text for Dorothy Rowe's comments on the removal of references to biochemical imbalances from the Royal College of Psychiatrists' website.
3. Jonah Lehrer, "Head fake: How Prozac sent the science of depression in the wrong direction", *Boston Globe*, 06 July 2008, http://www.boston.com/bostonglobe/ideas/articles/ 2008/07/06/ head_fake/, accessed 09 May 2014.
4. For information on Begging the Question logical fallacies see note 22 in the Notes to the Introduction.
5. For information on Weak Analogy logical fallacies see note 69 in the Notes to Chapter Five.
6. For information on Weak Analogy logical fallacies see note 69 in the Notes to Chapter Five.
7 Thomas Insel, "Rethinking Mental Illness", 2011 American Psychiatric Association annual meeting, Honolulu, 14 May 2011.
8. "'Psychiatry on Verge of New World', Says NIMH Director", 17 May 2011, in *Psychiatric News Alert: The Voice of the American Psychiatric Association and the Psychiatric Community*, http://alert.psychiatricnews.org/2011_05_01_archive.html, accessed 20 August 2014.
9. "'Psychiatry on Verge of New World', Says NIMH Director", 17 May 2011, in *Psychiatric News Alert: The Voice of the American Psychiatric Association and the Psychiatric Community*, http://alert.psychiatricnews.org/2011_05_01_archive.html, accessed 20 August 2014.
10. For information on Begging the Question logical fallacies see note 22 in the Notes to the Introduction.
11. Thomas Insel & Remi Quirion, "Psychiatry as a Clinical Neuroscience Discipline", *Journal of the American Medical Association* 294, no. 17, 2005, 2221-24.
12. Thomas Insel & Remi Quirion, "Psychiatry as a Clinical Neuroscience Discipline", *Journal of the American Medical Association* 294, no. 17, 2005, 2221-24.
13. The Merriam-Webster Dictionary definition of insight, http://www.merriam-webster.com/ dictionary/insight, accessed 20 August 2014.
14. For information on Begging the Question logical fallacies see note 22 in the Notes to the Introduction.
15. In Kirsten Weir, "The Roots of Mental Illness", American Psychological Association website, June 2012, Vol. 43, No. 6, http://www.apa.org/monitor/2012/06/roots.aspx, access-ed 15 April 2014.
16. Nancy Andreasen, *The Broken Brain: The Biological Revolution in Psychiatry*, New York: Harper & Row, 1984, p. viii.
17. Edward Shorter, *A History of Psychiatry: From the Era of the Asylum to the Age of Prozac*, New York: John Wiley, 1997, p. 296.
18. In Kirsten Weir, "The Roots of Mental Illness", American Psychological Association website, June 2012, Vol. 43, No. 6, http://www.apa.org/monitor/2012/06/roots.aspx, accessed 15 April 2014.
19. James Hunter & NIMH, "Research on Depression", http://psychcentral.com/disorders /depressionresearch.htm, accessed 15 April 2014.
20. Thomas Insel, "Transforming Diagnosis", 29 April 2013, http://www.nimh.nih.gov/about/ director/2013/transforming-diagnosis.shtml, accessed 15 April 2014.
21. Thomas Insel, "Transforming Diagnosis", 29 April 2013, http://www.nimh.nih.gov/about/ director/2013/transforming-diagnosis.shtml, accessed 15 April 2014.
22. Thomas Insel, "Transforming Diagnosis", 29 April 2013, http://www.nimh.nih.gov/about/ director/2013/transforming-diagnosis.shtml, accessed 15 April 2014.
23. D. G. Amen, *Healing the Hardwire of the Soul*, New York: Free Press, 2002.
24. Pam Belluck & Benedict Carey, "Psychiatry's Guide Is Out Of Touch With Science, Experts Say", *The New York Times*, 06 May 2013, http://www.nytimes.com/2013/05/07/health/psychiatrys-new-guide-falls-short-experts-say.html?pagewanted=all

25. Steven Hyman, "Psychiatric Drug Development: Diagnosing a Crisis", The Dana Foundation website, 02 April 2013, http://www.dana.org/cerebrum/2013/psychiatric_drug_development _diagnosing_a_crisis/.

16. THE CONSEQUENCES OF THE DEPRESSION CHEMICAL IMBALANCE DELUSION

There are many flaws within the medical understanding of depression, including its failure to provide anything other than a superficial and distorted understanding of depression. Tenaciously holding on to the biochemical brain imbalance falsehood is both an example and a consequence of this. Convinced by repeated authoritative statements from trusted figures, organizations and institutions, the general public's belief in the depression chemical imbalance delusion is understandable. Most people are unaware that this delusion keeps the understanding of depression at a surface level, a cul-de-sac upon which one inevitably runs out of road. Seeking a deeper understanding of the emotional and psychological aspects of depression is generally not encouraged, indeed it is often frowned upon. This artificial floor is where medical interest largely stops. It is not surprising that the interest of many members of the public stops there too.

The medical understanding of depression is by its very nature incomplete. The limited medical definition and understanding of depression has no space for many of the experiences that become swept into the domain of depression. The significance of these experiences is missed. Instead, they are reframed into the medical model rather than being seen for what they are in themselves. Their significance and meaning is usually either regularly missed or dismissed as irrelevant. The important clues they often provide are regularly missed because the experience itself is either misinterpreted or missed completely. Consequently, many recipients of a diagnosis of and treatment for depression are little wiser regarding what is happening to and within them. Often, the only piece of information they have been given—that their brain chemicals are low—is a falsehood.

Medicalizing experiences as evidence of a mental illness called depression caused by brain chemical imbalances disempowers many members of the general public from contributing to a better understanding of the experiences that have become known as depression. Translating and reframing the situation into the language of medicine rather than plain English keeps the subject elitist, beyond the understanding and input of the general public. It becomes more difficult for members of the public to examine depression for themselves or to question the experts on an equal footing. Potentially enlightening areas of knowledge and ideas such as philosophy, the humanities, sociology, psychology and psychotherapy are excluded from having any meaningful input into the debate about what depression really is. Most people defer to doctors and to the medical view as being the only real credible view because it is incorrectly claimed to be so scientific.

We may have collectively become comfortable with the medicalization of human experience and the creation of the depression brain chemical delusion, but that does not make the situation benign or without consequences. In their 2005 book *Depression: An Emotion not a Disease*, psychiatrist Michael Corry and GP Aine Tubridy described the major significance of so doing:

The moment depression is classified as a disease, the medical community, and then the public, seem to lose all clarity and become as duped as the hounds, and a wrong turn is taken. Once called a disease, a cure is called for. In this way it becomes a defining straitjacket in which the depressed person has to function. Diseases do not have meanings, therefore none are sought. By placing it solely within the realm of imbalanced chemistry, we distance it from the problems of living, lack of resources and our human responses, which are the primary cause. We have been misled, and it is time to find our way back to a true understanding of depression. [1]

Almost twenty years earlier, psychiatrist David Kaiser expressed similar concerns:

This identification as a biologically-impaired patient is one of the most destructive effects of biologic psychiatry . . . Now, if you are depressed or anxious, it has no real meaning, because as a biological process similar to say diabetes, it is separate from the world of real meaning and merely is . . . Modern psychiatry, under the guise of medical and "scientific" authority and legitimacy, has surpassed all past attempts by psychiatry to identify and control dissent and individual difference. It has done this by infiltrating the cultural psyche, a psyche already vulnerable to any kind of medical discourse, to the point where it is a generally accepted cultural notion now that, say, depression is an illness caused by a chemical imbalance. Now, when a person becomes depressed, for example, they are less able to read it or interpret it as a sign that there may be a problem in their life that needs to be looked at and addressed. They are less able to question their life choices, or question for example the institutions that surround them. They are less able to fashion their own personal or cultural critique which could potentially lead them to more fruitful directions. Instead they identify themselves as ill and submit to the correction of a psychiatrist, who promised to take away the depression so they can get back to their lives as they are. In short, the very meanings of unhappiness are being redefined as illness. In my view this is a dismaying cultural catastrophe. I do not mean to suggest that psychiatry is solely to blame for this, given how wide a cultural shift this is. However, I do think that psychiatry has not only not resisted its role here, but has actually fulfilled it with considerable hubris. [2]

The psychiatric preoccupation with biology, exemplified in the dominance of the chemical imbalance misunderstanding of depression within the mental health field for fifty years, has long diminished the focus on the role of other issues such as psychological and social factors in depression. In a 2005 *Wall Street Journal* article, Sharon Begley described some of the consequences of this narrow and distorted focus:

Most people treated for depression get pills rather than psychotherapy, and this week a study from Stanford University reported that drugs have been supplanting psychotherapy for depressed adolescents, despite the acknowledged risks. Clinical guidelines call for using both, and for psychotherapy to be the first-line treatment for most kids. Psychotherapy "can be as effective as medications" for major depression, concluded a study in April of 240 patients, in the *Archives of General Psychiatry*. Numerous other studies find the same. [3]

As neuroscientist Elliot Valenstein wrote in his 1998 book *Blaming the Brain: The Truth About Drugs and Mental Health*:

> A reductionist approach that studies only the properties of organs, neurotransmitters, cells or atoms cannot understand consciousness and thought. Moreover, it is impossible to understand consciousness and thought without considering the psychosocial context that not only shapes the content of thought, but also the physical structure of the brain . . . There is an appropriate level at which to study a phenomenon, and a reductionist approach may miss the whole point, at least, the most important point. [4]

In 1998 psychiatrist Loren Mosher resigned from the American Psychiatric Association. Mosher trained in psychiatry at Harvard University and lectured in psychiatry at Yale. He was a Professor of Psychiatry at the University of California, San Diego. In his letter of resignation, Loren Mosher referred to psychiatric preoccupation with neurotransmitters and its consequences:

> No longer do we seek to understand whole persons in their social contexts. Rather we are there to realign their neurotransmitters. [5]

In 2000 psychiatrist Elio Fratteroli spoke at the American Psychiatric Association's 52nd Institute on Psychiatric Services. Fratteroli was then Assistant Professor of Psychiatry at the University of Pennsylvania. During his talk, Fratteroli lamented the consequences of the dominance of biological emphasis in psychiatry, the brain chemical imbalance notion in particular:

> Over the last quarter century there has been a dramatic erosion of psychotherapeutic training and practice in psychiatry, caused largely by a change in our philosophical beliefs. Psychopharmacology has replaced psychotherapy because brain has replaced soul—i.e., chemical balance has replaced inner conflict—as the philosophical basis for psychiatric explanation. We no longer consider it important to trouble ourselves with the inner lives of our patients—the nuances of thought, feeling, impulse, and imagery in their minds and souls. We consider these private experiences that are of such deep concern to our patients to be largely irrelevant to their symptoms and personality problems, which we believe are caused directly by chemical imbalances in the brain. [6]

The aforementioned 2002 address to the Rocky Mountain Psychological Association in Park City, Utah, titled "Hook, Line and Sinker: Psychology's Uncritical Acceptance of Biological Explanation" by psychologists Professor Brent D. Slife and Dr. Colin M. Burchfield Ph.D. and psychiatrist Associate Professor Dawson W. Hedges, contained great concern regarding the consequences of the excessive focus on biology in mental health:

> Our uncritical adoption of the materialism of the natural sciences has come at an incredible price. Some of the most important aspects of our lives are not biological, at least not biological exclusively. [7]

Many psychiatrists claim that they use a bio-psycho-social approach, in which the person's biological, psychological and social states are of equal importance. In practice, the vast majority of people treated by psychiatrists experience primarily a biological approach, with little in-depth focus on the psychological and social aspects of their existence. The dominant position of the brain chemical imbalance delusion as the fundamental issue in depression has contributed greatly to this regrettable situation. When the head of the American Psychiatric Association speaks out against psychiatric practice, there is clearly a problem. In 2005, then president of the American Psychiatric Association Dr. Steven S. Sharfstein wrote:

> We must examine the fact that, as a profession, we have allowed the biopsychosocial model to become the bio-bio-bio-model. In a time of economic constraint, a "pill and an appointment" has dominated treatment. [8]

In his 2008 book *Music and Madness*, Irish psychiatrist and former professor of psychiatry at University College Dublin, Professor Emeritus Ivor Browne described the potentially malignant effect of the brain chemical imbalance delusion:

> If you believe there is such an entity as clinical depression that is biochemically determined, then there really is nothing the person himself can do to alleviate it. Now from a systems perspective, this is a lethal message. If self-organization is the essence of what it is to be healthy and alive, then to deprive a person of the very quality of being in control of himself is the worst thing that could be done to him. Yet this is what is happening every day of the week in psychiatric clinics. It is because of this, more than anything else, that many people are gradually led towards a pathway of illness. Seeing themselves as ill and helpless, they move imperceptibly into a state of chronic ill health. [9]

In his 1999 book *The Feeling Good Handbook*, American psychiatrist David Burns expressed similar concerns about the impact on patients of a brain chemical imbalance explanation for their problems:

> It may make at least some patients feel helpless—they may wrongly conclude that their depression results from chemical factors beyond their control that can only be treated with medications. This belief can act as a self-fulfilling prophecy. If you do not try to cope with the stressful events that may have triggered your depression, it is not likely that you will identify and resolve your problems. [10]

Psychiatrist Vivek Datta set out some major consequences of erroneously concluding that depression is caused by brain chemical abnormalities:

> Like the black unicorn, we have cultivated a dangerous mythology in the promotion of the notion that mental illnesses are due to chemical imbalances . . . this level of explanation is unhelpful because it ignores what our feelings and experiences of living mean, and ignores the context in which we experience joy, love, anger and fear. By convincing individuals that their problems are due to chemical imbalances, we have succeeded not only in creating a generation who has recoded their moods and feelings into neurochemicals, we have undermined their ability to manage these problems themselves. Most troubling of all, the notion of chemical imbalances has transformed mental illnesses from temporary aberrations of mental states understandable in a particular context, to permanent disorders of the self embedded in the brain . . . If it is a chemical problem, then it is largely outside of one's control. The source of distress is no longer rooted in the fabric of society, interpersonal discord, a life story punctuated by loss, trauma and abuse, but it is located within the individual. It is located within the brain. Suddenly, the problem is no longer unemployment, widening inequality, social disadvantage, or alienation: the problem is you. [11]

EXAGGERATED HOPE

The notion that depression and our moods are governed by brain chemical abnormalities can be dressed up to sound quite positive. It may fit into people's pre-existing concept of illness. This notion may sound reassuring for two dubious reasons. It implies that doctors understand the brain a great deal better than they actually do. It also implies that these supposed biochemical brain abnormalities are eminently treatable, a message that has been reinforced consistently by the pharmaceutical industry and the medical profession since the arrival of the SSRIs in the late 1980s. In practice, the drugs have not lived up to these expectations.

When a person is told by a doctor that they have an illness called depression that is caused by a chemical imbalance similar to what happens in diabetes, and that the doctor can and will prescribe medication to correct this chemical imbalance, this can seem reassuring. The person is given the impression that their supposed illness can be treated successfully. This may engender some hope, for a while at least. As time passes, for many people this optimism may change to fear and despair. If the medication doesn't seem to work very well or only transiently, anxiety levels may rise. Already fearful and pessimistic, not getting better on drugs they have heard such positive things about heightens fear and anxiety. They may conclude that their condition is so bad that even the clever doctors and their powerful potions cannot help them. Even when their medication does help, many feel that the drug is the only possible reason they feel better. Many feel disempowered, believing that they are only being held together for as long as they are taking the medication that they have been told balances their brain chemistry. After all, if you have been either specifically told by your doctor that you have a brain chemical deficiency that requires rebalancing, or you have come to believe this over the years because you have repeatedly heard it in conversations or in the media, you will likely believe that your problem lies in your brain chemicals, something that you yourself have little power over or potential to correct. Your dependency on yourself—which may already be in a delicate and reduced state—is further eroded, while your dependency on external agencies such as doctors and medication grows stronger. Especially if this situation continues long-term, this approach works counter to recovery, since becoming gradually more self-reliant is a key aspect of the recovery process for most people. This growth of external dependence and internal disempowerment and its significance is often completely missed by many doctors, as is the increased sense of self-efficacy that accompanies working and coming through challenging times without resorting to drugs. This is often one of the benefits of psychotherapy.

WHO BENEFITS AND WHO LOSES

Whenever an idea which has no basis in fact becomes widely accepted as a fact within society, some people are generally benefitting and others are losing out. The depression delusion has created many winners—some very big winners—and many losers. That many of the same names and groups appear in this section as in the "A perfect storm" section in chapter eleven is no coincidence.

Pharmaceutical companies have been major beneficiaries of the depression delusion. Antidepressant manufacturers have benefitted enormously, particularly since launch of Prozac in the late 1980s. Drug companies have amassed vast amounts of money from the sale of antidepressants, well in excess of 250 billion dollars during the past thirty-five years.

Psychiatry too has been a major beneficiary of the depression delusion. The exponential growth in the diagnosis of depression and in its perception as a disease like any other has produced many enormous benefits for psychiatry and for psychiatrists. The societal acceptance of depression and other psychiatric diagnoses has legitimized psychiatrists as real doctors treating real diseases, specialists at an equal level to other medical specialists. The depression delusion has resulted in an exponential increase in the workload of psychiatry. It is with good reason that depression has been called psychiatry's "bread and butter". [12] The number of psychiatrists has increased greatly in most Western countries. Psychiatrists' salaries are on a par with other medical specialists. The widespread societal acceptance of the notion that depression and other psychiatric diagnoses has a biological basis has greatly helped to place and to keep psychiatry at the top of the mental health tree.

The medical profession is generally a conformist system in which hierarchy matters greatly. GPs have not benefitted from the depression brain chemical imbalance delusion as much as psychiatrists, but they have benefitted. Being lower on the medical ladder, generalists compared to psychiatric specialists, GPs have been willing to accept the pronouncements of psychiatrists as truth. Being trained primarily in the diagnosis and treatment of physical, biological diseases, GPs are generally far more comfortable with depression as a biologically based illness than as a state comprised of primarily emotional and psychological experiences and behaviours. They are more comfortable dealing with situations where the prescription pad comes into play. Their status has increased as a consequence of depression being seen as a brain chemical imbalance for which they can prescribe correctional treatment. As doctors, they are seen as being a great deal more expert at dealing with emotional and mental health problems than they actually are. The brain chemical imbalance depression delusion has considerably raised the profile of GPs in the mental health field.

The status of some therapists is increased. A "clinical" psychologist is generally seen as better placed to work with a "clinical" depression that a supposedly non-clinical therapist. The supposed disease status of depression has provided an understanding that is welcomed by some patients and family members, who feel relieved that it is not their fault. This line is often rolled out when claims of brain chemical imbalance are made; "it's not your—or our—fault, you have a brain chemical imbalance". Such claims are a False Dilemma logical fallacy. [13] As I discussed in chapter four, there are other more accurate ways of understanding depression than just these two options. It is also a Begging the Question logical fallacy, since the premise upon which such arguments are built—that people with depression have a brain chemical imbalance—is itself merely unproven and indeed disproven conjecture. [14]

Being able to blame faulty chemistry in their brains is for some people preferable to taking ownership of their situation and their recovery. For society in general, the depression delusion allows us to blame our brains for our distress. We can distance ourselves from our own painful feelings and those of others. Some people say that the medical approach has helped them.

There are many losses and losers also. Many people say that the prevailing psychiatric approach has held them back and hindered their progress. The problem we refer to as depression cannot be addressed properly as long as we remain deluded regarding what the problem actually is. The numbers being diagnosed, the knock-on effects on employment and disability and the supposed chronicity of depression are all increasing, despite all the focus and attention than depression has received for over thirty years. The problem is not the amount but the type of attention depression receives. As long as our approach to depression remains deluded, we can expect poor results and the ongoing societal burden to continue to increase. Some people do benefit from the current system and approach, but the overall approach depression instils little confidence. As Robert Whitaker commented in 2010:

> In a short span of forty years, depression has been utterly transformed. Prior to the arrival of the (SSRI) drugs, it had been a fairly rare disorder, and outcomes generally were good. Today, the National Institute of Mental Health informs the public that depressive disorders afflict one in ten Americans every year, and that the long-term outlook for those it strikes is glum. [15]

Informed consent is a core principle of medical practice. Legal experts Hill and Hill define informed consent as:

> An agreement to do something or to allow something to happen only after all the relevant facts are known. In contracts, an agreement may be reached only when there has been full disclosure by both parties of everything each party knows which is significant to the agreement. [16]

According to *West's Encyclopedia of American Law*, 2nd edition, informed consent is:

> The name for a fundamental principle of law that a physician has a duty to reveal what a reasonably prudent physician in the medical community employing reasonable care would reveal to a patient . . . This disclosure must be afforded so that a patient . . . can intelligently exercise judgement by reasonably balancing the probable risks against the probable benefits . . . assent to permit an occurrence . . . . that is based on a complete disclosure of facts needed to make the decision intelligently. [17]

The legal right of people to be accurately informed regarding medical practice and treatment is generally taken very seriously by doctors and patients alike. The medical profession's approach to placebo use and informed consent is a good example of this. A placebo is a substance which has no therapeutic effect by way of direct biochemical action on the health problem in question, but may have a positive psychological impact on the person. The American Medical Association's position on placebos and informed consent is very clear. The use of a placebo is strictly prohibited unless the patient is informed that they are receiving a placebo, the details of placebo action and effectiveness are accurately explained to the patient, and being thus fully informed the patient agrees to take the placebo. In 2008 the American Medical Association published a report on placebo use in clinical practice. According to this report:

> The deception associated with placebo use is now widely viewed as problematic because it directly conflicts with contemporary notions of patient autonomy and the practice of shared decision making . . . the deceptive use of placebos is not ethically acceptable . . . This is particularly true in cases when placebos are utilized to serve the convenience of the physician rather than promote the welfare of the patient . . . Physicians must avoid deception when administering placebos by informing the patient that a placebo may be used . . . Physicians may use placebos for diagnosis or treatment only if the patient is informed of and agrees to its use.[18]

The medical position on the use of placebos is therefore very clear. The word "deception" appears three times in the passage above. Doctors cannot prescribe a placebo to a patient, in an attempt to help them feel better, without explaining that the drug is indeed a placebo. The fact that placebos—particularly active placebos—can have surprisingly beneficial effects does not matter. [19] Such standards of honesty and transparency contrast starkly with the everyday practice of psychiatrists and GPs who inform their patients that their depression is or is probably caused by a brain chemical imbalance, and that antidepressants work by "balancing" brain chemistry than has not even been found to be out of balance.

In 2003, Eaton T. Fores of the Eaton T. Fores Research Center wrote an article titled "There are no 'chemical imbalances'" which is published on the Academy for the Study of the Psychoanalytic Arts website. He addressed the chemical imbalance question and then posed some serious questions regarding informed consent (italics his):

> In contemporary culture, it is not uncommon for someone to return from a visit to the doctor with a prescription for an "antidepressant" drug and the notion that the doctor has diagnosed some kind of "chemical imbalance" in the extremely delicate process of neurotransmitter metabolism and release. Medical diagnoses are generally backed up by empirical facts: infection may be diagnosed when the patient has a fever and a high white blood cell count. Hyperthyroidism may be diagnosed by measuring circulating levels of thyroid hormones. Heart disease may be diagnosed by angioscopic visualization. How are the "chemical imbalances" which are the supposed basis for the prescription of "antidepressants" diagnosed? Is exploratory neurosurgery performed, using some technique that allows the surgeon to quantify synaptic transmitter levels? No, the very idea is absurd. Is a spinal tap, then, done to at least measure, on a gross scale, the distribution of neurotransmitter metabolites? Of course not. How many people have undergone spinal taps before receiving a prescription for Effexor? Is blood at least drawn, to test *something*? No. This diagnosis—the diagnosis of the most subtle of chemical disorders in the most complex organ in the body—is made on the patient's report of feeling sad and lethargic. Try to imagine a haematologist diagnosing leukemia this way to get a sense of just how ridiculous this idea is. The latest edition of one pharmacology text has this to say about the status of depression as a disease: "Despite extensive efforts, attempts to document the metabolic changes in human subjects predicted by these hypotheses have not, on balance, provided consistent or compelling corroboration". This is a complicated way of admitting that not even a scrap of evidence supports the idea that depression results from a "chemical imbalance" ... Yet patients are told every day—by their doctors, by the media, and by drug company advertising—that it is a *proven scientific fact* that depression has a known biochemical origin. It follows directly that *millions of Americans are being lied to by their doctors*; and people surely can't give informed consent for drug treatment when what they are being "informed by" is a fraud. These facts should have enormous social consequences, yet, for reasons that are unclear, they have no social or legal effects at all. [20]

In a May 2014 article titled "Psychiatry's Manufactured Consent: Chemical Imbalance Theory and the Antidepressant Explosion", American psychologist and author Bruce Levine equated the mass consumption of antidepressants—on the pretext that these substances correct an underlying brain chemical imbalance—with Edward Herman and Naom Chomsky's concept of manufacturing consent:

> Starting in the 1990s—despite research findings that levels of the neurotransmitter serotonin were unrelated to depression—Americans began to be exposed to highly effective television commercials for antidepressants that portrayed depression as being caused by a "chemical imbalance" of low levels of serotonin, and which could be treated with "chemically balancing" antidepressants . . . Why has the American public not heard psychiatrists in positions of influence on the mass media debunk the chemical imbalance theory? . . . Many psychiatrists . . . did not alert the general public because they believed that the chemical imbalance theory was a useful fiction to get patients to accept their mental illness and take their medication. In other words, the chemical imbalance theory was an excellent way to manufacture consent.
>
> Truly well-informed psychiatrists have long known that research showed that low serotonin (or other neurotransmitter) levels were not the cause of depression. . . But the vast majority of Americans . . . never heard this. Prior to the chemical imbalance campaign, many Americans were reluctant to take antidepressants—or to give them to their children. But the idea that depression is caused by a chemical imbalance which can be corrected with SSRI antidepressants sounded like taking insulin for diabetes. Correcting a chemical imbalance seemed like a reasonable thing to do, and so the use of SSRI antidepressants skyrocketed. [21]

These are very serious matters. The public have been misinformed for decades about brain chemical imbalances and depression. There are major question marks regarding whether people prescribed antidepressants are in a position to give informed consent. They are consenting to a treatment whose mode of action as explained to them by many doctors is a falsehood, for an imbalance that has not been shown to exist. It is because the brain chemical imbalance delusion is so widely accepted as truth that this unethical practice has been so widespread and not generally seen as wrong.

The medical obsession with biochemical abnormalities has greatly hindered the search for a deeper understanding of depression. A fundamental reappraisal of the understanding of and approach to depression is urgently required. A thorough independent examination of the dominant medical approach to depression is the necessary first step of this reappraisal, including the examination of the brain chemical imbalance notion I have undertaken in this book.

NOTES TO CHAPTER SIXTEEN

1. Michael Corry & Aine Tubridy, *Depression: An Emotion not a Disease*, Cork: Mercier Press, 2005, p.8.
2. David Keiser, "Commentary: Against Biologic Psychiatry", *Psychiatric Times*, Vol XIII, Issue 12, Dec 1996, http://www.psychiatrictimes.com/articles/commentary-against-biologic-psychiatry#sthash.9RYNROfF.dpuf, accessed 14 April 2014.
3. Sharon Begley, "Some Drugs Work to Treat depression, But It Isn't Clear How", *Wall Street Journal*, 18 November 2005, accessed 19 August 2014.
4. Elliot S. Valenstein, *Blaming the Brain: The Truth About Drugs and Mental Health*, New York: The Free Press, 1998, p. 140.
5. Loren Mosher's letter of resignation from the American Psychiatric Association, 1998, http://www.moshersoteria.com/articles/resignation-from-apa/, accessed 16 July 2014.
6. Elio Fratteroli, printed summary, 52nd Institute on Psychiatric Services, October 2000, p. 66, http://www.behaviorismandmentalhealth.com/wp-content/uploads/2014/06/Frattaroli.pdf, accessed 20 August 2014.
7. Brent D. Slife, Dr. Colin M. Burchfield &. Dawson Hedges, "Hook, Line and Sinker: Psychology's Uncritical Acceptance of Biological Explanation", Invited Address at the 2002 Rocky Mountain Psychological Association, Park City, Utah, U.S.A., http://brentslife.com/article/upload/biologization/Hook, line,andsinker.pdf, accessed 19 August 2014.
8. Steven Sharfstein, 2005, http://batstar.net/item/biobio.htm, accessed 24 December 2013.
9. Ivor Browne, *Music and Madness,* Cork: Cork University Press, 2008, pps. 261-262.
10. David Burns, *The Feeling Good Handbook*, New York: Plume, 1999.
11. Vivek Datta, "Chemical Imbalances and Other Black Unicorns", Mad in America website, 25 June 2012, http://www.madinamerica.com/2012/06/chemical-imbalances-and-other-black-unicorns/, accessed 27 February 2014.
12. For example, see Depression powerpoint presentation, slide 4, https://facultystaff.richmond.edu/~bmayes/Depression_6.ppt, accessed 12 April 2014.
13. For information on False Dilemma logical fallacies see note 38 in the Notes to Chapter Five.
14. For information on Begging the Question logical fallacies see note 22 in the Notes to the Introduction.
15. Robert Whitaker, *Anatomy of an Epidemic: Magic Bullets, Psychiatric Drugs and the Astonishing Rise of Mental Illness in America,* 2010, New York: Crown Publishers.
16. Gerard N. Hill and Kathleen T. Hill, 1981-2005, http://legal-dictionary.thefreedictionary.com/Informed+Consent, accessed 16 May 2014.
17. *West's Encyclopedia of American Law*, 2nd edition, The Gale Group Inc, 2008, definition of informed consent, The Free Dictionary website, http://legal-dictionary.thefreedictionary. com/Informed+Consent.
18. Nathan A. Bostick, Robert Sade, Mark A Levine & Dudley M. Stewart Jr., "Placebo Use in Clinical Practice: Report of the America Medical Association Council on Ethical and Judicial Affairs", *The Journal of Clinical Ethics* 19, no. 1 (Spring 2008): 58-61, http://academicde-partments.musc.edu/humanvalues/pdf/placebo.useinclinicalpractice.pdf, accessed 16 May 2014.
19. An active placebo is a substance used in research that has no effect on the condition being researched but does produce noticeable side effects, often similar to those of the drug to which it is being compared. Compared to an inactive placebo—such as a sugar pill—which produces no effects whatsoever, a person who experiences the effects of an active placebo may be more open to the possibility that this substance is an active drug for their condition. This expectation may then give rise to an enhanced placebo response.
20. Eaton T. Fores, "There are no 'chemical imbalances'", 2003, Academy for the Study of the Psychoanalytic Arts, http://www.academyanalyticarts.org/fores.htm, accessed 17 May 2014.
21. Bruce Levine, "Psychiatry's Manufactured Consent: Chemical Imbalance Theory and the Antidepressant Explosion", Mad in America website, 14 May 2014, https://www.madinamerica.com /2014/05/psychiatrys-manufacture-consent-chemical-imbalance-theory-antidepressant-explosion/, accessed 16 May 2014.

CONCLUSION

The selling of the brain chemical imbalance fiction story is one of the most remarkable public relations stories in the history of health care. By the mid-sixties a strong consensus that depression was caused by a chemical imbalance in the brain had been established within psychiatry. GPs too were seduced into accepting the depression brain chemical imbalance delusion as a fact. The consensus was that depression was caused by an abnormal chemical state consisting of reduced brain chemical levels. Over the next fifty years, the medical profession carried on as though this theory was an established fact. This delusional idea is now firmly engrained as a fact in the collective public mind.

Is focusing solely on the brain in depression really the only way forward? For the fifty years that it has dominated medical thinking on depression, the brain chemical imbalance delusion has had no accessible or practical role in everyday medical practice, other than misrepresenting depression as a known biological illness like any other and legitimising the widespread prescribing of antidepressants.

Many people recover from depression. People do not recover from conditions characterised by chemical abnormalities such as diabetes or an underactive thyroid gland. In twelve years providing a mental health service and working with hundreds of people diagnosed with depression, I regularly find that the medical focus on the brain and biochemical abnormalities is an irrelevant red herring, having no practical or useful application to everyday practice. This practical irrelevancy is true for all doctors, including those who believe in and regularly articulate the depression delusion to their patients. Since I have developed a deeper understanding of the emotional and psychological aspects of depression, not everything I see looks like a nail. Depression is a legitimate response to the stresses and difficulties of life. There is often potential for healing and recovery when the deeper issues that are generally present are properly considered.

According to the 2013 psychiatry textbook *The Oxford Handbook of Psychiatry* (brackets mine):

> Currently practicing psychiatrists are keenly aware of the deficiencies of current psychiatric practice. We lack knowledge of the aetiology (cause) and pathogenesis (how a disease develops) of most psychiatric disorders; we have no objective or prognostic investigations; and our drug and psychological treatments are often minimally or partially effective . . . we hope to join the other medical specialties in moving "from the descriptive to the analytical". [1]

If currently practicing psychiatrists are "keenly aware of the deficiencies of current practice", they rarely convey this message in their dealings with their patients or the public.

Meanwhile, psychiatry largely ignores one very valid possibility:

That existence, experience and life itself is at the heart of the human distress that doctors reframe as psychiatric diagnoses such as depression.

The cardinal medical error is a major exaggeration and distortion of assumed yet utterly unproven biological aspects of depression. Allied to this is a corresponding major underestimation of non-biological aspects of depression such as the emotional and psychological aspects. All else flows from this major cardinal error. Since society's responses to depression is determined by what depression is interpreted to be, this is a very serious matter.

It is potentially very dangerous to have a group with a major vested interest in drugs sales—drug companies—and a group that through self-interest is blinkered in its approach—psychiatry—leading the way in mental health. There is not and there never has been any direct verifying evidence that brain chemical imbalances are a known feature of depression. Every time people read or hear a comment that brain chemical imbalances are a known feature of depression, the delusion becomes reinforced. The major potential dangers of allowing the medical profession to dominate mental health care through public "trust without examination" is well articulated in the following passage from a 2014 article titled "The Chemical Imbalance Myth" on the website of The Sanctuary at Sedona Addictions, Recovery and Trauma Healing Center in Arizona:

There is no scientific evidence to support the claim that "chemical imbalances" cause depression, anxiety or similar illnesses. This is called the chemical imbalance myth. This truth of the chemical imbalance myth is well known by the mainstream medical and psychiatric profession . . . Belief in doctors . . . and the medications they prescribe . . . has clearly reached "religious" proportions. And sadly the medical profession, whether conscious of this fact or not, has exploited its faithful so thoroughly and completely to where they now enjoy authoritative monopoly over the individuals who entrust them with their health. In this way, it can at least be understood how "trust without examination" can have serious side effects. [2]

AN APPALLING VISTA

Some ideas are so globally accepted as truth and trustworthy that to even contemplate that they may not be true or trustworthy can spark immediate anxiety and a strong urge to dismiss the possibility. Such scenarios are sometimes known as appalling vistas. An appalling vista is a scenario or occurrence that is way out of line with what we have perceived as reality and truth. Collectively and individually, we create beliefs and views of ourselves, life and the world. These beliefs and views become fundamental to how we live. Any development that impacts greatly on something or someone we hold dear may create an appalling vista. Appalling vistas are inconvenient and distressing truths that may create within us many distressing emotions and thoughts.

Appalling vistas are unexpected and shocking occurrences that have the potential to rock an important presumption or belief—and therefore rock ourselves—to the core. We never imagined that such a thing could happen. To even consider that it could happen is beyond our comprehension. Fundamental perceptions, which we have taken for granted and that we want to believe in, are suddenly blown out of the water, often creating much uncomfortable cognitive dissonance within us. Appalling vistas generally involve the potential shattering of beliefs and perceptions that really matter to us. An appalling vista may appear so awful that there appears little scope for good emerging, certainly not in the initial stages.

The appalling vista that arises upon acknowledging that the depression chemical imbalance notion is a delusion includes many difficult truths; the reality that doctors and drug companies have been misinforming and misleading the public and their patients; the fact that in general doctors know far less about depression that they profess to; and the real possibility that our long-held collective understanding of depression is way off the mark.

Russian writer, philosopher and social activist Leo Tolstoy once wrote:

> I know that most men—not only those considered clever, but even those considered very clever and capable of understanding most difficult scientific, mathematical, or philosophic problems—can seldom discern even the simplest and most obvious truth if it be such as obliges them to admit the falsity of conclusions which they have formed, perhaps with much difficulty—conclusions of which they are proud, which they have taught to others, and on which they have built their lives. [3]

The concept of an appalling vista was brought into sharp focus in Britain, Ireland and beyond in 1980 by Lord Denning, then a senior judge and Master of the Rolls within the British legal system. Lord Denning was then presiding over the appeal of a group of men known as the Birmingham Six who were found guilty of the 1974 Birmingham bombings. This and other similar cases were the focus of considerable international attention for many years both before and after Lord Denning's judgement. Lord Denning dismissed the appeal. The following remarks formed a major part of Lord Denning's reasoning:

> If the six men win, it will mean that the police are guilty of perjury, that they are guilty of violence and threats, that the confessions were invented and improperly admitted as evidence and the convictions were erroneous . . . This is such an appalling vista that every sensible person in the land would say that it cannot be right that these actions should go any further. [4] . . . We shouldn't have all these campaigns to get the Birmingham Six released if they'd been hanged. They'd have been forgotten and the whole community would have been satisfied. [5]

On this basis, the appeal was rejected; better to not reassess the evidence, to risk wrongful conviction of innocent men and to deny them justice than to risk uncovering that a major miscarriage of justice had taken place. The Birmingham Six were forced to remain in prison for a further eleven years. Belatedly in 1991, a Court of Appeal quashed the convictions of the Birmingham Six. These six men spent sixteen years in jail, convicted of crimes they did not commit. A similar travesty of justice occurred in relation to four people referred to as the Guildford Four who were wrongly convicted of the 1974 bombings in Guildford, United Kingdom. When these convictions were finally overturned in 1989, Lord Denning remarked that they were probably guilty of murder anyway. [6]

Regarding the law, it is often said that it does not matter what one believes, only what one can prove. This position is the polar opposite of the brain biochemical imbalance delusion. This notion is totally grounded upon belief; there is no direct scientific proof of the existence of any such imbalances. In science as in law, evidence is supposed to be king. It does not matter to true scientists whether or not they like the evidence. It *is* the evidence, and as such is taken as real and true. In psychiatry, there is no evidence of brain chemical abnormalities. Where there is no evidence, there is no scientific validation.

It is said that nature hates a vacuum. Where there is no evidence, the resulting void tends to become filled with beliefs, hopes, biases, prejudices, personal preferences, individual and group dynamics. In depression and in psychiatry in general, these factors therefore play a far greater role than would be expected within a true science.

When basic principles of correct reasoning and science are applied to the brain chemical imbalance idea, the flaws and inconsistencies of this belief become obvious. When the depression brain chemical imbalance idea is rigorously examined, we find that like the emperor, it has no clothes. These flaws and inconsistencies were known prior to Prozac coming on stream in 1988. They were dismissed because they risked ruining a great story, from which many groups could profit enormously.

This whole scenario is an example of a common human phenomenon. When an idea gains traction and becomes familiar, critical discernment often diminishes. Ideas become accepted as truth, as fact, without any felt need to examine them. It is broadly and erroneously concluded that since the truth of these ideas has long been established, there is no need to question their validity.

Those in positions of power relevant to any collective delusion have a solemn and profound moral obligation to ensure that major falsehoods and delusions that affect the wellbeing of their citizens are addressed and the situation redressed fully, in the public interest. This issue is far too important to be left as merely an academic question, discussed only within academic and professional ivory towers. The importance of the depression delusion extends far beyond the confines of academia. It impacts directly on the lives of millions of people every day.

This issue requires urgent attention and redressing from within mainstream society. Since one side of the argument has a vested interest in maintaining the depression delusion, it is imperative that this matter is not left to the medical profession and the drug companies to resolve. There is too much at stake to let this delusion continue any longer.

NOTES TO THE CONCLUSION

1. David Semple & Roger Smyth, *The Oxford Handbook of Psychiatry*, 3rd edition, Oxford: Oxford University Press, 2013.

2. From the website of The Sanctuary at Sedona, Addictions, Recovery and Trauma Healing Center, "The Chemical Imbalance Myth", 28 August 2014, http://sanctuary.net/chemical-imbalance-myth/, accessed 25 November 2014.

3. Leo Tolstoy, translation of *What Is Art and Essays on Art*, Oxford University Press, 1930, translator Aylmer Maude, opening to chapter fourteen.

4. "Parliamentary Business", http://www.publications.parliament.uk/pa/cm199798/ cmhansrd/ vo980902/debtext/80902-26.htm, accessed 05 December 2014.

5. Clare Dyer, "Lord Denning, controversial 'people's judge' dies aged 100", 06 March 1999, *The Guardian,* http://www.theguardian.com/uk/1999/mar/06/claredyer1, accessed 05 December 2014.

6. Clare Dyer, "Lord Denning, controversial 'people's judge' dies aged 100", 06 March 1999, *The Guardian,* http://www.theguardian.com/uk/1999/mar/06/claredyer1, accessed 05 December 2014.

INDEX

a better way, 77
a vision for psychiatry
    Insel, Thomas, psychiatrist, director NIMH, 320
    Quirion, Remi, psychiatrist, 320
actions speak louder than words, 272
    Boyle, Mary, psychologist, 296
    Horgan, John, science writer, 272
    Santagato, Danny, 272
Agam, Galila, psychiatrist
    serotonin breakdown products, 51
alcohol, 6, 39
    vodka, 6
allaboutdepression website
    the *DSM*, 16
Alliance for Human Research Protection, 59, 209
    chemical imbalances, no evidence, 41
Amen, Daniel, psychiatrist
    brain chemicals misinformation, 99
America's Pharmaceutical Research Companies
    depression and diabetes, inappropriate comparison, 225
American Counseling Association
    concerns regarding *DSM-5*, 20
American Foundation for Suicide Prevention Research
    chemical imbalance misinformation, 183
American Medical Association
    brain, complexity, 64
    chemical imbalance misinformation, 130, 132
    logical fallacy, Begging the Question, 131
    logical fallacy, Red Herring, 131
    logical fallacy, Wishful Thinking, 132
American Psychiatric Association, 15, 20, 27, 28, 106, 107, 134, 180, 209, 213, 244, 251, 254, 267, 269, 298, 299, 309, 325, 329, 337
    chemical imbalance misinformation, 92, 99, 180
    deficit, losing members & drug co. money, 18, 24
    depression diagnosis criteria, 34
    DSM creators, 15
    president's reply to the American Counseling Association, 20
    promoted chemical imbalances, 73

American Textbook of Psychiatry
    chemical imbalances, no evidence, 55
amphetamine, 10-20-30-year cycle, 26
Andersen, Hans Christian
    The Emperor Has No Clothes, 302
Anderson, E., psychiatrist, 93, 134, 285
Andreasen, Nancy, psychiatrist, 74, 134, 286, 325
    brain, simplistic view, 65
    chemical imbalance misinformation, 95
    logical fallacy, Red Herring, 282
    psychiatry, revolution in?, 321
    psychotherapy undervalued, 95
Angell, Marcia, 28, 59, 134, 266
Angell, Marcia, physician, pathologist, 14
    chemical imbalances notion, 7
    chemical imbalances, no evidence, 7, 43
    drug company criticism, 239
    logic, great leap, 7
    medical mindset, 91
    New York Review of Books, 7
    psychiatrist's bible, the *DSM*, 22
antidepressants, brain action, no idea
    Carlat, Daniel, psychiatrist, 246
antidepressants, effectiveness exaggerated, 287
    Coppen, Alec, psychiatrist, 243
    Malhi, G.S., psychiatrist, 103
    Rottenberg, Jonathan, psychology professor, 296
antidepressants, misinformation
    Azmitia Efrain C., neuroscientist, 70
    Eli Lilly, 70
    Glenmullen, Joseph, psychiatrist, 71
    Shorter, Edward, psychiatrist, 70
anxiety
    chemical imbalances, no evidence, 39
    in depression, 85
appalling vista, 341
    Birmingham Six, 341
    chemical imbalance delusion, 341
    Guildford Four, 342
    inconvenient truths, 340
    Lord Denning, 341
    Tolstoy, Leo, social activist, 341
Appeal to Authority logical fallacy. *See* logical fallacy, Appeal to Authority
Aristotle, 8

arm-bands, depression and, 86
Astra-Zeneca, decreased psychiatric research, 23
Athlone Literary Festival
  Lynch, Terry, GP & psychotherapist, 124
Attention Deficit Disorder
  chemical imbalances, no evidence, 39
avoidance
  in depression, 85
avoidance, in depression, 84
Aware
  chemical imbalance misinformation, 144
  mental health organization, 145
aware, refusing to be
  Rowe, Dorothy, psychologist, 294
Azmitia Efrain C., neuroscientist
  antidepressants, misinformation, 70
Balanced Mind Parent Network
  chemical imbalance misinformation, 184
  Scientific Advisory Council, 184
Baldessarini, Ross, psychiatrist
  chemical imbalances, no evidence, 37
barbiturates, 10-20-30 year cycle, 26
Barry, Harry, general practitioner
  brain, simplistic view, 67
  chemical imbalance misinformation, 127
  depression and diabetes, inappropriate
    comparison, 227
  depression, assumed biological basis, 128
  logical fallacy, Begging the Question, 127
  logical fallacy, False Cause, 127
  logical fallacy, Weak Analogy, 227
  psychotherapy, a biological treatment, 254
  Raggy Doll Club, 128
Barry, Siobhan, psychiatrist, 192
  chemical imbalance misinformation, 104, 192
  logical fallacy, Begging the Question, 104
Basco, Monica Ramirez, psychologist
  logical fallacy, Red Herring, 282
Bates, Tony, psychologist
  chemical imbalance misinformation, 163
Beating Stress, Anxiety and Depression
  chemical imbalance misinformation, 168
Begley, Sharon, journalist, 41
  chemical imbalances delusion,
    consequences, 328
  chemical imbalances notion, hegemony, 310
belief system, psychiatry, 301
belief, fixed
  depression, biological disorder, 77

beliefs, fixed
  medical profession, 78
Belmaker, R.H., psychiatrist
  serotonin breakdown products, 51
Bentall, Richard, psychology professor
  chemical imbalances, based on deduction, 49
  chemical imbalances, marketing, 241
  chemical imbalances, no evidence, 49
benzodiazepine tranquillisers
  10-20-30 year cycle, 26
  addiction, 26
Beyond Blue, mental health organization
  chemical imbalance misinformation, 202
Beyond Prozac
  misgivings re depression approach, 33
Beyond Prozac, Healing Mental Distress
  diagnostic approach questioned, 34
  Lynch, Terry, GP & psychotherapist, 33
bias, biological research
  Hyman, Steven, psychiatrist, ex-director
    NIMH, 324
  Insel, Thomas, psychiatrist, director NIMH, 324
bias, confirmation
  Buffett, Warren, investor, 130
  Houston, Muiris, general practitioner, 130
biobabble
  Scull, Andrew, sociology professor, 239
bio-bio-bio model
  Sharfstein, Steven, president, American
    Psychiatric Association, 330
biochemistry, definition, 52
Biochemistry: Molecules, Cells and the Body
  chemical imbalances, no evidence, 52
biological answers
  Scull, Andrew, sociology professor, 276
biological evidence
  just around the corner, 276
biological markers
  definition, 17, 45
  none in DSM-3, 19
  play no part in diagnosis, 17, 32, 165
bipolar disorder
  chemical imbalance misinformation, 96
  chemical imbalances, no evidence, 39
Birmingham Six
  appalling vista, 341
Birthistle, Ian, psychologist
  chemical imbalance misinformation, 170
black cloud
  in depression, 88

Bloch, Douglas, counsellor
  chemical imbalance misinformation, 174
blood glucose deficiency. *See* hypoglycemia
blood test, ask for
  Leifer, Ron, psychiatrist, 40
  Leo, Jonathan, neuroanatomy professor, 40
Bolenius, Emma Miler
  delusion, mass, 293
Boston Globe
  delusions, new replacing old, 317
  logical fallacy, Begging the Question, 317
  logical fallacy, Weak Analogy, 317
Bouchez, Colette, medical journalist
  chemical imbalance misinformation, 201
Boyle, Mary, psychologist
  actions speak louder than words, 296
  groupthink, 292
brain
  complexity, 9
  master of the mind?, 65
Brain Basics, NIMH website
  chemical imbalance misinformation, 179
brain chemicals, breakdown products
  Moncrieff, Joanna, psychiatrist, 50
brain chemicals, depletion studies, 67
brain diseases, mental diseases are,
  Griesinger, Wilhelm, 306
brain diseases, who treats?, 271
  do GPs treat brain diseases?, 279
  do psychiatrists treat brain diseases?, 271
brain scans and depression, 273
brain, assessment
  absent in psychiatry, 272
brain, complexity, 63, 66
  American Medical Association, 64
  Azmitia, Efrain C., neuroscientist, 70
  Carlat, Daniel, psychiatrist, 66
  Greenberg, Gary, psychotherapist, 65
  Hyman, Steven, psychiatrist, ex-director
    NIMH, 63
  Shorter, Edward, psychiatrist, 65
  Valenstein, Elliot, neuroscientist, 64, 71
  Whitaker, Robert, journalist, author, 66
brain, simplistic view
  Andreasen, Nancy, psychiatrist, 65
  Barry, Harry, general practitioner, 67
brain, who are the experts?, 271
Brainphysics.com
  chemical imbalance misinformation, 203
  logical fallacy, Red Herring, 284
breakdown products. *See* serotonin,
  breakdown products
Breggin, Peter, psychiatrist

chemical imbalances, discredited, 68
chemical imbalances, no evidence, 36, 42
propaganda, 307
seminal moments, 10
British Medical Association
  chemical imbalance misinformation, 109,
    110
  endorses depression delusion, 109
  logical fallacy, Red Herring, 283
British Psychological Society, 7, 14, 27
  depression, assumed biological basis, 20
  disease model, 7
  DSM-5 Position Statement, 7, 20
  paradigm shift, need for, 7
bromides, 10-20-30-year cycle, 26
Browne, Ivor, 59, 140, 337
Browne, Ivor, psychiatry professor
  chemical imbalance delusion, consequences,
    330
  chemical imbalances, no evidence, 43
  denying demonstrable imbalances?, 129
  evangelical?, 130
  Toibin, Colm, author, 130
Browne, Vincent, broadcaster, 130
  chemical imbalance misinformation, 192
Buffett, Warren, investor, 130
  confirmation bias, 130
BUPA
  chemical imbalance misinformation, 208
  logical fallacy, Begging the Question, 208
  logical fallacy, False Cause, 208
Burchfield, Colin, psychologist, 160, 329
  chemical imbalances, discredited, 160
  consequences of biological focus, 329
Burns, David, psychiatrist
  chemical imbalance delusion, consequences,
    330
  chemical imbalance delusion, importance,
    240
  chemical imbalances, no evidence, 32, 39,
    41
  marketing, chemical imbalances, 240
  theory confused with fact, 38
Cantopher, Tim, psychiatrist
  chemical imbalance misinformation, 107,
    187
Caplan, Paula, psychologist
  diagnoses by consensus, 21
  mental disorders, no scientific basis, 21
  resignation from *DSM*, 20
Carlat, Daniel, 28, 58, 59, 60, 61, 74, 75, 135,
    137, 139, 212, 233, 266, 269, 285, 299
Carlat, Daniel, psychiatrist, 58

antidepressants action, no idea, 246
brain, complexity, 66
Carlat, Daniel, psychiatrist, *(continued)*,
    chemical imbalance misinformation, 105,
        239
    chemical imbalances, based on deduction,
        48, 49
    chemical imbalances, discredited, 71
    chemical imbalances, doctors misinforming
        patients, 246
    chemical imbalances, marketing, 241
    chemical imbalances, no evidence, 33, 44,
        67, 96
    chemical imbalances, wishful thinking, 105
    depression, assumed biological basis, 246
    depression, biological, what else could it
        be?, 254
    depression, pathophysiology, 4
    depression, why 5 criteria?, 34
    diagnostic labels, consequences, 23
    ignorance, regarding psychiatric disorders,
        263
    law of the instrument, 256
    logic, flawed, 241, 255
    mass delusion in psychiatry, 297
    misinformation for patients' sake, 246
    neurotransmitter wizards, 105, 228, 248
    serotonin breakdown products, 50
    what psychiatrists do, 274
Caro, Janice E.,psychologist
    chemical imbalance misinformation, 162
Cartesian split
    psychiatry, 302
Carver, Joseph, psychologist, 199
    chemical imbalance misinformation, 164,
        165, 166, 167
    logical fallacy, Begging the Question, 165
Casey, Patricia, psychiatry professor
    depression, assumed biological basis, 10
    seminal moments, 10
Castello, Greg, general practitioner
    chemical imbalance misinformation, 119,
        120, 122
    flawed logic, 123, 124
Channel 5, *GPs: Behind Closed Doors*,
    chemical imbalance misinformation, 116
Chat magazine
    chemical imbalance misinformation, 189
chemical imbalance. *See also* chemical
    imbalances, *See also* chemical imbalances
chemical imbalance delusion. *See also* chemical
    imbalances delusion
chemical imbalance delusion, consequences

Browne, Ivor, psychiatry professor, 330

chemical imbalance notion
    a placebo, 238
chemical imbalance, delusion, importance
    Burns, David, psychiatrist, 240
chemical imbalance, myth
    The Sanctuary at Sedona, 340
chemical imbalances
    discredited, 12
    drug companies move from, 25
    endogenous depression, 85
    little white lie, 73
    no practical application, 73
    pseudoscience, 72
chemical imbalances delusion, 1
    appalling vista, 341
    appears familiar, reasonable, 6
    Corry, Michael, psychiatrist, 44
    doctors portrayed positively, 77
    dominated thinking x 50 years, 77
    embedded within society, 4
    embraced by medical profession, 77
    emperor without clothes, 342
    grounded on belief, not evidence, 342
    ingrained in our psyche, 3
    marketing, 241, 309
    misrepresented as fact, 12
    propaganda, 339
    trust in doctors, 72
    vested interests, 77
chemical imbalances delusion, consequences,
    327
    Begley, Sharon, journalist, 328
    Burns, David, psychiatrist, 330
    Datta, Vivek, psychiatrist, 331
    distorted understanding, 327
    Fratteroli Elio, psychiatrist, 329
    hope, exaggerated, 331
    inner conflict replaced, 329
    inner life hardly relevant, 329
    Kaiser, David, psychiatrist, 328
    Mosher, Loren, psychiatrist, 329
    most important point missed, 329
    psychosocial factors undermined, 328
    public disempowered, 327
    responses limited, 328
    self-empowerment diminished, 330, 331,
        332
    Valenstein, Elliot, neuroscientist, 329
    wrong turn, Corry, Michael, psychiatrist,
        328

wrong turn, Tubridy, Aine general
    practitioner, 328

chemical imbalances delusion, importance
    Cohen, David, social work professor, 240
    Moncrieff, Joanna, psychiatrist, 240
chemical imbalances delusion, widely believed
    Scientific American, 1
chemical imbalances, no evidence
    Humphreys, Tony, psychologist, 38
chemical imbalances, a lie
    Gotzcshe, Peter, physician, 229
chemical imbalances, accepted as fact
    Goldacre, Ben, physician, science writer,
        241
chemical imbalances, based on deduction
    Carlat, Daniel, psychiatrist, 48, 49
    Hicks, James W., psychiatrist, 49
    Kirsch, Irving, psychologist, 50
    Lacasse, Jeffrey, social work professor, 48
chemical imbalances, breakdown products
    The Shorter Oxford Textbook of Psychiatry, 51
    Whitaker, Robert, journalist, author, 51
chemical imbalances, cause depression
    Hicks, James W., psychiatrist, 49
chemical imbalances, cause or consequence
    logical fallacy, Begging the Question, 12
    logical fallacy, Red Herring, 12
chemical imbalances, credence given
    *The Human Brain, An introduction To Its
        Functional Anatomy*, 56
chemical imbalances, culture
    affecting outcomes, 89
chemical imbalances, deception
    Tores, Eaton T., Research Center, 335
chemical imbalances, delusional
    Corry, Michael, psychiatrist, 43
chemical imbalances, discredited, 63
    brain complexity, 63
    Breggin, Peter, psychiatrist, 68
    Burchfield, Colin, psychologist, 160
    Carlat, Daniel, psychiatrist, 71
    Dawson W
        Slife, Brent D., psychology professor, 160
    Glenmullen, Joseph, psychiatrist, 71
    Hardon, Anita, anthropology professor, 237
    Hedges, Dawson W., psychiatry professor,
        160
    Hook, Line and Sinker, 160
    Jackson, Grace, psychiatrist, 71
    Kety, Seymour, psychiatrist, 69
    Kirsch, Irving, psychologist, researcher, 48,
        50

Lacasse, Jeffrey, social work professor, 48
Leo, Jonathan, neuroanatomy professor, 48
Levine, Bruce, psychologist, 336
Maitre, Laurent, research scientist, 69
Medawar, Charles, Social Audit UK, 237
Puech, Alain, pharmacist, 69
Shorter, Edward, psychiatrist, 70, 235
Snyder, S.H., neuroscientist, 70
Valenstein, Elliot, neuroscientist, 63, 235
Whitaker, Robert, journalist, author, 73
chemical imbalances, doctors misinforming
    patients, 84, 87, 88
    Carlat, Daniel, psychiatrist, 246
    Goodman, Wayne, psychiatrist, 245
chemical imbalances, fabrication, 73
chemical imbalances, false premises
    Ellison, Shane, research chemist, 243
chemical imbalances, fictitious notions, 79
chemical imbalances, hypothesis
    fifty years, no evidence, 47
    Schildkraut, Joseph, psychiatrist, 46
chemical imbalances, inappropriate
    comparison
    hormone replacement therapy, Steele,
        Chris, 113
    thyroid deficiency, Dr. Greg Castello, 121
chemical imbalances, inappropriate metaphor,
    245
    Goodman, Wayne, psychiatrist, 244
    Moncrieff, Joanna, psychiatrist, 244
chemical imbalances, lying
    Reidbord, Steven, psychiatrist, 244
chemical imbalances, marketing, 245
    Bentall, Richard, psychology professor, 241
    Carlat, Daniel, psychiatrist, 241
    Datta, Vivek, psychiatrist, 242
    Healy, David, psychiatrist, 242
    Kirsch, Irving, psychologist, researcher, 241
    Shipko, Stuart, psychiatrist, 242
    Shorter, Edward, psychiatrist, 242
    Sommers-Flanagan, John, counsellor
        education professor, 243
chemical imbalances, misinformation
    "How Prozac works" website, 142
    Amen, Daniel, psychiatrist, 99
    American Foundation for Suicide
        Prevention Research, 183
    American Medical Association, 131, 132
    American Psychiatric Association, 92, 99,
        180
    Andreasen, Nancy, psychiatrist, 95
    anonymous, 198
    Aware, 144

Balanced Mind Parent Network, 184
Barry, Harry, general practitioner, 127
Barry, Siobhan, psychiatrist, 104, 192
Bates, Tony, psychologist, 163
Beating Stress, Anxiety and Depression, 168
chemical imbalances, misinformation,
   (continued),
   Beyond Blue, mental health organization,
      202
   bipolar disorder, 96
   Birthistle, Ian, psychologist, 170
   Bloch, Douglas, counsellor, 174
   Bouchez, Colette, medical journalist, 201
   Brain Basics, NIMH website, 179
   Brainphysics.com, 203
   British Medical Association, 109, 110, 111
   Browne, Vincent, broadcaster, 192
   BUPA, 208
   Cantopher, Tim, psychiatrist, 107, 187
   Carlat, Daniel, psychiatrist, 105, 239
   Caro, Janice E., psychologist, 162
   Carver, Joseph, psychologist, 164, 165, 166,
      167
   Castello, Greg, general practitioner, 119,
      120, 121, 122
   Channel 5, *GPs
      Behind Closed Doors, 116*
   Chat magazine, 189
   Crockett, Molly, neuroscientist, TED talk,
      133
   Crowe, Jonathan, science editor, 194, 195
   Daly, Robert, psychiatry professor, 189
   D'Arcy, Ray, broadcaster, 193
   Davidson's Principles and Practice of Medicine,
      256, 257
   Dealing with Depression in 12-Step Recovery, 172
   *Dealing with Depression: Understanding and
      Overcoming the Symptoms of Depression*, 125
   Depression and Bipolar Support Alliance,
      184, 185
   *Depression, Cognitive Behaviour Therapy with
      Children and Young People*, 170
   depression-guide website, 205, 206
   DesJardins Financial Security, 144
   Desmaisons, Kathleen PhD, author, 220
   Devon, Michelle L., freelance writer, 196
   direct-to-consumer advertising, 152
   doctors misinforming patients, 82, 84, 85
   Dosani, Sabina, psychiatrist, 102
   Duke, Sean, science journalist, 207
   East Coast FM radio, 207
   Edwards, Virginia, psychiatrist, 100
   Effexor, 152

Eli Lilly, 141, 142
eMedTV, 203, 204
Erdelyi, Matthew H., psychology professor,
   161

European Depression Association, 144
Farrell, Elaine, author, 181
Fennell, Leonie, mental health advocate,
   115
Food and Drug Administration, 152
Forest Pharmaceuticals, 148, 149, 150
Fox-Spencer, Rebecca, neurochemist, 103
Francis-Cheung, Theresa, health writer, 207
Friedman, Richard, psychiatry professor,
   104
Fryer, LaShon, freelance writer, 196
Gilbert, Paul, psychology professor, 170
GlaxoSmithKline, 145, 147
Gotzcshe, Peter, physician, 229
GPs stay silent, 188
Grey, Robin, psychotherapist, 207
Harding, Richard, psychiatrist, 99
Harper, Dawn, general practitioner, 116
Healing from Depression, 174
Heaton-Harris, Nicolette, author, 193
hegemony, 305
Hicks, James W., psychiatrist, 101
Holford, Patrick, nutritionist, author, 215,
   216, 217
Houston, Muiris, general practitioner, 129,
   226
importance to drug companies, 141
in *Prozac Nation*, 264
Introduction to Psychology, 161
Irish Medicines Board, 153
irishhealth.com, 107, 108, 109
ITV, *Loose women*, 185
ITV, *This Morning*, 111, 116
Jowit, Juliette, journalist, 187
Kenny, Mary, journalist, 189
Keyes, Marian, author, 186
kidshealth website, 205
Kimmelman, Michael, *New York Times*, 253
Kresser, Chris, integrative medicine
   practitioner, 152
Leonovs, Julie, mental health activist, 113
Lieberman, Jeffrey, psychiatry professor,
   106
Lipton, Morris, psychiatry professor, 93
Living with Depression, 171
Lundbeck, 143, 144
Lustral, 150
Malhi, G.S., psychiatrist, 103

Mayo Clinic, 94
McEvoy, Mary, actress, 193
McKenzie, Kwame, psychiatry professor, 109, 110

chemical imbalances, misinformation, *(continued)*,
McMaster, Norman, hypnotherapist, 172
Men and Depression, What to Do When the Man You Care About is Depressed, 207
Mental Health America, 184
MIND, UK, 181
Mohl, P., psychiatrist, 254
Moncrieff, Joanna, psychiatrist, 115
Mondimore, Francis, psychiatrist, 96, 103
Murtagh's General Practice, 280, 281
National Alliance for Research on Schizophrenia and Depression, 183
National Alliance on Mental Illness, 180
National Institute of Mental Health, 173, 179
Nazario, Brunilda, MD, 201
neurologists stay silent, 188
New York Times, depression In-Depth Report, 195
Newsweek, 2001, 146
Norden, Michael J., psychiatrist, 97, 98
Nottinghamshire Healthcare NHS Trust, 180
O, Jack, therapist, 172
O'Callaghan, Gareth, broadcaster, 191, 265
Opong, Dr., general practitioner, 117
Osbourne, Sharon, TV personality, 186
O'Shaughnessy, Kevin, medical editor, 111
Oster, Gerald D., psychologist, 162
O'Sullivan, Ronnie, snooker player, 191
Overcoming Depression, A Self-Help Guide Using Cognitive Behavioural Techniques, 169
Patrick, Diane, governor's wife, 265
paxilcr.com website, 147
Pert, Candace, neuroscientist, 133
Pfizer, 150, 151
Pittsburgh Tribune, 192
Plant, Jane, CBE, environmental geochemistry professor, 168, 169
Portland Psychotherapy Depression Treatment Program, 172
Potatoes Not Prozac, 220
promoted by psychiatry, 252
propaganda, 305
Prozac Diary, 96
Psychcentral website, 199
Psychology Information Online, 171

Ramirez, Monica, psychologist, 100
RBC Insurance, 144
Redman, Nick, Bristol Healing Voices Network, 113
Reidbord, Steven, psychiatrist, 244
Rethink Mental Illness, 182
Royal College of Psychiatrists, 92, 93
Sawalha, Nadia, TV presenter, 186
schizophrenia, 96
Serani, Deborah, psychologist, 171
Sharfstein, Steven, president, American Psychiatric Association, 244
Shepherd, Charles, M.E. Association Medical Director, 133
Short Hills Pharmacy, New Jersey, 155
Shreeve, Caroline, general practitioner, 125
Slater, Lauren, author, *Prozac Diary*, 96
SmithKlineBeecham, 147
Solomon, Andrew, author, 190
sophistry, 305
Spiegel, Alix, NPR correspondent, 247
spunout.ie, 185
Standard Life, 144
Steele, Chris, general practitioner, 111, 112, 114
Stephenson, Janet, psychologist, 168, 169
Stoppard, Miriam, general practitioner, 133
Stotland, Nada L, psychiatry professor, 100
Textbook of Medicine, 133
The Complete Book of Men's Health, 206
The Complete Guide to Mental Health, 181
The Guardian, 187
The Human Brain, An Introduction to its Functional Anatomy, 56
Tighe, Sophie, Senior Reporter, Yahoo Lifestyle UK, 207
tryptophan, 217
U.S. Pharmacist, 155
Valenstein, Elliot, neuroscientist, 141
Verduyn, C., Rogers, J. & Wood, A., psychologists, 170
WebMD website, 199, 201
Weil, Andrew, physician, 265
Westen, Drew, psychology professor, 168
WONCA, 144
World Federation for Mental Health, 144
World Organization of Family Doctors,144
Wright, Jesse, psychiatrist, 100
Writing, Alexis, 199
Wurtzel, Elizabeth, author, 264
Wyeth, 152
Yahoo, 207
Zoloft, 150

chemical imbalances, misinformation, drug
    companies' fault
    Graff, Mark, psychiatrist, 251
    Pies, Ronald, psychiatry professor, 251
chemical imbalances, misinformation, for
    patients' sake
    Carlat, Daniel, psychiatrist, 246
chemical imbalances, misinformation, for
    patients' sake, (continued),
    Fieve, Ronald, psychiatrist, 249
    Frazer, Alan, psychiatry professor, 248
    Freedman, Robert, psychiatry professor,
        249
    Murtagh's General Practice, 251
    Pies, Ronald, psychiatry professor, 249
chemical imbalances, misinformation, little
    white lie
    Hickey, Phil, psychologist, 252
    Pies, Ronald, psychiatry professor, 252
chemical imbalances, no evidence, 35
    Alliance for Human Research Protection,
        41
    American Textbook of Psychiatry, 55
    Angell, Marcia, physician, pathologist, 7, 43
    any mental illness, 39
    Attention Deficit Disorder, 39
    Baldessarini, Ross, psychiatrist, 37
    Bentall, Richard, psychology professor, 49
    Biochemistry: Molecules, Cells and the Body, 52
    bipolar disorder, 39
    Breggin, Peter, psychiatrist, 36, 42
    Browne, Ivor, psychiatry professor, 43
    Burns, David, psychiatrist, 32, 39, 42
    Carlat, Daniel, psychiatrist, 33, 67, 96
    Clinical Chemistry
        Principles, Procedures and Correlations, 52
    Cohen, David, social work professor, 42
    Colbert, Ty C., psychologist, 38
    College of Psychiatrists website changes, 42
    Corry, Michael, psychiatrist, 43
    Datta, Vivek, psychiatrist, 45
    Delgado, Pedro, psychiatrist, 47
    Drummond, Edward, psychiatrist, 32
    Essentials of Preventive Medicine, 55
    Fennell, Leonie, mental health activist, 115
    Fiddaman, Bob, mental health activist, 115
    Fores, Eaton, T., Research Center, 335
    Functional Neuroanatomy
        An Interactive Text and Manual, 54
    Glenmullen, Joseph, psychiatrist, 38
    Goodman and Gilman's The Pharmacological
        Basics of Therapeutics, 36
    Healy, David, psychiatrist, 41

Horgan, John, science writer, 32
Hyman, Steven, psychiatrist, ex-director
    NIMH, 38
Insel, Thomas, psychiatrist, director NIMH,
    42
Institute of Psychiatry, 42
Irish Medicines Board, 39
journalists shocked, 40
Kaiser, David, psychiatrist, 31
Kendler, Kenneth, 40
Kirsch, Irving, psychologist, researcher, 43,
    91
Lacasse, Jeffrey, social work professor, 41,
    195, 247
Lecture Notes
    Clinical Biochemistry, 53
Lecture Notes on Clinical Chemistry, 52
Leifer, Ron, psychiatrist, 40
Leo, Jonathan, neuroanatomy professor, 39,
    41, 195, 247
Leonovs, Julie, mental health activist, 113,
    115
Levine, Bruce, psychologist, 32, 39
Lipowski, Z.J., psychiatrist, 31
Lowe, Derek, medicinal chemist, 4
Lynch, Terry, GP & psychotherapist, 121,
    122, 124
Maddock, Mary, Mindfreedom Ireland, 46
Mark's Basic Medical Biochemistry
    A Clinical Approach, 53
McCarter, Gordon, biological sciences
    professor, 41
McLaren, Niall, psychiatrist, 44
Medical Biochemistry, 53
Medical Sciences, 55
Memorising Medicine, A Revision Guide, 54
Moncrieff, Joanna, psychiatrist, 40, 42, 43,
    115
Moore, Thomas J., Health Policy expert, 37
Morena, Francisco, psychiatrist, 47
Neuroscience in Medicine, 54
Nierenberg, Andrew, psychiatrist, 37
obsessive-compulsive disorder, 39
Paykel, Eugene, psychiatrist, 46
personality disorder, 39
post mortem, inconclusive findings, 124
Practical General Practice, 281
Principles of Anatomy and Physiology, 54
Ratna, L., psychiatrist, 36
Reidbord, Steven, psychiatrist, 45
Ross, Colin, psychiatrist, 36
Rottenberg, Jonathan, psychology
    professor, 44

Rowe, Dorothy, psychologist, 22, 42
Royal College of Psychiatrists, 42
Sanghavi, Darshak, 40
schizophrenia, 39
Shorter, Edward, psychiatrist, 45
Stahl, Stephen M., psychiatrist, 38
Szasz, Thomas, psychiatrist, 32, 39
chemical imbalances, no evidence, *(continued)*,
   Textbook of Biochemistry with Clinical
     Correlations, 53
   The Science of Laboratory Diagnosis, 57
   U.S. Congress Office of Technology, 36
   Valenstein, Elliot, neuroscientist, 32, 37
   Wakefield, Jerome, social work &
     psychiatry professor, 44
   Watson, Toby, psychologist, 115
chemical imbalances, no imbalance, 31
chemical imbalances, no tests, 113
chemical imbalances, notion, 20
   Angell, Marcia, physician, pathologist, 7
   hegemony, 310
   hegemony, Begley, Sharon, journalist, 310
   sophistry, 311
chemical imbalances, pseudoscience, 72
chemical imbalances, sloppy thinking
   Reidbord, Steven, psychiatrist, 244
chemical imbalances, urban legend
   Pies, Ronald, psychiatry professor, 72
chemical imbalances, venerable status
   Kresser, Chris, integrative medicine
     practitioner, 3
chemical imbalances, wishful thinking
   Carlat, Daniel, psychiatrist, 105
chemical imbalances, wizards of
   Carlat, Daniel, psychiatrist, 105
Child and Adolescent Bipolar Foundation. *See*
   Balanced Mind Parent Network
Chomsky, Naom, philosopher, logician
   consent, manufactured, 336
Clinaero, 203
Clinical Chemistry, Principles, Procedures and
   Correlations
   chemical imbalances, no evidence, 52
CNN
   depression and diabetes, inappropriate
     comparison, 230
cnsdiseases website
   chemical imbalance misinformation, 206
   logical fallacy, Begging the Question, 206
cocaine, 10-20-30-year cycle, 26
Cochrane Centre, Nordic
   depression and diabetes, inappropropriate
     comparison, 229

Coffey, Calvin, surgery professor
   saving my life, 309
Cohen, David, social work professor
   chemical imbalance importance, 240
   chemical imbalances, no evidence, 42
   propaganda, 307
Colbert, Ty C., psychologist
   chemical imbalances, no evidence, 38
collective delusion. *See* delusion, mass
collegiality before truth, 256
   Davidson's Principles and Practice of Medicine,
     256
Columbus, Christopher
   delusion, mass, 293
consensus
   agreement in mental disorders, 16, 17
   and the *DSM*, 16
   diagnoses based on, 17
   manufacturing, 16
consensus approach to diagnosis
   collapsing, 18
consensus not science, product of
   Diagnostic and Statistical Manual of Mental
     Disorders-3, 19
consent, informed
   "physicians must avoid deception", 334
   American Medical Association, 334
   placebo, 334
   placebo, deception, 334
consent, informed, definition
   Hill & Hill, legal experts, 334
   West's Encyclopedia of American Law, 334
consent, manufactured
   Chomsky, Naom, philosopher, logician, 336
   Herman, Edward, finance professor, 336
   Levine, Bruce, psychologist, 335
Conspiracy of Goodwill
   Medawar, C. & Hardon, A., 238
Copernicus
   delusion, mass, 293
Coppen, Alec, psychiatrist
   antidepressants effectiveness exaggerated,
     243
   logic, flawed, 243
Corry, Michael, 59, 266, 337
Corry, Michael, psychiatrist
   chemical imbalance delusion, consequences,
     328
   chemical imbalances delusion, 44
   chemical imbalances, no evidence, 43
   pharmaceutical industry, 240
Council for Evidence-based Psychiatry, 229
   doctors misinforming patients, 119

Council for Evidence-Based Psychiatry, 119
Cresswell, Mark, sociologist
  psychiatric hegemony, 308
Crockett, Molly, neuroscientist
  chemical imbalances misinformation, TED
    talk, 133
  logical fallacy, Begging the Question, 133
  logical fallacy, False Cause, 133

Crowe, Jonathan, science editor
  chemical imbalance misinformation, 194,
    195
  logical fallacy, Begging the Question, 195
Daly, Robert, psychiatry professor
  chemical imbalances misinformation, 189
D'Arcy, Ray, broadcaster
  chemical imbalance misinformation, 193
Datta, Vivek, psychiatrist, 44
  chemical imbalances delusion,
    consequences, 331
  chemical imbalances, marketing, 242
  chemical imbalances, no evidence, 45
  dangerous mythology, 331
  mythology, dangerous, 331
  self-empowerment diminished, 331
David Burns, 57, 59, 266
Davidson's Principles and Practice of Medicine
  chemical imbalance misinformation, 256,
    257
  collegiality before truth, 256
  logical fallacy, Appeal to Authority, 260
  logical fallacy, Begging the Question, 259
  logical fallacy, Circular Reasoning, 259
  logical fallacy, False Cause, 257
  logical fallacy, Hasty Generalisation, 258
Davies, James, psychologist
  Allen Frances interview, 19
  mental disorders, contrived, in DSM, 19
  Robert Spitzer, psychiatrist, interview, 19
Dealing with Depression in 12-Step Recovery
  chemical imbalance misinformation, 172
Dealing with Depression: Understanding and
  Overcoming the Symptoms of Depression
  chemical imbalance misinformation, 125
DeAngelis, Catherine, physician
  drug company influence, 241
deception, 305
deduction, the only "evidence"
  Bentall, Richard, psychology professor, 49
  Carlat, Daniel, psychiatrist, 48, 49
  Hicks, James W., psychiatrist, 49
  Kirsch, Irving, psychologist, researcher, 50
  Lacasse, Jeffrey, social work professor, 48

Leo, Jonathan, neuroanatomy professor, 48
defence mechanisms, 83
  depression, core component, 79, 80, 85, 89,
    255
  depression, core components, 84
defence mechanisms, in depression, 84
Delgado, Pedro, psychiatrist
  chemical imbalances, no evidence, 47
delusion, characteristics, 13
delusion, chemical imbalance, 1
  sounds familar, reasonable, 6
delusion, chemical imbalances
  Corry, Michael, psychiatrist, 44
delusion, definition
  Diagnostic and Statistical Manual of Mental
    Disorders-5, 287, 289
  dictionary.com website, 287
  McKenzie, Kwame, psychiatry professor,
    288
  Meerloo, A.M., psychiatrist, 288
  Shorter Oxford Textbook of Psychiatry, 288, 290
delusion, depression. See also depression
  delusion
delusion, depression, beneficiaries
  general practitioners, 332
  pharmaceutical companies, 332
  psychiatry, 332
  some therapists, 333
delusion, mass, 111
  Bolenius, Emma Miler, 293
  Columbus, Christopher, 293
  Copernicus, 293
  Goebbels, Joseph, propaganda officier, 293
  Lenin, Vladimir, Marxist, 293
  Meerloo, A.M., psychiatrist, 293
  Wilson, Charles, Abacus news
    correspondent, 293
delusion, mass, in psychiatry
  Carlat, Daniel, psychiatrist, 297
  Foudraine, Jan, psychiatrist, 297
delusions
  Encyclopaedia Britannica, 289
  National Institute of Mental Health, 13
delusions, consequences
  Meerloo, A.M., psychiatrist, 288
delusions, new replacing old, 315
  Boston Globe, 316, 317
  Duman, Ronald, psychiatry professor, 317,
    318
  from chemicals to genetics, 316
  Insel, Thomas, psychiatrist, NIMH director,
    319
  National Institute of Mental Health, 13, 319

delusions, purpose
  Frances, Allen, lead *DSM-4* psychiatrist,
    289
  Meerloo, A.M., psychiatrist, 289
delusions, widespread, 289
  Science Brainwaves website, 288
  Stanford Encyclopedia of Philosophy, 288
depression
  a protective reaction, 88
depression, *(continued)*,
  a supposedly biological disease, 13
  absence of lab tests, 57
  anxiety, 85
  assumed biological basis, 2, 91
  avoidance, 85
  black cloud, 88
  chemical imbalances, no evidence, 39
  core aspects, 13, 84
  distress, 84, 85
  experiences and behaviour real, 287
  grief, 85, 87
  habits and patterns, 84
  legitimate response to life, 339
  loss, 87
  mass delusion, 1
  medical mindset, 91
  no known chemical abnormalities, 31
  not caused by serotonin depletion, 67
  perverse implantation, 311
  psychosocial causal factors, 7
  self-doubt, 89
  serotonin breakdown products, 50
  supposed genetic nature, 13
  tears, 85
  unresolved shock, 84
  withdrawal, 85
  wounding, 84
Depression and Bipolar Support Alliance
  chemical imbalance misinformation, 184,
    185
  Scientific Advisory Board, 185
depression and diabetes, inappropriate
    comparison, 13, 35
  America's Pharmaceutical Research
    Companies, 225
  anonymous, 198
  Barry, Harry, general practitioner, 227
  CNN, 230
  Cochrane Centre, Nordic, 229
  Devon, Michelle L., freelance writer, 231
  Francis-Cheung, Theresa, health writer, 230
  Gotzcshe, Peter, physician, 229
  Grey, Robin, psychotherapist, 230

  Harper, Dawn, general practitioner, 226
  Houston, Muiris, general practitioner, 226
  Levine, Bruce, psychologist, 336
  marketing strategy, 229
  McEvoy, Mary, actress, 231
  *Men and Depression, What to Do When the Man
    You care About is Depressed*, 230
  National Alliance on Mental Illness, 225
  Wade, Alan, general practitioner, 226
depression and the DSM, 33
depression delusion, 1, 289
  accepted as truth, 2
  beliefs and ideas, no evidence, 1
  deconstructing, 6, 8
  described, 294
  Goldacre, Ben, physician, science writer,
    295
  logic, flawed, 290
  propaganda, 339
  seeing through it, 3
depression delusion, endorsed by
  British Medical Association, 109
depression recovery
  small steps, 87
depression, a brain disorder?
  what else could it be?, 320
depression, abuse and neglect, 78
depression, arm-bands and, 86
depression, assumed biological basis, 151,
    160, 254, 303, 321, 340
  Barry, Harry, general practitioner, 128
  beyond questioning, 96
  British Psychological Society, 20
  Carlat, Daniel, psychiatrist, 246
  Casey, Patricia, psychiatry professor, 10
  fact or hypothesis?, 11
  Goodman, Wayne, psychiatrist, 245
  Greenberg, Gary, psychotherapist, 5
  groupthink, 292
  Hicks, James W., psychiatrist, 101
  Hyman, Steven, psychiatrist, ex-director
    NIMH, 24
  Insel, Thomas, psychiatrist, director NIMH,
    319, 321, 324
  Klein, D.F., psychologist, 163
  National Alliance on Mental Illness, 180
  National Institute of Mental Health, 173,
    319
  never-changing, 315
  psychiatry, 302
  psychiatry's identity, 275
  Thompson, C., psychiatrist, 98
  vital to psychiatry, 321

WebMD website, 200
Wender, P.H., psychologist, 163
depression, avoidance, 84
depression, biological disorder
    fixed belief, 77
depression, biological, what else could it be?
    Carlat, Daniel, psychiatrist, 254
*Depression, Cognitive Behaviour Therapy with
    Children and Young People*
    chemical imbalance misinformation, 170

depression, core component
    distress, 82, 85
    woundedness, 84, 89
depression, core components, 79
    defence mechanisms, 79, 80, 84, 85, 89, 255
    distress, 79, 80, 84, 89, 197
    selfhood reduction, 79, 80, 83, 84, 89, 255
    self-protection strategies, 255
    shock, 79, 80, 89
    woundedness, 79, 80, 82, 85, 255
depression, defence mechanisms, 84
depression, diagnosis
    science plays no part, 33
depression, distorted understanding
    medical profession, 77
depression, endogenous, 85
    a psychiatrist's diagnosis, 85
    chemical imbalances, 85
depression, fundamentals misconceived
    Rottenberg, Jonathan, psychology
        professor, 295
depression, grief and, 84
depression, loss and, 84
depression, medical approach
    hegemony, 309
depression, monoamine theory of, 7, 41, 42,
    43, 46, 50, 257
depression, nine cases, 80
depression, pathophysiology
    Carlat, Daniel, psychiatrist, 4
depression, prognosis
    worse rather than better, 333
depression, shutdown in, 84
depression, why 5 criteria?
    Carlat, Daniel, psychiatrist, 34
    Lynch, Terry, GP & psychotherapist, 34
    Spitzer, Robert, lead *DSM-3* psychiatrist, 34
depression-guide website
    chemical imbalance misinformation, 205
    logical fallacy, Begging the Question, 205
DesJardins Financial Security
    chemical imbalance misinformation, 144

Desmaisons, Kathleen PhD
    chemical imbalances, misinformation, 220
Devon, Michelle L., freelance writer
    chemical imbalance misinformation, 196
    depression and diabetes, inappropriate
        comparison, 231
    False Dilemma logical fallacy, 196
    flawed logic, 196
    Weak Analogy logical fallacy, 231
diabetes and depression, misinformation. *See*
    depression and diabetes, misinformation
diagnoses by consensus
    Caplan, Paula, psychologist, 21
diagnosis
    and ideology, 277
    without investigations, 273
diagnosis by flipping a coin
    Mayberg, Helen, psychiatrist, 322
*Diagnostic and
    Statistical Manual of Mental Disorders-5. See
Diagnostic and Statistical Manual of Mental
    Disorders*, 15, 16, 17, 22, 207, 298, 299, 323
    "totally wrong model", ex-director NIMH,
        18
    aura of science and authority, 15
    collection of opinions, 22
    cost, 18
    depression, 33
    nine depression criteria, 33
    psychiatrist's bible, 22, 23
    validity 0%, Insel, Thomas, psychiatrist,
        director, NIMH, 323
    validity questioned, 18, 20
    validity, Dorothy Rowe, psychologist, 22
*Diagnostic and Statistical Manual of Mental
    Disorders-3*
    product of consensus not science, 19
*Diagnostic and Statistical Manual of Mental
    Disorders-4*, 16
*Diagnostic and Statistical Manual of Mental
    Disorders-5*, 16
    British Psychological Society Position
        Statement, 20
    British Psychological Society's response to,
        7
    delusion, definition, 287, 289
    validity, 12
dictionary.com website
    delusion, definition, 287
direct-to-consumer advertising
    chemical imbalance misinformation, 152
Discovering Nutrition, 218
disease model

British Psychological Society, 7
distress
    interpretation of, 4
    medicalisation of, 119
    repackaged as mental illness, 77
distress, in depression, 84, 85
    core component, 79, 82, 84, 85, 89, 197,
        255
    core components, 80
distress, medicalisation of
    Humphreys, Tony, psychologist, 287
distress, medicalisation of, *(continued)*,
    Smith, Richard, physician, editor, 287
Dobelli, Rolf, author
    confirmation basis, 130
doctors know best, 77
doctors misinforming patients
    chemical imbalances, 85, 87
    Council for Evidence-based Psychiatry, 119
doctors portrayed positively
    chemical imbalance delusion, 77
doctors, majority
    well-intentioned but misguided, 3
dopamine, 174
Dosani, Sabina, psychiatrist
    chemical imbalance misinformation, 102
drug companies
    chemical imbalances, misinformation, 141
    moving from chemical imbalances, 25
    withdrawal from psychiatric research, 9
drug companies, misinformation. *See*
    individual companies
drug companies, reduced research, 23
    Astra-Zeneca, 23
    Friedman, Richard, psychiatry professor, 24
    GlaxoSmithKline, 23
    Hyman, Steven, psychiatrist, ex-director
        NIMH, 23
    Paul, Steven, psychiatry professor, 24
    Pfizer, 23
    Whitaker, Robert, journalist, author, 25
drug company criticism
    Angell, Marcia, physician, pathologist, 239
drug company influence
    DeAngelis, Catherine, physician, 241
drug cycles, 10-20-30 year patterns, 25
    Medawar, Charles, Social Audit UK, 26
Drug Regulatory authorities
    and misinformation, 152
Drummond, Edward, psychiatrist
    chemical imbalances, no evidence, 32
DSM-3, 17, *See Diagnostic and Statistical Manual
    of Mental Disorders-3*

DSM-3, no biological markers
    Spitzer, Robert, lead *DSM-3* psychiatrist, 19
DSM-4, 18, *See Diagnostic and Statistical Manual
    of Mental Disorders-4, See*
*DSM-5. See Statistical Manual of Mental
    Disorders-5, See Diagnostic and Statistical
    Manual of Mental Disorders-5*
DSM-5 Position Statement
    British Psychological Society, 7, 20
DSM-5, secretive approach to
    Spitzer, Robert, lead *DSM-3* psychiatrist, 19

Duke, Sean, science journalist
    chemical imbalance misinformation, 207
Duman, Ronald, psychiatry professor
    delusions, new replacing old, 317, 318
    logical fallacy, Weak Analogy, 318
East Coast FM radio
    chemical imbalance misinformation, 207
Edmunds, Dan, psychotherapist
    psychiatry, belief system, 301
Edwards, Virginia, psychiatrist
    chemical imbalance misinformation, 100
Effexor
    chemical imbalance misinformation, 152
    mode of action misrepresented, 152
electroconvulsive therapy, 82, 83
Eli Lilly
    antidepressants, misinformation, 70
    chemical imbalance misinformation, 141
Ellison, Shane, research chemist
    chemical imbalances, false premises, 243
eMedTV
    chemical imbalance misinformation, 203,
        204
    flawed logic, 204
    logical fallacy, Red Herring, 284
emotions
    education about, 89
    time to decriminalise, 5
emperor without clothes
    chemical imbalance delusion, 342
Encyclopaedia Britannica
    delusions, 289
Erdelyi, Matthew H., psychology professor
    chemical imbalance misinformation, 161
Essentials of Human Nutrition, 218
Essentials of Preventive Medicine
    chemical imbalances, no evidence, 55
estrogen. *See* oestrogen
European Depression Association
    chemical imbalance misinformation, 144
Evans-Prichard, E.E., anthropologist

why untruths persist, 297
existence, understanding
    importance diminished, 78
fabrication
    chemical imbalances, 73
fact, confused with theory
    Burns, David, psychiatrist, 38
fact, errors of
    Harding, Richard, psychiatrist, 99
    in medical approach to depression, 8
    Lieberman, Jeffrey, psychiatry professor,
        106
Fallacist's Fallacy. *See* logical fallacy, Fallacist's
    Fallacy
false knowledge system
    Moncrieff, Joanna, psychiatrist, 295
false premises
    Ellison, Shane, research chemist, 243
family doctor. *See* general practitioner
family doctors. *See* general practitioners
family physician. *See* general practitioners
family practitioner. *See* general practitioner
Farrell, Elaine, author
    chemical imbalances misinformation, 181
Fennell, Leonie, mental health activist
    chemical imbalance misinformation, 115
Fiddaman, Bob, mental health activist
    chemical imbalance misinformation, 115
Fieve, Ronald, psychiatrist
    chemical imbalances, misinformation, for
        patients' sake, 249
    logic, flawed, 249
Finucane, Marian, broadcaster, 186
food
    as comfort, 82
Food and Drug Administration
    chemical imbalance misinformation, 152
Fores, Eaton, T., Research Center
    chemical imbalances, no evidence, 335
Forest Pharmaceuticals
    chemical imbalance misinformation, 148,
        149, 150
    logical fallacy, Begging the Question, 149
Foucault, Michael, philosopher
    perverse implantation, 311
Foudraine, Jan, psychiatrist
    mass delusion in psychiatry, 297
Fox-Spencer, Rebecca, neurochemist
    chemical imbalance misinformation, 102
Frances, Allen, lead *DSM-4* psychiatrist
    delusions, purpose, 289
    DSM lacks evidence, 19
    DSM-5 criticism, 18

Francis, Cheung, Theresa, health writer
    depression and diabetes, inappropriate
        comparison, 230
Francis-Cheung, Theresa, health writer
    chemical imbalance misinformation, 207
Franklin, Donald J., psychologist, 171
Fratteroli, Elio, psychiatrist
    chemical imbalances delusion,
        consequences, 329
Frazer, Alan, psychiatry
    chemical imbalance misinformation, for
        patints' sake, 248
Freedman, Robert, psychiatry professor
    chemical imbalances, misinformation, for
        patients' sake, 249
Friedman, Richard, psychiatry professor
    chemical imbalance misinformation, 104
    logical fallacy, Begging the Question, 104
    reduced drug company research, 24
Fryer, LaShon, freelance writer
    chemical imbalance misinformation, 196
    logical fallacy, Begging the Question, 197
*Functional Neuroanatomy: An Interactive Text and
    Manual*
    chemical imbalances, no evidence, 54
general practitioners
    delusion, depression, beneficiaries, 332
    do they treat brain disorders?, 279
genetics, "our best hope"
    Hyman, Steven, psychiatrist, ex-director
        NIMH, 324
Gilbert, Paul, psychology professor
    Begging the Question logical fallacy, 170
    chemical imbalance misinformation, 169
    flawed logic, 170
Glasser, William, psychiatrist
    seminal moments, 10
GlaxoSmithKline
    chemical imbalance misinformation, 145,
        147
    psychiatry labs closed, 23
Glenmullen, Joseph, 29, 58, 75
Glenmullen, Joseph, psychiatrist, 14
    10-20-30 year drug cycles, 25
    antidepressants, misinformation, 71
    chemical imbalances, discredited, 71
    patients seriously misled, 9
Goebbels, Joseph, propaganda officer
    delusion, mass, 293
    lies becoming truth, 293
Goldacre, Ben, physician, science writer
    chemical imbalances, accepted as fact, 241
    depression delusion, 295

Goldberg, Michael Lewis
  hegemony, 308
Gombos, Gabor, mental health campaigner,
  14, 176
  mistakes, with helping attitude, 3
Goodman and Gilman's The Pharmacological Basics
  of Therapeutics
  chemical imbalances, no evidence, 36
Goodman, Wayne, psychiatrist
  chemical imbalance, inappropriate
    metaphor, 244

Goodman, Wayne, psychiatrist, *(continued),*
  chemical imbalances, doctors misinforming
    patients, 245
  depression, assumed biological basis, 245
  logical fallacy, Begging the Question, 245
Gotzcshe, Peter, physician
  chemical imbalance lie, 229
  chemical imbalance misinformation, 229
  depression and diabetes, inappropriate
    comparison, 229
  erroneous myths of psychiatry, 229
Gould, Donald, physiology professor, 14
  medical ignorance, mental health, 4
  medical paternalism, 5
GP. *See* general practitioner
Graff, Mark, psychiatrist
  chemical imbalances misinformation, drug
    companies' fault, 251
Gramsci, Antonio, social theorist
  hegemony, 308
  hegemony, definition, 308
Greenberg, Gary, psychotherapist, 14, 19, 27,
  57, 74, 299
  brain, complexity, 65
  psychiatry's lack knowledge, 31
  should psychiatry manage suffering?, 5
Greenblatt, David, psychiatrist
  no case of benzo addiction?, 26
Grey, Robin, psychotherapist
  chemical imbalance misinformation, 207
  depression and diabetes, inappropriate
    comparison, 230
grief, 44, 84
  depression component, 83
grief, in depression, 84, 85, 87, 197
Griesinger, Wilhelm
  mental diseases are brain diseases, 306
groupthink
  Boyle, Mary, psychologist, 292
  characteristics, in psychiatry, 292
  definition, 291

depression, assumed biological basis, 292
Janis, Irving, social psychologist, 291
Wilson, Charles, Abacus news
  correspondent, 293
Guildford Four
  appalling vista, 342
hallmark, of a true scientist, 305
Hamlet
  protesting too much, 321
Harding, Richard, psychiatrist
  chemical imbalance misinformation, 99
  errors of fact, 99
  flawed logic, 99
  logical fallacy, False Dilemma, 99
Hardon, Anita, anthropology professor
  chemical imbalances discredited, 237
Harper, Dawn, general practitioner, 116, 138,
  233
  chemical imbalance misinformation, 116
  depression and diabetes, inappropriate
    comparison, 226
  logical fallacy, Begging the Question, 116
  logical fallacy, False Cause, 116
  logical fallacy, Weak Analogy, 226
Hasty Generalisation logical fallacy. *See* logical
  fallacy, Hasty Generalisation
Healing from Depression
  chemical imbalance misinformation, 174
Healy, David, psychiatrist
  chemical imbalances, marketing, 242
  chemical imbalances, no evidence, 41
Heaton-Harris, Nicolette, author
  chemical imbalance misinformation, 193
Hedges, Dawson, psychiatrist, 160
  chemical imbalances, discredited, 160
  consequences of biological focus, 329
hegemony, 305
  chemical imbalance misinformation, 305
  chemical imbalances notion, 310
  depression, medical approach, 309
  Goldberg, Michael Lewis, 308
  Gramsci, Antonio, social theorist, 308
  Jackson, Grace, psychiatrist, 311
  Johnstone, Lucy, psychologist, 310
  New York Times, 308
  Valenstein, Elliot, neuroscientist, 311
hegemony, definition
  wisegeek website, 308
hegemony, psychiatric
  Cresswell, Mark, sociologist, 308
  Kaiser, David, psychiatrist, 310
Herman, Edward, finance professor
  consent, manufactured, 336

Hickey, Phil, psychologist
    chemical imbalances, misinformation, little
        white lie, 252
Hicks, James W., psychiatrist
    chemical imbalance misinformation, 102
    chemical imbalances, based on deduction,
        49
    depression, assumed biological basis, 101
Hill & Hill, legal experts
    consent, informed, definition, 334
*Histology and Cell Biology: An Introduction to
    Pathology*, 54
Holford, Patrick, nutritionist, author
    Begging the Question, logical fallacy, 215
Holford, Patrick, nutritionist, author,
    (continued),
    chemical imbalance misinformation, 215,
        216, 217
homosexuality
    abolition as a mental illness, 17
    as mental illness, 16
    aversion therapy for, 17
Hook, Line and Sinker
    chemical imbalances discredited, 160
    consequences of biological focus, 329
Horgan, John, science writer
    actions speak louder than words, 272
    chemical imbalances, no evidence, 32
Houston, Muiris, general practitioner, 140,
        233
    chemical imbalance misinformation, 129,
        226
    depression and diabetes, inappropriate
        comparison, 226
human beings
    multidimensional nature, 301
Humphreys, Tony, 58, 298
Humphreys, Tony, psychologist
    chemical imbalances, no evidence, 38
    distress, medicalisation of, 287
Hunter, James, NIMH
    research misinformation, 322
Hyman, Steven, psychiatrist, ex-director
    NIMH
    bias, biological research, 324
    brain, complexity, 63
    chemical imbalances, no evidence, 38
    decreased drug company research, 23
    depression, assumed biological basis, 24
    genetics, "our best hope", 324
    logical fallacy, Begging the Question, 24
hypothesis, discredited
    promoted as fact, 13

hypothesis, unconfirmed, 2
ICD. See International Classification of Diseases, See
ideology, psychiatric, 78, 301
ignorance, regarding psychiatric disorders
    Carlat, Daniel, psychiatrist, 263
importance diminished
    understanding existence, 78
    understanding life, 78
Insel, Thomas, 27, 59, 325
Insel, Thomas, psychiatrist, director NIMH,
        17, 322
    a vision for psychiatry, 320
    Begging the Question logical fallacy, 320
    bias, biological research, 324
    chemical imbalances, no evidence, 42
    delusions, new replacing old, 319
    depression, assumed biological basis, 321,
        324
    DSM, zero percent validity, 323
    flawed logic, 320
    interesting pronouncements, 323
    logical fallacies, Begging the Question, 320
    no cures, no vaccines, 319
    predicting the future, 321
    psychiatry, revolution in?, 321
    reading the future, 324
    Research Domain Criteria, remarkable
        claims, 323
    stating the obvious, 324
insight, definition
    Merriam-Webster Dictionary, 320
Institute of Psychiatry
    chemical imbalances, no evidence, 42
International Classification of Diseases (ICD),
        15
    British Psychological Society statement, 7
Introduction to Psychology
    chemical imbalances, misinformation, 161
investigations, diagnostic
    absent in psychiatry, 273
Irish Medicines Board, 39, 154, 157, 262
    chemical imbalance misinformation, 153
    chemical imbalances, no evidence, 39
    communications with me, 153
irishhealth.com
    chemical imbalances, misinformation, 107,
        108, 109
    logical fallacy, Begging the Question, 108
ITV, *Loose Women*
    chemical imbalance misinformation, 185
ITV, *This Morning*
    chemical imbalance misinformation, 111,
        116

Jackson, Grace, psychiatrist
    chemical imbalances, discredited, 71
    hegemony, 311
Janis, Irving, social psychologist
    groupthink, 291
Johnstone, Lucy, psychologist
    hegemony, 310
Jowett, Garth
    propaganda, definition, 306
Jowit, Juliette, journalist
    chemical imbalance misinformation, 187
Kabat-Zinn, Jon, psychologist, 174
Kahneman, Daniel, economist, 75
    trust and credibility, 72
Kaiser, David, psychiatrist
    chemical imbalances delusion,
        consequences, 328
    chemical imbalances, no evidence, 31
    hegemony, psychiatric, 310
Kelly, Dee
    ITV's *This Morning*, 112
Kendler, Kenneth, psychiatrist
    chemical imbalances, no evidence, 40
Kenny, Mary, journalist
    chemical imbalance misinformation, 189
Kety, Seymour, psychiatrist
    chemical imbalances, discredited, 69
Keyes, Marian, author
    blaming the person, 236
    chemical imbalance misinformation, 186
kidshealth website
    chemical imbalance misinformation, 205
Kimmelman, Michael, *New York Times*
    chemical imbalances, misinformation, 253
Kinsey, Alfred, 16
Kirsch, Irving, psychologist, researcher
    chemical imbalances, based on deduction,
        50
    chemical imbalances, discredited, 48, 50
    chemical imbalances, marketing, 241
    chemical imbalances, no evidence, 43
Klein, D.F., psychologist
    depression, assumed biological basis, 163
Kramer, Peter, psychiatrist
    brain functioning theories wrong, 48
Krause, Robert, nursing tutor
    depression, a perverse implantation, 312
Kresser, Chris, integrative medicine
    practitioner, 14
    chemical imbalance misinformation, 152
    chemical imbalances, venerable status, 3
laboratory tests
    depression, absence of, 57

Lacasse, Jeffrey, 60, 137
Lacasse, Jeffrey, social work professor
    chemical imbalances, based on deduction,
        48
    chemical imbalances, discredited, 48
    chemical imbalances, no evidence, 41, 195,
        247
language
    medical, 2, 5
law of the instrument
    Carlat, Daniel, psychiatrist, 256
    Maslow, Abraham, psychologist, 255
Lean on me campaign
    chemical imbalance misinformation, 144

Lecture Notes on Clinical Chemistry
    chemical imbalances, no evidence, 52
Lecture Notes: Clinical Biochemistry
    chemical imbalances, no evidence, 53
Leifer, Ron, psychiatrist
    ask for blood test, 40
Lenin, Vladimir, Marxist
    delusion, mass, 293
    lies becoming truth, 293
Leo, Jonathan, 59, 60, 137, 157, 269, 285
Leo, Jonathan, neuroanatomy professor
    ask for blood test, 40
    chemical imbalances, based on deduction,
        48
    chemical imbalances, discredited, 48
    chemical imbalances, no evidence, 39, 41,
        247
    contradictions, 275
Leonovs, Julie, mental health activist, 114, 138
    chemical imbalance misinformation, 113,
        115
Levine, Bruce, 28, 57, 58, 75, 337
Levine, Bruce, psychologist
    chemical imbalances, discredited, 336
    chemical imbalances, no evidence, 32, 39
    consent, manufactured, 335
    depression and diabetes, inappropriate
        comparison, 336
    psychiatry wrong, 72
lie, little white
    chemical imbalances, 73
    Hickey, Phil, psychologist, 252
    Pies, Ronald, psychiatry professor, 252
Lieberman, Jeffrey, psychiatry professor
    chemical imbalance misinformation, 106
    flawed logic, 106
    logical fallacy, Begging the Question, 106
    logical fallacy, Weak Analogy, 106

lies becoming truth, 293
  Goebbels, Joseph, propaganda officer, 293
  Lenin, Vladimir, Marxist, 293
lies, some professionals lie
  Rowe, Dorothy, psychologist, 73
life, understanding
  importance diminished, 78
Lipowski, Z.J., psychiatrist
  chemical imbalances, no evidence, 31
Lipton, Morris, psychiatry professor
  chemical imbalance misinformation, 93
LiveScience website
  science based on fact, 304
Living with Depression
  chemical imbalance misinformation, 171
Locke, Don, president, American Counseling
  Association
  DSM-5 concerns, 20
logic, 135
logic, errors. See logic, flawed
logic, flawed, 263
  Carlat, Daniel, psychiatrist, 241, 255
  Castello, Greg, general practitioner, 123,
    124
  Cohen, David, social work professor, 42
  common, in delusions, 8
  Coppen, Alec, psychiatrist, 243
  depression delusion, 290
  Devon, Michelle L., freelance writer, 196
  eMedTV, 204
  Fieve, Ronald, psychiatrist, 249
  Gilbert, Paul, psychology professor, 170
  Harding, Richard, psychiatrist, 99
  Insel, Thomas, psychiatrist, director NIMH,
    320
  Lieberman, Jeffrey, psychiatry professor,
    106
  Lustral, 151
  Mayo Clinic, 94
  Moncrieff, Joanna, psychiatrist, 42
  Mondimore, Francis, psychiatrist, 96
  National Alliance on Mental Illness, 225
  Newsweek, 2001, 146
  Pfizer, 151
  Writing, Alexis, 198
  Zoloft, 151
logic, great leap
  Angell, Marcia, physician, pathologist, 7
logical fallacies, 135, 136, 137, 138, 139, 140,
    157, 176, 177, 209, 211, 212, 213, 232, 233,
    267, 269, 285, 286, 325, 337
logical fallacies, Begging the Question
  Fryer, LaShon, freelance writer, 197

logical fallacy, 14, 28, 62, 135, 137, 140, 183,
    231, 269
logical fallacy, Appeal to Authority
  Davidson's Principles and Practice of Medicine,
    260
logical fallacy, Begging the Question, 333
  American Medical Association, 131
  Barry, Harry, general practitioner, 127
  Barry, Siobhan, psychiatrist, 104
  Boston Globe, 317
  BUPA, 208
  Carver, Joseph, psychologist, 165
  chemical imbalances, cause or
    consequence?, 12
  cnsdiseases website, 206
  Crockett, Molly, neuroscientist, TED talk,
    133
  Crowe, Jonathan, science editor, 195
  Davidson's Principles and Practice of Medicine,
    259
  depression-guide website, 205
  DesMaisons, Kathleen, PhD, 222
  Forest Pharmaceuticals, 149
  Francis-Cheung, Theresa, health writer, 230
  Friedman, Richard, psychiatry professor,
    104
  Fryer, LaShon, freelance writer, 197
  Gilbert, Paul, psychology professor, 170
  Goodman, Wayne, psychiatrist, 245
  Grey, Robin, psychotherapist, 230
  Harper, Dawn, general practitioner, 116
  Hicks, James W., psychiatrist, 101
  Holford, Patrick, nutritionist, author, 215
  Hyman, Steven, psychiatrist, ex-director
    NIMH, 24
  Insel, Thomas, psychiatrist, director NIMH,
    320
  irishhealth.com, 108
  Lieberman, Jeffrey, psychiatry professor,
    106
  Men and Depression, What to Do When the Man
    You Care About is Depressed, 230
  New York Times, In-Depth Report, 195
  Norden, Michael J., psychiatrist, 98
  Nottinghamshire Healthcare NHS Trust,
    181
  O'Callaghan, Gareth, broadcaster, 266
  Oxford Handbook of Psychiatry, 274
  Patrick, Diane, governor's wife, 266
  Potatoes Not Prozac, 222
  Quirion, Remi, psychiatrist, 320
  Short Hills Pharmacy, New Jersey, 156
  Shreeve, Caroline, general practitioner, 126

SmithKline Beecham, 146
Steele, Chris, general practitioner, 112, 113
Thompson, C., psychiatrist, 98
Verduyn, C., Rogers, C & Wood, A.,
    psychologists, 170
WebMD website, 202
logical fallacy, Circular Reasoning. *See also*
    logical fallacy, Begging the Question
    Davidson's Principles and Practice of Medicine,
    259
logical fallacy, definition, 8
logical fallacy, Fallacist's Fallacy, 8
logical fallacy, False Cause, 104
    Barry, Harry, general practitioner, 127
    BUPA, 208
logical fallacy, False Cause, *(continued)*,
    Crockett, Molly, neuroscientist, TED talk,
    133
    Davidson's Principles and Practice of Medicine,
    257
    Forest Pharmaceuticals, 150
    Friedman, Richard, psychiatry professor,
    104
    Harper, Dawn, general practitioner, 116
    Lieberman, Jeffrey, psychiatry professor,
    106
    New York Times, In-Depth Report, 195
    Ramirez, Monica, psychologist, 100
    Short Hills Pharmacy, New Jersey, 156
    Steele, Chris, general practitioner, 112, 113
    Wright, Jesse, psychiatrist, 100
    Wright, Jesse, psychiatrist, 100
logical fallacy, False Dilemma, 333
    Devon, Michelle L., freelance writer, 196
    Francis-Cheung, Theresa, health writer, 230
    Grey, Robin, psychotherapist, 230
    Harding, Richard, psychiatrist, 99
    McCartney, Margaret, general practitioner,
    279
    National Alliance for Research on
    Schizophrenia and Depression, 183
    Pittsburgh Tribune, 192
    Shreeve, Caroline, general practitioner, 126
logical fallacy, Hasty Generalisation
    Davidson's Principles and Practice of Medicine,
    258
logical fallacy, Proof of Tradition
    Thompson, C., psychiatrist, 98
logical fallacy, Red Herring, 56, 282
    American Medical Association, 131
    Andreasen, Nancy, psychiatrist, 282
    anonymous, 198
    Basco, Monica Ramirez, psychologist, 282

Brainphysics.com, 284
British Medical Association, 283
chemical imbalances, cause or
    consequence?, 12
eMedTV, 284
McKenzie, Kwame, psychiatry professor,
    110, 283
New York Times, Depression In-depth
    Report, 283
Shreeve, Caroline, general practitioner, 284
Understanding Depression, 283
Wright, Jesse, psychiatrist, 282
logical fallacy, Straw Man
    Houston, Muiris, general practitioner, 130
logical fallacy, Subjectivist Fallacy, 9

logical fallacy, Weak Analogy
    anonymous, 198
    Barry, Harry, general practitioner, 227
    Boston Globe, 317
    Devon, Michelle L., freelance writer, 231
    Duman, Ronald, psychiatry professor, 318
    Francis-Cheung, Theresa, health writer, 230
    Grey, Robin, psychotherapist, 230
    Harper, Dawn, general practitioner, 226
    Houston, Muiris, general practitioner, 226
    Lieberman, Jeffrey, psychiatry professor,
    106
    McCartney, Margaret, general practitioner,
    278
    *Men and Depression, What to Do When the Man
    You Care About is Depressed*, 230
    Murtagh's General Practice, 280
    National Alliance on Mental Illness, 225
    Wade, Alan, general practitioner, 227
logical fallacy, Wishful Thinking, 62, 140, 263,
    269
    American Medical Association, 132
    *The Human Brain, An Introduction to its
    Functional Anatomy*, 56
Loose Women, ITV programme
    chemical imbalance misinformation, 185
Lord Denning
    appalling vista, 341
loss
    in depression, 87, 197
loss, and depression, 84
love, 5, 81
Lowe, Derek, 14
Lowe, Derek, medicinal chemist
    no more knowledge than jack, 4
Lundbeck

chemical imbalance misinformation, 143,
144
chemical imbalances misinformation, 143
Lustral
chemical imbalance misinformation, 150
flawed logic, 151
Lynch, Terry, GP & psychotherapist
Athlone Literary Festival, 124
Beyond Prozac, Healing Mental Distress, 33
MacCarthy, John, mental health activist, 14
is it time?, 5
Mad Pride Ireland, 5
Maddock, Jim, Mindfreedom Ireland, 45
Maddock, Mary, 60
Maddock, Mary, Mindfreedom Ireland
chemical imbalances, no evidence, 45
Maitre, Laurent, research scientist
chemical imbalances, discredited, 69
Malhi, G.S., psychiatrist
antidepressants,effectiveness exaggerated,
103
chemical imbalance misinformation, 103
*Mark's Basic Medical Biochemistry: A Clinical
Approach*
chemical imbalances, no evidence, 53
marketing
chemical imbalance delusion, 241, 309
marketing strategy
depression and diabetes, inappropriate
comparison, 229
marketing, chemical imbalances. *See* chemical
imbalances, marketing
Burns, David, psychiatrist, 240
Maslow, Abraham, psychologist
law of the instrument, 255
mass delusion. *See* delusion, mass
depression, 1
mass thinking. *See also* groupthink
Meerloo, A.M., psychiatrist, 294
masturbation
as mental illness, 16
Mayberg, Helen, psychiatrist
flipping a coin, 322
Mayo Clinic
chemical imbalances, misinformation, 94
flawed logic, 94
McCarter, Gordon, biological sciences
professor
chemical imbalances, no evidence, 40
McCartney, Margaret, general practitioner
logical fallacy, False Dilemma, 279
logical fallacy, Weak Analogy, 278
on depression, 278

McEvoy, Mary, actress
chemical imbalance misinformation, 193
depression and diabetes, inappropriate
comparison, 231
McKenzie, Kwame, 285, 286
McKenzie, Kwame, psychiatry professor, 109,
138, 285, 298
chemical imbalance misinformation, 109
delusion, definition, 288
logical fallacy, Red Herring, 110, 283
McKeon, Pat, psychiatrist, 145
McLaren, Niall, psychiatrist
chemical imbalances, no evidence, 44
McMaster, Norman, hypnotherapist
chemical imbalance misinformation, 172
Medawar, Charles, Social Audit UK
chemical imbalances discredited, 237
drug, 10-20-30 year cycles, 26
making the same mistakes, 26
Medical Biochemistry
chemical imbalances, no evidence, 53
medical mindset
Angell, Marcia, physician, pathologist, 91
depression, 91
medical paternalism
Gould, Donald, physiology professor, 5
medical profession
depression, distorted understanding, 77
fixed beliefs, 78
Medical Sciences
chemical imbalances, no evidence, 55
medicalisation
of loss and distress, 119
Smith, Richard, physician, editor, 287
medication, 8
Meerloo, A.M., psychiatrist
delusion, definition, 288
delusion, mass, 293
delusions, purpose, 289
lies becoming truth, 293
Memorising Medicine, A Revision Guide
chemical imbalances, no evidence, 54
*Men and Depression, What to Do When the Man
You Care About is Depressed*
chemical imbalance misinformation, 207
mental disorders
by consensus agreement, 16
definition of, 20
homosexuality, 16
masturbation, 16
no definition of, 19
no scientific verification, 16
mental disorders, "bullshit"

Frances, Allen, lead *DSM-4* psychiatrist, 19
mental disorders, can't test definition
    Regier, Darrel, psychiatrist, vice-chair *DSM-5*, 19
mental disorders, contrived, in *DSM*
    Davies, James, psychologist, 19
mental disorders, no scientific basis
    Caplan, Paula, psychologist, 21
Mental Health America
    chemical imbalance misinformation, 184
mental health organizations. *See also* individual
    organizations
    misinformation, 13
meprobamate, 10-20-30 year cycle, 26
metaphor, definition, 245
metaphor, mixed, definition, 245
mind
    servant of the brain?, 65
MIND, UK
    chemical imbalance misinformation, 181
Mindfreedom Ireland, 45
mind-reading
    erroneous conclusions, 82
misinformation
    from media sources, 13
    Insel, Thomas, psychiatrist, director NIMH,
        321
    mental health organizations, 13
    the general public, 13
misinformation, research
    Hunter, James, NIMH, 322
    National Institute of Mental Health, 322
misleading patients, seriously
    Glenmullen, Joseph, psychiatrist, 9
Modern Nutrition in Health and Disease, 217
Mohl, P., psychiatrist
    chemical imbalance misinformation, 254
    psychotherapy, a biological treatment, 254
Moncrieff, Joanna, psychiatrist
    brain chemicals, breakdown products, 50
    chemical imbalance importance, 240
    chemical imbalance misinformation, 115
    chemical imbalance, inappropriate
        metaphor, 244
    chemical imbalances, 35
    chemical imbalances, no evidence, 40, 42,
        43
    false knowledge system, 295
    longstanding psychiatric model, 315
    propaganda, 306, 307
    serotonin breakdown products, 50
Mondimore, Francis, psychiatrist
    chemical imbalances, misinformation, 103

flawed logic, 96
Moore, Thomas J., Health Policy expert
    chemical imbalances, no evidence, 37
Morena, Francisco, psychiatrist
    chemical imbalances, no evidence, 47
Mosher, Loren, psychiatrist
    chemical imbalances delusion,
        consequences, 329
multidisciplinary teams, 5
Murtagh's General Practice
    chemical imbalance misinformation, 280,
        281
    chemical imbalances, misinformation, for
        patients' sake, 251
    logical fallacy, Weak Analogy, 280
mythology, dangerous
    Datta, Vivek, psychiatrist, 331
myths
    Oxford Handbook of Psychiatry, 303
myths of psychiatry, erroneous
    Gotzcshe, Peter, physician, 229
myths, scientists
    Sheldrake, Rupert, author, lecturer, 305
National Alliance for Research on
    Schizophrenia and Depression
    chemical imbalance misinformation, 183
    logical fallacy, False Dilemma, 183
National Alliance on Mental Illness
    chemical imbalance misinformation, 180
    depression and diabetes, inappropriate
        comparison, 225
    depression, assumed biological basis, 180
    flawed logic, 225
    logical fallacy, Weak Analogy, 225
    moral authority, 309
National Institute of Mental Health, 27, 179,
    208, 319
    buying time and money, 323
    chemical imbalance misinformation, 173,
        179
    delusions, 13
    delusions, new replacing old, 13, 319
    depression, a brain disorder, 275
    depression, assumed biological basis, 319
    distancing from *DSM-5*, 17
    research misinformation, 322
Nazario, Brunilda, MD
    chemical imbalance misinformation, 201
Nelson, Richard, mass communications
    professor
    propaganda, definition, 305
neuroscience, 54
Neuroscience in Medicine

chemical imbalances, no evidence, 54
neurotransmitter chatter
Shorter, Edward, psychiatrist, 34
neurotransmitter wizards
Carlat, Daniel, psychiatrist, 228, 248
New York Review of Books, 14, 22, 28, 43, 59,
91, 134, 239, 240, 253, 266
Angell, Marcia, physician, pathologist, 7
New York Times
hegemony, 308
New York Times, depression In-Depth Report
chemical imbalance misinformation, 195
logical fallacy, Begging the Question, 195
logical fallacy, False Cause, 195
logical fallacy, Red Herring, 283
Newsweek
chemical imbalance misinformation, 146
flawed logic, 146
Nierenberg, Andrew, psychiatrist
chemical imbalances, no evidence, 37
NIMH. See National Institute of Mental
Health
no cures, no vaccines
Insel, Thomas, psychiatrist, director NIMH,
319
noradrenaline, 61
Norden, Michael J., psychiatrist
chemical imbalance misinformation, 97, 98
logical fallacy, Begging the Question, 98
Valenstein, Elliot, neuroscientist, 98
norepinephrine. See noradrenaline
Nottinghamshire Healthcare NHS Trust
chemical imbalance misinformation, 180
logical fallacy, Begging the Question, 181
Nutrition: A Health Promotion Approach, 218
O, Jack, therapist
chemical imbalance misinformation, 172
O'Sullivan, Ronnie, snooker player
chemical imbalances misinformation, 191
obsessive-compulsive disorder
chemical imbalances, no evidence, 39
O'Callaghan, Gareth, broadcaster
chemical imbalance misinformation, 191,
265
logical fallacy, Begging the Question, 266
occupational therapy, 5
O'Donnell, Victoria
propaganda, definition, 306
Oldham, John, psychiatrist
president, American Psychiatric
Association, 20
O'Meara, Kelly Patricia, investigative reporter
absence of diagnostic tests, 273

opiates, 10-20-30-year cycle, 26
Opong, Dr., general practitioner
chemical imbalance misinformation, 117
Osbourne, Sharon
chemical imbalance misinformation, 186
O'Shaughnessy, Kevin, medical editor
chemical imbalance misinformation, 111
Oster, Gerald D., psychologist
chemical imbalance misinformation, 162
outcomes
chemical imbalances, 89
Overcoming Depression, A Self-Help Guide Using
Cognitive Behavioural Techniques
chemical imbalance misinformation, 169
Oxford Handbook of Psychiatry
logical fallacy, Begging the Question, 274
paradigm shift, need for
British Psychological Society, 7

paradigm, new
of understanding, 8
pathophysiology, 55, 66, 96, 103, 276
absence of, 4
definition, 4, 37
Patrick, Diane, governor's wife
chemical imbalance misinformation, 265
logical fallacy, Begging the Question, 266
Paul, Steven, psychiatry professor
reduced drug company research, 24
Paxil, 145
Paxil CR website
chemical imbalance misinformation, 147
Paykel, Eugene, psychiatrist
chemical imbalances, no evidence, 46
pellagra, 217
People magazine
1998 Prozac advertisement, 141
personality disorder
chemical imbalances, no evidence, 39
persuasion, 305
Pert, Candace, neuroscientist
chemical imbalance misinformation, 133
perverse implantation
depression, 311
Foucault, Michael, philosopher, 311
perverse implantation, depression
Krause, Robert, nursing tutor, 312
Pfizer
chemical imbalance misinformation, 150,
151
decreased research, 23

pharmaceutical companies. *See* drug
    companies
    delusion, depression, beneficiaries, 332
    financial muscle, 309
pharmaceutical industry
    hijacked science, 240
pharmacodynamics
    definition, 37
Pies, Ronald, psychiatry professor, 268
    chemical imbalance misinformation, little
        white lie, 252
    chemical imbalances misinformation, drug
        companies' fault, 251
    chemical imbalances misinformation, for
        patients' sake, 249
    chemical imbalances, urban legend, 72
Pittsburgh Tribune
    chemical imbalance misinformation, 192
placebo
    consent, informed, 334
Plant, Jane, CBE, environmental geochemistry
    professor
    chemical imbalance misinformation, 168,
        169
Plato, 8
Plomin, Robert, psychologist
    biology dominant in psychology, 161
Portland Psychotherapy Depression
    Treatment Program
    chemical imbalance misinformation, 172
Potatoes Not Prozac
    chemical imbalances, misinformation, 220
    logical fallacy, Begging the Question, 222
Practical General Practice
    chemical imbalances, no evidence, 281
practices, questionable
    psychiatry, 13
predicting the future
    Insel, Thomas, psychiatrist, director NIMH,
        321
Principles of Anatomy and Physiology
    chemical imbalances, no evidence, 54
promoted chemical imbalances
    American Psychiatric Association, 73
propaganda, 305
    Breggin, Peter, psychiatrist, 307
    chemical imbalance misinformation, 305
    chemical imbalances, 339
    Cohen, David, social work professor, 307
    depression delusion, 339
    Moncrieff, Joanna, psychiatrist, 306, 307
    Shorter, Edward, psychiatrist, 307
    Valenstein, Elliot, neuroscientist, 306

Whitaker, Robert, journalist, author, 309
Propaganda and Persuasion
    propaganda, definition, 306
propaganda, definition
    Jowett & O'Donnell, 306
    Nelson, Richard, mass communications
        professor, 305
    Oxford dictionary, 305
protective reaction
    depression, 88
Prozac, 141
Prozac Diary
    chemical imbalance misinformation, 96
Prozac Nation. See also, Wurtzel, Elizabeth
    chemical imbalance misinformation, 264
pseudoscience
    chemical imbalances, 72
Psychcentral website
    chemical imbalance misinformation, 199
psychiatric diagnoses
    arbitrary nature, 24
psychiatric drugs
    10-20-30 year cycle, 12
psychiatrist's bible, the *DSM*
    Angell, Marcia, physician, pathologist, 22
    Rowe, Dorothy, psychologist, 22
psychiatrist's bible
    *Diagnostic and Statistical Manual of Mental
        Disorders*, 22, 23
psychiatry
    belief system, 301
    between a rock and a hard place, 275
    Cartesian split, 302
    delusion, depression, beneficiaries, 332
    depression, assumed biological basis, 302
    filters and radars, 77
    groupthink characteristics, 292
    ideology, 301
    narrow biological perspective, 302
    no organ of expertise, 274
    primarily one-dimensional, 302
    questionable practices, 13
    Scientific Method, 304
    standards, low, 13
    survival of, 277
    survivors, 291
    valid possibilities ignored, 340
psychiatry wrong
    Levine, Bruce, psychologist, 72
    Whitaker, Robert, journalist, author, 72
psychiatry, 19th century medicine
    Shorter, Edward, psychiatrist, 322
psychiatry, belief system

Edmunds, Dan, psychotherapist, 301
psychiatry, deficiencies
  Oxford Handbook of Psychiatry, 339
psychiatry, fixed belief
  biology most important, 9
psychiatry, revolution in?
  Andreasen, Nancy, psychiatrist, 321
  Insel, Thomas, psychiatrist, director NIMH,
    321
psychology, 5, 44, 160, 161
  biologized, 161
Psychology Information Online
  chemical imbalance misinformation, 171
psychology, mass
  Meerloo, A.M., psychiatrist, 294
psychotherapy, a biological treatment
  Barry, Harry, general practitioner, 254
  Mohl, P., psychiatrist, 254
psychotherapy, undervalued
  Andreasen, Nancy, psychiatrist, 95
Puech, Alain, pharmacist
  chemical imbalances, discredited, 69
Quirion, Remi, psychiatrist
  a vision for psychiatry, 320
  Begging the Question logical fallacy, 320
Ramirez, Monica, psychologist
  chemical imbalance misinformation, 100
  logical fallacy, False Cause, 100
rapport, building, 79
Ratna, L., psychiatrist
  chemical imbalances, no evidence, 36
RBC Insurance
  chemical imbalance misinformation, 144
reasoning, flawed. See logic, flawed, See
recovery journey, 83
Red Herring logical fallacy. See logical fallacy,
  Red Herring
Redman, Nick
  Bristol Hearing Voices Network, 113
  chemical imbalance misinformation, 113
Regier, Darrel, psychiatrist, vice-chair DSM-5
  mental disorders, impossible to test, 19
  on mental disorders, 19
regulatory bodies
  failure, 12
Reidbord, Steven, psychiatrist, 60, 276, 285
  chemical imbalances, lying, 243
  chemical imbalances, misinformation, 244
  chemical imbalances, no evidence, 45
  chemical imbalances, sloppy thinking, 244
relationships, high quality, 81, 83
Research Domain Criteria
  no solid evidence, 323

Research Domain Criteria, remarkable claims
  Insel, Thomas, psychiatrist, director NIMH,
    323
research, misinformation
  Hunter, James, NIMH, 322
  National Institute of Mental Health, 322
reserpine
  depressive effects exaggerated, 68
  importance to medical model, 67
Rethink Mental Illness
  chemical imbalance misinformation, 182
Richard Bentall, psychologist, 60, 267
Rogers, Julia, psychologist
  chemical imbalances misinformation, 170
Rosewater, Lynn, psychologist
  DSM-3 meeting, 21
Ross, Colin, psychiatrist
  chemical imbalances, no evidence, 36
Rottenberg, Jonathan, psychology professor
  chemical imbalances, no evidence, 44
  depression, fundamentals misconceived,
    295
Rowe, Dorothy, psychologist
  chemical imbalances, no evidence, 22, 42
  doctors, refusing to be aware, 294
  DSM not valid, 22
  lies, some professionals lie, 73
  on Terry Lynch, 294
  untruths, why they persist, 297
Royal College of Psychiatrists
  chemical imbalance misinformation, 93
  chemical imbalances, no evidence, 42
Royal College of Psychiatrists, website
  changes
  chemical imbalances, no evidence, 42
sadness
  in depression, 85, 87
safe space, 81
Sangavi, Darshak, Harvard clinical fellow
  chemical imbalances, no evidence, 40
Santagato, Danny
  actions speak louder than words, 272
Sawalha, Nadia, TV presenter
  chemical imbalance misinformation, 186
Schildkraut, Joseph, psychiatrist
  chemical imbalances, hypothesis, 46
schizophrenia
  chemical imbalance misinformation, 96
  chemical imbalances, no evidence, 39
Science Brainwaves website
  delusions, widespread, 288
science, based on facts
  LiveScience website, 304

science, hijacked
  pharmaceutical industry, 240
science, objectivity in
  Sheldrake, Rupert, author, lecturer, 304
Scientific American
  chemical imbalances delusion, widely
    believed, 1
Scientific Method
  definition, 303
  Oxford Handbook of Psychiatry, 303
  psychiatry, 304
scientist, hallmark, 305
scientists, objectivity, 320
Scull, Andrew, sociology professor
  biobabble, 239
  waiting for biological evidence, 276
self-doubt
  in depression, 89
selfhood, 79, 89
selfhood reduction
  depression, core component, 79, 80, 83, 84,
    89, 255
self-protection strategies
  depression, core components, 255
seminal moments, 10
  Breggin, Peter, psychiatrist, 10
  Casey, Patricia, psychiatry professor, 10
  Glasser, William, psychiatrist, 10
  Whitaker, Robert, journalist, author, 10
Serani, Deborah, psychologist
  chemical imbalance misinformation, 171
serotonin, 50, 59, 61, 62, 156, 174, 209, 267,
    268
serotonin breakdown products
  Agam, Galila, psychiatrist, 51
  Belmaker, R.H., psychiatrist, 51
  depression, 50
  Mancrieff, Joanna, psychiatrist, 50
  Shorter Oxford Textbook of Psychiatry, 51
  Valenstein, Elliot, neuroscientist, 50
  Whitaker, Robert, journalist, author, 51
serotonin depletion
  does not cause depression, 67
serotonin imbalances. *See* chemical imbalances
serotonin, breakdown products
  Carlat, Daniel, psychiatrist, 50
Seroxat, 145
Shannon, Bill, professor in general practice
  on GPs' skills and resources, 281
Sharfstein, Steven, president, American
    Psychiatric Association
  bio-bio-bio model, 330
  chemical imbalances misinformation, 244

Sheldrake, Rupert, author, lecturer
  myths, scientists, 305
  science, objectivity in, 304
Shepherd, Charles, M.E. Association Medical
    Director
  chemical imbalances misinformation, 133
Shipko, Stuart, psychiatrist
  chemical imbalances, marketing, 242
shock
  depression, core component, 79, 80, 85, 89
shock, unresolved
  in depression, 84
Short Hills Pharmacy, New Jersey
  chemical imbalance misinformation, 155
  logical fallacy, False Cause, 156
Shorter Oxford Textbook of Psychiatry
  delusion, definition, 288, 290
  serotonin breakdown products, 51
Shorter, Edward, psychiatrist
  antidepressants, misinformation, 70
  brain, complexity, 64
  chemical imbalances discredited, 235
  chemical imbalances, marketing, 242
  chemical imbalances, no evidence, 45
  neurotransmitter chatter, 34
  propaganda, 307
Shreeve, Caroline, general practitioner
  chemical imbalance misinformation, 125
  logical fallacy, Begging the Question, 126
  logical fallacy, False Dilemma, 126
  logical fallacy, Red Herring, 284
shutdown, in depression, 84
Slater, Lauren, author, *Prozac Diary*
  chemical imbalance misinformation, 96
Slife, Brent, psychology professor
  chemical imbalances, discredited, 160
  consequences of biological focus, 329
Smith, Richard, physician, editor
  distress, medicalisation of, 287
SmithKline Beecham
  logical fallacy, Begging the Question, 146
Snyder, S.H., neuroscientist
  chemical imbalances discredited, 70
social work, 5, 59
Solomon, Andrew, author
  chemical imbalance misinformation, 189,
    190
Sommers-Flanagan, John, counsellor
    education professor
  chemical imbalances, marketing, 243
sophistry, 305
  chemical imbalance misinformation, 305
  chemical imbalances notion, 311

sophistry, definition
    Free Online Dictionary, 311
Spiegel, Alix, NPR correspondent
    chemical imbalance misinformation, 247
Spitzer, Robert, lead *DSM-3* psychiatrist, 19
    depression, why 5 criteria?, 34
    DSM-3, no biological markers, 19
    DSM-5, secretive approach to, 19
spunout.ie
    chemical imbalance misinformation, 185
Stahl, Stephen M., psychiatrist
    chemical imbalances, no evidence, 38
Standard Life
    chemical imbalance misinformation, 144
standards, low
    psychiatry, 13
Stanford Encyclopedia of Philosophy:
    delusions, widespread, 288
Steele, Chris, general practitioner, 111
    chemical imbalance misinformation, 111,
        112, 114
    logical fallacy, Begging the Question, 112,
        113
    logical fallacy, False Cause, 112, 113
Stephenson, Janet, psychologist
    chemical imbalances misinformation, 168,
        169
Stoppard, Miriam, general practitioner, 140
    chemical imbalance misinformation, 133
Stotland, Nada L, psychiatry professor
    chemical imbalance misinformation, 100
Subjectivist Fallacy
    see logical fallacy, Subjectivist Fallacy, 9
support, 83
supports, 89
survival, of psychiatry, 277
survivors, of psychiatry, 291
Szasz, Thomas, 58
Szasz, Thomas, psychiatrist
    chemical imbalances, no evidence, 32, 39
tears
    depression recovery, 84
    in depression, 85
Teasdale, John, psychologist, 174
tests, diagnostic
    absence, O'Meara, Kelly Patricia, 273
Textbook of Biochemistry with Clinical Correlations
    chemical imbalances, no evidence, 53
Textbook of Medicine:
    chemical imbalance misinformation, 133
The Complete Book of Men's Health
    chemical imbalance misinformation, 206
The Complete Guide to Mental Health

chemical imbalance misinformation, 181
The Emperor's New Clothes
    Andersen, Hans Christian, 302
The Guardian
    chemical imbalance misinformation, 187
*The Human Brain, An Introduction to its
    Functional Anatomy*
    chemical imbalances, misinformation, 56
    logical fallacy, Wishful Thinking, 56
The Sanctuary at Sedona
    chemical imbalance myth, 340
The Science of Laboratory Diagnosis
    chemical imbalances, no evidence, 57
theory confused with fact
    Burns, David, psychiatrist, 38
Thompson, C., psychiatrist
    depression, assumed biological basis, 98
    logical fallacy, Begging the Question, 98
    logical fallacy, Proof of Tradition, 98
Tighe, Sophie, Senior Reporter, Yahoo
    Lifestyle UK
    chemical imbalance misinformation, 207

Toibin, Colm, author
    Ivor Browne, psychiatrist, 130
Tolstoy, Leo, social activist
    appalling vista, 341
Tores, Eaton T., Research Center
    chemical imbalances, deception, 335
tranquillisation
    on hospital wards, 274
Trethowen,W., psychiatrist, 93
trust and credibility
    Kahneman, Daniel, psychologist, 72
trust in doctors
    chemical imbalance delusion, 72
trust, betrayal of
    Whitaker, Robert, journalist, author, 72, 73
trust, building, 79
truth, 14, 28, 75, 266, 320
tryptophan
    chemical imbalance misinformation, 217
    precursor of serotonin, 67
Tubridy, Aine, GP & psychotherapist
    chemical imbalance delusion, consequences,
        328
    pharmaceutical industry, 240
U.S. Congress Office of Technology
    chemical imbalances, no evidence, 36
U.S. Pharmacist
    chemical imbalance misinformation, 155
Understanding Depression

logical fallacy, Red Herring, 283
Understanding Nutrition, 219
University of Limerick library, 52, 53, 280
untruths, why they persist
    Evans-Prichard, E.E., anthropologist, 297
    Rowe, Dorothy, psychologist, 297
Valenstein, Elliot, neuroscientist
    brain, complexity, 64, 70
    chemical imbalance misinformation, 141
    chemical imbalances delusion,
        consequences, 329
    chemical imbalances discredited, 63, 235
    chemical imbalances, no evidence, 32, 37
    hegemony, 311
    on Norden, Michael J., psychiatrist, 98
    propaganda, 306
    serotonin breakdown products, 50
validity
    *Diagnostic and Statistical Manual of Mental
        Disorders-5*, 12
Verduyn, Chrissie, psychologist
    chemical imbalances misinformation, 170

vested interests
    chemical imbalance delusion, 77
Wade, Alan, general practitioner
    depression and diabetes, inappropriate
        comparison, 226
    logical fallacy, Weak Analogy, 227
Wakefield, Jerome, social work & psychiatry
    professor
    chemical imbalances, no evidence, 44
Watson, Toby, psychologist, 115
    chemical imbalances, misinformation, 115
Wax, Ruby
    antidepressant overprescribing, 278
Weak Analogy logical fallacy. *See* logical
    fallacy, Weak Analogy
WebMD website
    chemical imbalance misinformation, 199,
        201
    depression, assumed biological basis, 200
    logical fallacy, Begging the Question, 202
Weil, Andrew, physician
    chemical imbalances, misinformation, 265
Wender, P.H., psychologist
    depression, assumed biological basis, 163
West's Encyclopedia of American Law
    consent, informed, definition, 334

Westen, Drew, psychology professor
    chemical imbalance misinformation, 168
Whitaker, Robert, journalist, author
    brain, complexity, 66
    chemical imbalances, discredited, 73
    powerful voices, 309
    propaganda, 309
    psychiatry wrong, 72
    reduced drug company research, 25
    seminal moments, 10
    serotonin breakdown products, 51
    trust, betrayal of, 73
Williams, Mark, psychologist, 174
Wilson, Charles, Abacus news correspondent
    delusion, mass, 293
    groupthink, 293
wisegeek website
    hegemony, definition, 308
Wishful Thinking logical fallacy. *See* logical
    fallacy, Wishful Thinking
withdrawal
    in depression, 85
Wood, Alison, psychologist
    chemical imbalances misinformation, 170
World Federation for Mental Health
    chemical imbalance misinformation, 144
World Organization of Family Doctors
    chemical imbalance misinformation, 144
woundedness
    depression, core component, 79, 80, 82, 84,
        85, 89, 255
wounding
    in depression, 84
Wright, Jesse, psychiatrist
    chemical imbalance misinformation, 100
    logical fallacy, False Cause, 100
    logical fallacy, Red Herring, 282
Writing, Alexis
    chemical imbalances, misinformation, 199
    flawed logic, 198
Wurtzel, Elizabeth, author
    chemical imbalance misinformation, 264
Wyeth
    chemical imbalance misinformation, 152
Yahoo
    chemical imbalance misinformation, 207
Zoloft
    chemical imbalance misinformation, 150
    flawed logic, 151
    mode of action misrepresented, 150

Sign up to Terry Lynch's newletter

Over the next decade, Terry Lynch intends to write 10-15 further books on important mental health topics including depression, anxiety, bipolar disorder, schizophrenia, OCD, eating disorders and suicide. To get news and updates, sign up for Terry's newsletter at www.doctorterrylynch.com.